Neurobiology, Diagnosis and Treatment in Autism

An Update

Mariani Foundation Paediatric Neurology Series
Editorial Board

Giuliano Avanzini, Milan, Italy
Philippe Evrard, Paris, France
Raoul Hennekam, Amsterdam, The Netherlands
Eugenio Mercuri, Rome, Italy
Fabio Sereni, Milan, Italy
Lawrence Wrabetz, Buffalo, NY, USA

Fondazione Pierfranco e Luisa Mariani
Viale Bianca Maria 28
20129 Milan, Italy

Telephone: +39 02 795458
Fax: +39 02 76009582
e-mail: publications@fondazione-mariani.org
www.fondazione-mariani.org

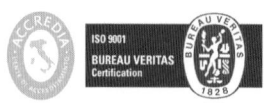

Fondazione con SGQ certificato

Neurobiology, Diagnosis and Treatment in Autism

An Update

Edited by

Daria Riva, Sara Bulgheroni and Michele Zappella

Mariani Foundation Paediatric Neurology Series: 26
Series Founder: Maria Majno
Associate Editor: Valeria Basilico

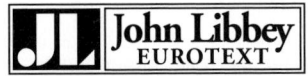

ISSN: 0969-0301
ISBN: 978-2-7420-0836-0

Cover illustration: Fanciulla con fico d'india, Thirties-Ferrara Fondazione Cavallini-Sgarbi.
By courtesy of Ilisso Edizioni.
From the volume *Coroneo. L'opera di due sorelle artiste-artigiane*, V. Sgarbi, M. Peri, Nuoro, Ilisso, 2009.

Technical and language editor: Justine Cullinan.

Published by

Éditions John Libbey Eurotext
127, avenue de la République, 92120 Montrouge, France
Tél. : +33 (0)1 46 73 06 60
Fax : +33 (0)1 40 84 09 99
e-mail : contact@jle.com
www.jle.com

© 2013 John Libbey Eurotext. All rights reserved.

Unauthorized duplication contravenes applicable laws.

It is prohibited to reproduce this work or any part of it without authorization of the publisher or of the Centre Français d'Exploitation du Droit de Copie (CFC), 20, rue des Grands Augustins, 75006 Paris, France.

Contents

Chapter 1	Neurobiology, diagnosis, and treatment in autism: an introduction *Daria Riva*	1

Neurobiology

Chapter 2	New diagnostic instruments and methods for autism spectrum disorders *So Hyun Kim*	13
Chapter 3	Conventional neuroimaging in autism *Alessandra Erbetta*	19
Chapter 4	Multimodal imaging of brain connectivity in autism spectrum disorders: an overview *Patrizia Chiesa and Ludovico Minati*	25
Chapter 5	Autism: the genetic viewpoint *Orsetta Zuffardi*	37
Chapter 6	Gene–environment interactions in autism spectrum disorder *Antonio M. Persico*	43
Chapter 7	GABA is essential for the construction of neuronal circuits early in development: dysfunction in autism spectrum disorders *Rocco Pizzarelli and Enrico Cherubini*	51
Chapter 8	The role of the immune response in autism spectrum disorders *Paul Ashwood and Milo Careaga*	65

Psychopharmacology

Chapter 9	New prospects towards more effective medication for ASDs *Roberta Zanni, Silvia Petza and Alessandro Zuddas*	81
Chapter 10	Pharmacologic treatment of autism in clinical practice *Gabriele Masi*	93

Rehabilitation

Chapter 11	The TEACCH approach to working with individuals on the autism spectrum: understanding, educating, empowering *Steven E. Kroupa*	107
Chapter 12	Experience using the TEACCH program at the Autism Center of AO San Paolo in Milan: applications and critical aspects *Monica Saccani*	121
Chapter 13	Applied Behaviour Analysis and the analysis of verbal behaviour in treating autism *Judah B. Axe*	127
Chapter 14	Applied Behaviour Analysis: the Italian experience of the Scuolaba Model for children with autism spectrum disorders *Lucia D'Amato*	139
Chapter 15	DIR–Developmental, Individual Difference, Relationship-Based Model: the sensory-motor affect connection to progress *Serena Wieder*	147
Chapter 16	The DIR model in treating autism: an Italian experience *Filippo Muratori and Giulia Campatelli*	155
Chapter 17	Imitation in autism spectrum disorders: from research to treatment *Giacomo Vivanti*	161
Chapter 18	Speech and language therapy intervention from the perspective of a multi-professional approach *Luciano Destefanis and Giuseppe Maurizio Arduino*	169
Chapter 19	Early psychomotor intervention in the treatment of young children with autism spectrum disorder *Roberto Militerni, Alessandro Frolli, Giovanna Gison, Guido Militerni and Ivana Sozio*	187
Chapter 20	Social skill training in autism spectrum disorders *Massimo Molteni and Sara Forti*	195

Complementary and alternative therapies

Chapter 21   A review of methods for facilitating speech in nonverbal children with ASD
Allison Landers, Gottfried Schlaug and Catherine Y. Wan   203

Chapter 22   Complementary and alternative medicine in treating autism: myths and reality
Laurence Robel   217

Chapter 1

Neurobiology, diagnosis, and treatment in autism: an introduction

Daria Riva

Developmental Neurology Division, Fondazione IRCCS Istituto Neurologico 'Carlo Besta', via Celoria 11, 20133 Milan, Italy

Introduction to the subject

Autism spectrum disorder (ASD) is a heterogeneous, behaviourally-defined neurodevelopmental disorder for which there are, to date, no biomarkers. The variability of the symptoms reflects the multiple biological and environmental influences that are unique to each individual's brain and that shape its abnormal and unique developmental trajectory (Silver & Rapin, 2012). The disorder's core symptoms are synthesized in the well-known triad of impairments identified in 1979 by the pioneering British autism researchers Lorna Wing and Judith Gould; this triad consists of deficits in social interaction and verbal and nonverbal communication and restricted or stereotyped patterns of behaviours and interests. The most frequent comorbidity is that of intellectual disability, which presents in approximately 70–85 per cent of cases (Fombonne, 2009). It is still being debated, however, whether intellectual deficit should be considered a symptom of autism itself or rather an associated disorder. Even the incidence of electroencephalographic abnormalities is rather high, as approximately 30 per cent of children with autism have epilepsy by adolescence (Tuchman *et al.*, 2009). A magnetoencephalographic study found epileptiform abnormalities in almost all subjects with early-onset autism, despite their normal standard scalp EEGs (Munoz *et al.*, 2008). The co-existence of concurrent psychiatric disorders, in particular anxiety and mood disorders, needs also be mentioned (Rosenberg *et al.*, 2011).

The different combinations of these multiple factors result in a marked phenotypic heterogeneity configured in a spectrum that can be classified into a set of three axes: symptom severity, its neurologic and psychiatric comorbidity, and temporal variability (Amaral, 2008). A *continuum* takes shape at the extremes of this spectrum: there are, on the one hand, situations that are close to normality and, on the other, serious neurodevelopmental disorders, such as severe developmental delay or intellectual disabilities, and it is at times extremely difficult to form a differential diagnosis between ASD and no spectrum-disorders. It is important to cite here the neurodiversity movement (Sinclair, 1993), according to which autism is not an illness or disease, but merely an atypical, alternative way of being and functioning that society should accept just as it accepts diversity in culture, religion, sexual orientation, and personality. The supporters of the neurodiversity movement argue that people with autism are not incapable of learning certain skills or participating in social interactions. These abilities must simply be learned and practiced in a different way (Walsh, 2011). This certainly represents a fascinating perspective as it recognizes the right of free expression to ASDs, but it could be dangerous because it underestimates the serious impact of this condition on the life of individuals with intellectual impairment and the extreme solitude of high-functioning autistics; in addition, such an attitude provides a disincentive to research.

From a nosographic viewpoint, the current version of the *Diagnostic and Statistical Manual of Mental Disorders* includes 'autistic disorder', 'Asperger's disorder', and 'pervasive developmental disorder not otherwise specified' (PDD–NOS) as subtypes of autism. Research has thus far failed to map these clinical phenotypes onto a specific aetiology or developmental pathway leading to each disorder. Today there is an increasing appreciation of the heterogeneity in the disorder's expression along numerous phenotypic dimensions, which overlap with those found in other conditions and in the general population. As a result, the next edition of the *Diagnostic and Statistical Manual of Mental Disorders*, to be released in 2013, will replace current categorical 'subtypes' with a single category labelled 'autism spectrum disorder' (Silver & Rapin, 2012).

Geschwind and Levitt have argued in 2007 that autism should not be considered a single disorder but, rather, as 'the autisms'. These authors suggested that there is a potential unifying model, called developmental disconnection, according to which higher-order association areas of the brain that normally connect to the frontal lobe are partially disconnected during development. According to that hypothesis, underconnectivity changes with age in children with ASD because the poorly developed cortical regions of the brain do not produce the *stream* of external and internal impulses which generate the right connections, and the lack of information flow does not produce a shaping effect on the brain cortices, impeding them from reaching the specialization they were destined for (Lee *et al.*, 2009).

Prevalence

Epidemiologic studies have demonstrated a dramatic increase in prevalence. Studies carried out during the 1970–80s indicated 5 cases out of 10,000, but according to recent studies the prevalence is between 1 in every 152 to 1 in every 100 (Leonard *et al.*, 2011; Fombonne, 2009). One epidemiologic study reported that the prevalence of autism in California has risen from 5.8 per 10,000 in 1987 to 14.9 per 10,000 in 1994 (Hertz-Picciotto & Delwiche, 2009). It is improbable that we are witnessing an epidemic, but rather the effect of younger ages at diagnosis, changes in diagnostic criteria, and inclusion of milder cases.

Behavioural correlation – cerebral processing areas

Thanks to the clinical acumen of some child psychiatrists such as Leo Kanner (1943), who coined the expression 'early infantile autism', a rather accurate description of the disorder's cognitive-behavioural phenotype, psychological hypotheses and theories were outlined that are still considered relevant today. I would also like to mention the 'theory of the mind' (Baron-Cohen *et al.*, 1985) and the 'weak central coherence theory' (Frith, 1989), which found its continuation in the current underconnectivity theory and in diffusion tensor imaging (DTI) studies (see the chapter in this volume by Chiesa & Minati) because the abnormal flow of information does not render stimuli integration *coherent* (Just et al., 2004; Kana et al., 2011).

Recently, cognitive neuropsychology and neuroscience have integrated a viewpoint according to which higher cognitive functions and complex behaviours are the final product of associative connections between specialized cortical areas, the locus of sensory motor elaborations which work together and constitute a complex, widely distributed network in the brain.

Given the extreme variability of the cognitive-behavioural phenotype of ASD, it is unlikely that there is a single neuroanatomic phenotype to which the disorder's aetiology can be attributed. It can, instead, be hypothesized that it involves complex networks with deficits caused by different subcircuits. Impaired reciprocal social interaction remains the pathognomonic characteristic of ASD and is the expression of a disruption in a discrete set of structures and their connections (*i.e.*, the 'social brain') which produce social behaviour and are shaped by it during development in a complex interaction between genes, brain, and the environment (Pelphrey et al., 2011). Bauman & Kemper's meta-analysis in 2005 and Amaral's review in 2008 concluded that the network *principally* includes the frontal lobes, the cerebellum, the limbic system (in particular the hippocampus and the amygdala), and obviously the white matter, which represents the connections that permit the system to work coherently and in synchrony.

Currently, one of the most prominent theories concerning the neuropathology of autism is that the brain undergoes a period of precocious growth during early postnatal life followed by a deceleration in age-related growth (Courchesne et al., 2003). A recent longitudinal MRI study on cortical development throughout early childhood (1.5–5 years) has confirmed that by the time the children being studied were 2 and a half years old, both cerebral gray and white matter volumes were enlarged in 41 autistic toddlers, with the most severe enlargement occurring in frontal temporal and cingulate cortices (Schumann et al., 2010). According to cross-sectional MRI studies, the enlargement concerns the total cerebral volume of the gray matter, but to a larger extent of the white matter of the frontal lobes and the radial cortical/subcortical intra-hemispheric areas, in particular the long connections (*i.e.*, those between the frontal lobes and the basal ganglia and the interhemispheric ones). The largest and most consistent increases have been reported in the frontal lobes. While there is some evidence of greater increases in the dorsolateral prefrontal and medial frontal cortex, there are no differences or decreases in the orbitofrontal cortex (Amaral et al., 2008).

Let us now take a look at the cerebral areas that are most frequently impaired in ASD.

The *frontal lobes* are associative areas *par excellence*; they regulate metacognition and meta-representation. There is an internal modularity, and the crucial areas, as far as ASD is concerned, are the associative ones, where complex integration and elaboration are carried out, that is, Brodmann areas 9 and 46, which process executive functions and sustain flexibility of thought, the capacity to quickly jump from one stimulus to another, to rapidly elaborate new stimuli, taking in information and putting pieces together, and attributing mental states to others (*i.e.*, the 'theory of the mind', which is often impaired in ASD). Studies on brain lesions confirm that children with tumors, congenital malformations, or tuberous sclerosis in frontal regions fail in frontal tests, particularly in the presence of clinical or subclinical epileptic foci (Hashimoto et al., 2001). In ASD the increase in gyration (Hardan et al., 2004; Jou et al., 2010a, 2010b) as well as in white matter volume has been demonstrated during the first years of life especially in the frontal regions (Amaral, 2008). fMRI studies, using 'theory of mind' paradigms, recently carried out found the recruitment of superior and middle frontal, in addition to anterior cingulate, insula and fusiform gyrus, in healthy subjects (Polosan *et al.*, 2011) and a lower activation in frontal and temporal regions, which is associated with a significantly weaker functional connectivity between the temporoparietal junction (TPJ) and motor areas, in ASD population (Kana *et al.*, 2012).

The role played by the limbic system and in particular the hippocampus and the amygdala is crucial. The hippocampus is an associative structure capable of integrating different stimuli and organizing them in constructs of superior order. The role of the limbic system includes that of acquiring and consolidating memories and learning and processing episodic memory, particularly autobiographic memory, which contextualizes personal memories in space and time. Neuropathologic alterations in the form of increased, although not consistently, neuronal packing in the hippocampal structures (Bauman & Kemper, 1994; Kemper & Bauman, 1998), an increase in the hippocampal dentate gyrus (declarative memory) (Saitoh *et al.*, 2001), and the presence of precocious mesial temporal sclerosis (DeLong & Heinz, 1997) have been reported in the hippocampus.

The amygdala is linked to decoding emotions, facial expressions, and rapid processing of behaviour consequent to emotional stimuli; for example, rapid decoding of an expression of fear sets into motion behaviours that are functionally valid from both a behavioural and a vegetative viewpoint.

Structural lesions, tumors, or encephalitis could cause a disturbance in recognizing facial emotions and 'reading' someone's thoughts/emotions through their eyes, as confirmed by experimental lesions in animals. Kemper & Bauman (1993) analyzed six post-mortem cases of autism in individuals between 9 and 29 years old (5/6 with mental retardation, 4/6 with seizure disorder), and they reported that the neurons of amygdala appeared unusually small and more densely packed with respect to those in age-matched controls. Sparks *et al.* (2002) showed an abnormal enlargement of the volume of amygdala in young children with ASD aged 36–56 months in comparison with both the typical developing sample (16.67 per cent on the right side and 13.64 per cent on the left side) and delayed developing group (16.67 per cent on the right side and 17.53 per cent on the left side). In a stereological study Schumann & Amaral (2006) estimated the number and the size of neurons in the amygdala of nine persons with autism aged between 10 and 44 years who did not have seizures compared to ten typically-developing age-matched male controls; they found significantly fewer neurons in the total amygdala and in the lateral nucleus of the subjects than were found in the controls, but not increased neuronal density or decreased neuronal size.

Those alterations were nonetheless found in extremely different age groups from youngest childhood to adulthood studied cross-sectionally. Since autism is a neurodevelopmental disorder it would seem logical that only samples of subjects with homogeneous ages studied longitudinally can provide conclusive data. Findings gathered until now have uncovered a similar pattern between abnormal growth of the head and growth of the amygdala in subjects from 12 months until 5 years of age. In children between 1 and 5 years old an enlargement of the amygdala is associated with antisocial behaviour (Schumann & Amaral, 2006; Courchesne *et al.*, 2007), while in adolescents/adults, a diminution in dimensions of the amygdala is associated with gaze avoidance (Nacewicz *et al.*, 2006). It should be remembered that decoding facial expressions is extremely complex and makes use of integrated network processes, which involve even the fusiform gyrus (constant facial characteristics) and the superior temporal sulcus (variable facial characteristics such as expression, gaze, and movement of the lips) (Calder & Young, 2005).

Let us now consider the cerebellum, an associative area that was previously considered crucial only for processing and learning complex motor activities. Today its ability to coordinate cognitive social and emotional behaviour of a higher order by means of its widespread connections with supratentorial cortical associative structures is unanimously recognized. Malfunction of this system causes the 'cognitive-affective syndrome', first theorized in 1998 by researchers in Boston (Schmahmann & Sherman, 1998), who described patients with cerebellar pathology. The subjects presented different clinical pictures depending on the intracerebellar localization of their lesion: vermal lesions caused affective and relational disorders, while lesions particularly of the lateral part of the cerebellar hemispheres were related to cognitive deficits. Brain lesion studies have confirmed these data (Schmahmann & Pandya, 2008; Levisohn *et al.*, 2000; Riva & Giorgi, 2000).

In a study we carried out in 2000, we described a 9-year-old girl with an enormous medulloblastoma cerebellar vermis, whose removal made necessary demolition of the 6th, 7th, and 8th lobes of the vermis (Riva & Giorgi, 2000). After the operation the child presented autistic-like behaviour, that is, she avoided eye contact, refused to be touched, and showed complex stereotyped motor and vocal mannerisms. She also presented a serious agrammatic language disorder typical of the frontal lesion, and while there was some improvement, the patient never returned to her normal state.

Since the 1990s the structure most cited in the literature as being altered in autistic persons is the cerebellum (Courchesne *et al.*, 1994); in particular, the 6th and 7th vermal lobules are hypoplastic, especially in young patients and in subjects with mental retardation and epilepsy (Stanfield *et al.* 2008), even in the context of a cerebellum of increased dimensions until the age of 5. In 1993 Kemper and Bauman found fewer Purkinje cells in the brains they examined and, according to Fatemi *et al.* (2002), the volume of the Purkinje cells was reduced. It is still not clear if the alteration in the number of those cells was due to the fact that fewer are produced or to a precocious apoptosis (Rout & Dhossche, 2008). In effect, the expression of reelin, which controls migration, was decreased by 40 per cent (Fatemi *et al.*, 2001) and BEL 12, which regulates apoptosis, was decreased by 34 to 51 per cent (Verhoeven *et al.*, 2010).

From an immunologic point of view, the presence of antibodies from the mother or from the infant itself against neurons of the cerebellum, including Purkinje cells, is a rather frequent finding. Immunologic processes can alter synaptogenesis and neuronal migration and thus have a significant impact on cortical organization. The link is not easy to establish but a recent study reported that the infants with anticerebellar autoantibodies had the most serious clinical symptoms (Goines *et al.*, 2011).

These data seem to confirm that there is a real anatomic–functional correlation between cerebral areas of the frontal–limbic–cerebellar network and typically altered functions in ASD. Subsequent meta-analyses of neuroanatomic and neuroimaging studies seemed nevertheless to demonstrate that many more areas can be involved (Abrahams & Geschwind, 2010; Amaral *et al.*, 2008). The ASD phenotypic heterogeneity is so vast that the underlying network must necessarily be extremely widespread. It follows that it will be possible to obtain consistent neuroradiologic data only starting from an accurate clinical characterization of large cohorts of subjects.

Our recent voxel-based morphometry (VBM) study (Riva *et al.*, 2011) comparing ASD children with intellectual disability with typically-developing subjects found reduced volumes of areas of the brain, including the *basal forebrain*, in ASD. The basal forebrain comprises a group of structures located in the medial and ventral surface of the frontal lobe, which provide projections to a variety of neocortical fields and limbic structures implicated in many cognitive functions and social behaviour patterns (Lam et al., 2006). The basal forebrain activates areas of the cerebral cortex and facilitates learning by using acetylcholine as a prominent neurotransmitter. Volume loss in the basal forebrain is consistent with the hypothesis proposed by Perry et al. (2001), according to which, in autism, the cholinergic system of the basal forebrain is impaired.

Another underactive system in autism is that of 'mirror neurons', which involve the inferior frontal gyrus, the inferior parietal lobule, and the insula. The mirror neurons are implicated in the comprehension of others' actions, intentions, and emotions through connections with the limbic system by means of the accumbens nucleus (Gallese, 2003; Leslie et al., 2004; Rizzolatti et al., 1996). By 1991, Rogers and Pennington hypothesized that the autistic impaired social interaction was due to an imitation deficit. Dysfunctioning of the mirror neuron system has been confirmed by fMRI (Dapretto, 2006) and VBM studies (Riva et al., 2011).

The important role of white matter in modulating information flow (the developmental disconnection or underconnectivity theory already cited) should also be mentioned. Brain connectivity in children is different from that in adults as early in development the sensory, motor, and perceptual homomodal areas (i.e., of the same kind) are connected to each other, and later, with brain maturation, the connections between homomodal areas and the heteromodal areas increase, and constitute the substrate for the processing of complex behaviours. A resting-state fMRI study demonstrated that higher-level associative areas are activated in the adult, while homomodal primary brain regions are activated in children (Uddin & Menon, 2010).

Disrupted brain connectivity is considered a possible cause of the autistic disorder: loss of long connections between distant areas of the brain (disconnections) determines an increase in the local connectivity, which often provokes an unruly hyperspecialization (distortions) (Wass, 2011). These perturbations of typical developmental trajectories are affected not only by multiple genetic factors, but also by a wide range of nongenetic, casual, epigenetic environmental risk factors, which interact according to a still undefined modality.

In order to synthesize and to render more comprehensible the factors influencing the ASD phenotype, I would like to mention a recent article by Rubenstein (2010) which reviewed the genetic mechanisms known to predispose to ASD, attempting to consolidate many of these within cellular/molecular pathways that regulate development of neural systems that underlie cognition and social behaviours. The author hypothesized that there are three additional mechanisms that may contribute to ASD: evolutionary-driven expansion of cerebral and cerebellar size; imbalance in the excitatory/inhibitory ratio in local and extended circuits, which reduces the ability to detect salient signals from noise signals; and the hormonal effects of the male genotype.

About the first mechanism, defects of distributed development are those that cause defective growth of connection systems represented by abnormalities in axon growth, dendrite growth, and synaptogenesis. These *abnormalities are distributed* because they involve different sectors of the brain, altering connectivity, and are caused by genes that encode for proteins of axonal growth, such as protocadherin, neurexin, and neuroligin. Local development defects of both connectivity (selective diminution of the corpus callosum of mutated mice [Paul et al., 2007] or of the internal capsule of rats [Garel & Rubenstein, 2004]) are associated with gene mutations that are expressed in neuron populations which share common characteristics, such as GABergic neurons of the basal forebrain and glutamatergic neurons (Long et al., 2009).

In addition to those listed, there are groups of genes that *regulate the development of specific cerebral regions* that are involved in the disease. The FGF genes are regulatory genes endowed with organizational properties across the frontal cortex (Grove & Fukuchi-Shimogori, 2003) and the cerebellum (Xu *et al.*, 2000), crucial areas for malfunction of the frontal-limbic-cerebellar network implicated in ASD. The most extraordinary change in the development of the human brain is represented by the increase in the surface of the neocortex and a parallel increase in laminar complexity.

The second mechanism is represented by the fact that the synapses are poorly developed and are thus unable to select the most salient signal to send to the cortex with respect to the background noise. Molecular alterations would alter the development and function of the synapses in their diversification in inhibitory, excitatory and modulating activities, with consequent modification in the balance between excitatory and inhibitory functions and thus the inability to uncover salient signals. This is the minicolumn hypothesis of Casanova *et al.* (2002), according to which the minicolumn structure of neurocortex would constitute a self-contained ecosystem of neurons and their afferent, efferent, and interneuronal connections. The minicolumn is a basic functional unit of the brain which processes sensory information. Minicolumns are found in the frontal and temporal lobes. Minicolumns in the brains of autistic patients are narrower, with an altered internal organization; more specifically, their minicolumns reveal less peripheral neuropil space, but increased spacing among their constituent cells. The peripheral neuropil space of the minicolumn is the conduit for inhibitory local circuit projections. A defect in these GABAergic fibres may correlate with the increased prevalence of seizures among autistic patients. Specificity of GABAergic inhibition in the neocortex is focused around its mini- and macrocolumnar organization. GABAergic interneurons are vital to proper minicolumnar differentiation and signal processing (*e.g.*, filtering capacity of the neocortex), thus providing a supposed correlate to autistic symptoms.

Finally, with regard to the strong male prevalence of the disorder, in 2005 Baron-Cohen and colleagues published his drastic hypothesis in *Science* that autism is an extreme form of the male brain. Males, in fact, have a greater capacity for concentration, do not love to talk, and are not disposed to understand the mental state of others, whereas women tend to be more intuitive and empathetic. Baron-Cohen affirmed that there is an increased susceptibility for autism to develop in the male brain. Despite the fact that many susceptibility genes such as *ARX*, *FMR 1*, *MECP 2*, and neuroligin are present on chromosome X, this does not account for the strong prevalence of ASD in males. It has been hypothesized that hormones are partly responsible for this prevalence. Hormones, especially the androgens that are transformed into estrogens, are powerful in conformations of the synapses and cortex and also control the GABAergic inhibitory effect. It is possible then that the hormonal effect contributes to the male prevalence of ASD, and it is possible that modulation of sexual male steroids could have a therapeutic value in severe forms of ASD (Rubenstein, 2010).

Conclusions

To conclude, there is an enormous hetero- as well as endophenotypic variability with regard to autism: The symptoms point to a pathologic disconnection of a widely distributed network of interconnected specialized areas. More than a lesion, it can be described as a complex, altered development of the brain that changes over time. Genetics and environment also shape the alteration in a dynamic perspective whose mechanisms are complex, intrinsically correlated, and still largely unknown. The efforts of researchers need to be part of a virtuous circle of transactional research, which first provides an accurate phenotype of the illness, then goes on to examine its neuropathology, to identify genes, and to study animal models and cell pathophysiology, and then moves in the direction of identifying pathologic targets that could be modified by therapy, and finally arrives at a treatment based on molecular mechanisms – all of these actions combine to restore health and wholeness to the autistic child and is the heart, soul and aim of all our work.

Conflicts of interest: The author declares no conflicts of interest.

References

Abrahams, B.S. & Geschwind, D.H. (2010): Connecting genes to brain in the autism spectrum disorders. *Arch Neurol.* **67**, 395–399.

Amaral, D.G., Schumann, C.M. & Nordahl, C.W. (2008): Neuroanatomy of autism. *Trends Neurosci.* **31**, 137–145.

Baron-Cohen, S., Leslie, A.M. & Frith, U. (1985): Does the autistic child have a 'theory of mind'? *Cognition* **21**, 37–46.

Baron-Cohen, S., Knickmeyer, R.C. & Belmonte, M.K. (2005): Sex differences in the brain: implications for explaining autism. *Science* **310**, 819–823.

Bauman, M. & Kemper, T.L. (1994): Neuroanatomic observations of the brain in autism. In: *The Neurobiology of Autism*, eds. M. Bauman & T.L. Kemper, pp. 119–145. Baltimore, MD: Johns Hopkins University Press.

Bauman, M.L. & Kemper, T.L. (2005): Neuroanatomic observations of the brain in autism: a review and future directions. *Int. J. Dev. Neurosci.* **23**, 183–187.

Calder, A.J. & Young, A.W. (2005): Understanding the recognition of facial identity and facial expression. *Nat. Rev. Neurosci.* **6**, 641–651.

Casanova, M.F., Buxhoeveden, D.P., Switala, A.E. & Roy, E. (2002): Minicolumnar pathology in autism. *Neurology* **58**, 428–432.

Courchesne, E., Townsend, J. & Saitoh, O. (1994): The brain in infantile autism: posterior fossa structures are abnormal. *Neurology* **44**, 214–223.

Courchesne, E., Carper, R. & Akshoomoff, N. (2003): Evidence of brain overgrowth in the first year of life in autism. *JAMA* **290**, 337–344.

Courchesne, E., Pierce, K., Schumann, C.M., *et al.* (2007): Mapping early brain development in autism. *Neuron* **56**, 399–413.

Dapretto, M., Davies, M.S., Pfeifer, J.H., *et al.* (2006): Understanding emotions in others: mirror neuron dysfunction in children with autism spectrum disorders. *Nat. Neurosci.* **9**, 28–30.

DeLong, G.R. & Heinz, E.R. (1997): The clinical syndrome of early-life bilateral hippocampal sclerosis. *Ann. Neurol.* **42**, 11–17.

Fatemi, S.H., Stary, J.M., Halt, A.R. & Realmuto, G.R. (2001): Dysregulation of reelin and Bcl-2 proteins in autistic cerebellum. *J. Autism Dev. Disord.* **31**, 529–535.

Fatemi, S.H., Halt, A.R., Realmuto, G., Earle, J., Kist, D.A., Thuras, P. & Merz, A. (2002): Purkinje cell size is reduced in cerebellum of patients with autism. *Cell. Mol. Neurobiol.* **22**, 171–175.

Fombonne, E. (2009): Epidemiology of pervasive developmental disorders. *Pediatr. Res.* **65**, 591–598.

Frith, U. (1989): *Autism: Explaining the Enigma.* Oxford, U.K.: Blackwell.

Gallese, V. (2003): The roots of empathy: the shared manifold hypothesis and the neural basis of intersubjectivity. *Psychopathology* **36**, 171–180.

Garel, S. & Rubenstein, J.L. (2004): Intermediate targets in formation of topographic projections: inputs from the thalamocortical system. *Trends Neurosci.* **27**, 533–539.

Geschwind, D.H. & Levitt, P. (2007): Autism spectrum disorders: developmental disconnection syndromes. *Curr. Opin. Neurobiol.* **17**, 103–111.

Goines, P., Haapanen, L., Boyce, R., *et al.* (2011): Autoantibodies to cerebellum in children with autism associate with behavior. *Brain Behav. Immun.* **25**, 514–523.

Grove, E.A. & Fukuchi-Shimogori, T. (2003): Generating the cerebral cortical area map. *Annu. Rev. Neurosci* **26**, 355–380.

Hardan, A.Y., Jou, R.J., Keshavan, M.S., Varma, R. & Minshew, N.J. (2004): Increased frontal cortical folding in autism: a preliminary MRI study. *Psychiatry Res.* **131**, 263–268.

Hashimoto, T., Sasaki, M., Sugai, K., Hanaoka, S., Fukumizu, M. & Kato, T. (2001): Paroxysmal discharges on EEG in young autistic patients are frequent in frontal regions. *J. Med. Invest.* **48**, 175–180.

Hertz-Picciotto, I. & Delwiche, L. (2009): The rise in autism and the role of age at diagnosis. *Epidemiology* **20**, 84–90.

Jou, R.J., Minshew, N.J., Keshavan, M.S., Vitale, M.P. & Hardan, A.Y. (2010a): Enlarged right superior temporal gyrus in children and adolescents with autism. *Brain Res.* **1360**, 205–212.

Jou, R.J., Minshew, N.J., Keshavan, M.S. & Hardan, A.Y. (2010b): Cortical gyrification in autistic and Asperger disorders: a preliminary magnetic resonance imaging study. *J. Child Neurol.* **25**, 1462–1467.

Just, V.L., Cherkassky, T.A., Keller, N.J. & Minshew, N.J. (2004): Cortical activation and synchronization during sentence comprehension in high-functioning autism: evidence of underconnectivity. *Brain* **127**, 1811–1821.

Kana, R.K., Libero, L.E. & Moore, M.S. (2011): Disrupted cortical connectivity theory as an explanatory model for autism spectrum disorders. *Phys. Life Rev.* **8**, 410–437.

Kana, R.K., Libero, L.E., Hu, C.P., Deshpande, H.R. & Colburn, J.S. (2012): Functional brain networks and white matter underlying theory-of-mind in autism. *Soc. Cogn. Affect. Neurosci.* [E-pub ahead of print].

Kanner, L. (1943): Autistic disturbances of affective contact. *Nervous Child* **2**, 217–250.

Kemper, T.L. & Bauman, M.L. (1993): The contribution of neuropathologic studies to the understanding of autism. *Neurol. Clin.* **11**, 175–187.

Kemper, T.L. & Bauman, M. (1998): Neuropathology of infantile autism. *J. Neuropathol. Exp. Neurol.* **57**, 645–652.

Lam, K.S., Aman, M.G. & Arnold, L.E. (2006): Neurochemical correlates of autistic disorder: a review of the literature. *Res. Dev. Disabil.* **27**, 254–289.

Lee, P.S., Yerys, B.E., Della Rosa, A., *et al.* (2009): Functional connectivity of the inferior frontal cortex changes with age in children with autism spectrum disorders: a fcMRI study of response inhibition. *Cereb. Cortex* **19**, 1787–1794.

Leonard, H., Glasson, E., Nassar, N., *et al.* (2011): Autism and intellectual disability are differentially related to sociodemographic background at birth. *PLoS One* **6**, e17875.

Leslie, A.M., Friedman, O. & German, T.P. (2004): Core mechanisms in 'theory of mind'. *Trends Cogn. Sci.* **8**, 528–533.

Levisohn, L., Cronin-Golomb, A. & Schmahmann, J.D. (2000): Neuropsychological consequences of cerebellar tumour resection in children: cerebellar cognitive affective syndrome in a paediatric population. *Brain* **123**, 1041–1050.

Long, J.E., Swan, C., Liang, W.S., Cobos, I., Potter, G.B. & Rubenstein, J.L. (2009): Dlx1&2 and Mash1 transcription factors control striatal patterning and differentiation through parallel and overlapping pathways. *J. Comp. Neurol.* **512**, 556–572.

Munoz-Yunta, J.A., Ortiz, T., Palau-Baduell, M., *et al.* (2008): Magnetoencephalographic pattern of epileptiform activity in children with early-onset autism spectrum disorders. *Clin. Neurophysiol.* **119**, 626–634.

Nacewicz, B.M., Dalton, K.M., Johnstone, T., *et al.* (2006): Amygdala volume and nonverbal social impairment in adolescent and adult males with autism. *Arch. Gen. Psychiatry* **63**, 1417–1428.

Paul, L.K., Brown, W.S., Adolphs, R., *et al.* (2007): Agenesis of the corpus callosum: genetic, developmental and functional aspects of connectivity. *Nat. Rev. Neurosci.* **8**, 287–299.

Pelphrey, K.A., Shultz, S., Hudac, C.M. & VanderWyk, B.C. (2011): Research review: constraining heterogeneity: the social brain and its development in autism spectrum disorder. *J. Child Psychol. Psychiatry* **52**, 631–644.

Perry, E.K., Lee, M.L., Martin-Ruiz, C.M., *et al.* (2001): Cholinergic activity in autism: abnormalities in the cerebral cortex and basal forebrain. *Am. J. Psychiatry* **158**, 1058–1066.

Polosan, M., Baciu, M., Cousin, E., Perrone, M., Pichat, C. & Bougerol, T. (2011): An fMRI study of the social competition in healthy subjects. *Brain Cogn.* **77**, 401–411.

Riva, D. & Giorgi, C. (2000): The cerebellum contributes to higher functions during development: evidence from a series of children surgically treated for posterior fossa tumours. *Brain* **123**, 1051–1061.

Riva, D., Bulgheroni, S., Aquino, D., Di Salle, F., Savoiardo, M. & Erbetta, A. (2011): Basal forebrain involvement in low-functioning autistic children: a voxel-based morphometry study. *AJNR Am. J. Neuroradiol.* **32**, 1430–1435.

Rizzolatti, G., Fadiga, L., Gallese, V. & Fogassi, L. (1996): Premotor cortex and the recognition of motor actions. *Brain Res. Cogn. Brain Res.* **3**, 131–141.

Rosenberg, R.E., Kaufmann, W.E., Law, J.K. & Law, P.A. (2011): Parent report of community psychiatric comorbid diagnoses in autism spectrum disorders. *Autism Res. Treat.* [E-pub 18 Aug 2011].

Rout, U.K. & Dhossche, D.M. (2008): A pathogenetic model of autism involving Purkinje cell loss through anti-GAD antibodies. *Med. Hypotheses* **71,** 218–221.

Rubenstein, J.L. (2010): Three hypotheses for developmental defects that may underlie some forms of autism spectrum disorder. *Curr. Opin. Neurol.* **23,** 118–123.

Saitoh, O., Karns, C.M. & Courchesne, E. (2001): Development of the hippocampal formation from 2 to 42 years: MRI evidence of smaller area dentata in autism. *Brain* **124,** 1317–1324.

Schmahmann, J.D. & Sherman, J.C. (1998): The cerebellar cognitive affective syndrome. *Brain* **121,** 561–579.

Schmahmann, J.D. & Pandya, D.N. (2008): Disconnection syndromes of basal ganglia, thalamus, and cerebrocerebellar systems. *Cortex* **44,** 1037–1066.

Schumann, C.M. & Amaral, D.G. (2006): Stereological analysis of amygdala neuron number in autism. *J. Neurosci.* **19,** 7674–7679.

Schumann, C.M., Bloss, C.S., Barnes, C.C., *et al.* (2010): Longitudinal magnetic resonance imaging study of cortical development through early childhood in autism. *J. Neurosci.* **30,** 4419-4427.

Silver, W.G. & Rapin, I. (2012): Neurobiological basis of autism. *Pediatr. Clin. N. Amer.* **59,** 45–61.

Sinclair, J. (1993): Don't mourn for us. Autism Network International Newsletter, *Our Voice,* Vol. **1,** 3.

Sparks, B.F., Friedman, S.D., Shaw, D.W., *et al.* (2002): Brain structural abnormalities in young children with autism spectrum disorder. *Neurology* **59,** 184–192.

Stanfield, A.C., McIntosh, A.M., Spencer, M.D., Philip, R., Gaur, S. & Lawrie, S.M. (2008): Towards a neuroanatomy of autism: a systematic review and meta-analysis of structural magnetic resonance imaging studies. *Eur. Psychiatry* **23,** 289–299.

Tuchman, R., Moshe, S.L. & Rapin, I. (2009): Convulsing toward the pathophysiology of autism. *Brain Dev.* **31,** 95–103.

Uddin, L.Q. & Menon, V. (2010): Introduction to special topic: resting-state brain activity: implications for systems neuroscience. *Front. Syst. Neurosci.* **4.** pii: 37.

Verhoeven, J.S., De Cock, P., Lagae, L. & Sunaert, S. (2010): Neuroimaging of autism. *Neuroradiology* **52,** 3–14.

Walsh, M.B. (2011): The top 10 reasons children with autism deserve ABA. *Behav. Anal. Pract.* **4,** 72–79.

Wass, S. (2011): Distortions and disconnections: disrupted brain connectivity in autism. *Brain Cogn.* **75,** 18–28.

Wing, L. & Gould, J. (1979): Severe impairments of social interaction and associated abnormalities in children: epidemiology and classification. *J. Autism Dev. Disord.* **9,** 11–29.

Xu, J., Liu, Z. & Ornitz, D.M. (2000): Temporal and spatial gradients of Fgf8 and Fgf17 regulate proliferation and differentiation of midline cerebellar structures. *Development* **127,** 1833–1843.

Neurobiology

Chapter 2

New diagnostic instruments and methods for autism spectrum disorders

So Hyun Kim

*Yale Child Study Center, Yale University School of Medicine,
New Haven, Connecticut 06510, USA*
so-hyun.kim@yale.edu

Summary

Autism spectrum disorder (ASD) is a neurobiological disorder that is defined purely by observable behaviours since reliable biomarkers have not yet been found. Standard diagnostic instruments that have been used widely for the comprehensive assessment of ASD combine information from multiple sources such as caregiver interviews and direct clinical observations. Recently proposed changes in the major framework of ASD diagnostic criteria are discussed in this chapter. With the newly developed and refined methods now available, the results of studies of individuals with ASD will contribute to more reliable and valid diagnosis of ASD.

Introduction

Core features of ASD include impairments and delays in social and communication skills as well as the presence of restricted and repetitive behaviours (RRBs; American Psychiatric Association, 1994). Communication deficits in ASD go beyond language delays since they include a variety of impairments such as the use of stereotyped speech or delayed echolalia (*e.g.*, repeating lines from a TV show) and difficulties initiating and maintaining meaningful back-and-forth conversation (*e.g.*, being preoccupied with certain topics and dominating conversations without responding to others' questions or leads). Moreover, other aspects of communication skills such as eye contact, gestures, and facial expressions that are commonly used to compensate for language delays by other populations are also impaired in individuals with ASD. Social deficits include the failure to develop peer relationships appropriate to developmental level and a lack of spontaneous seeking to share enjoyment or interests with others. Examples of RRBs include a very broad category of behaviours such as repetitive motor actions (*e.g.*, hand flapping and finger flicking), preoccupation with *parts* of objects (*e.g.*, peering at the wheels of toy cars while spinning them), and restricted patterns of interest (*e.g.*, having very specific knowledge about the New York City subway system), and adherence to specific, nonfunctional routines (*e.g.*, insisting on taking a certain route to go home).

Past studies have consistently suggested that individuals with ASD show tremendous heterogeneity in manifestation of the symptoms mentioned above. Heterogeneity in behavioural manifestations of autism symptoms is affected by variability in factors, including but not restricted to developmental trajectories, level of language, cognitive ability, gender, adaptive behaviours, and sensory and motor impairments (see Kim & Lord, in press). For instance, nonverbal toddlers with ASD may show kinds of social deficits that are different from those of older children with ASD whose language skills are fluent. Toddlers with ASD may use the body of another person to communicate without integrated look or vocalization, while adults with ASD may have difficulty having back-and-forth conversations with others because they are preoccupied with highly unusual and specific conversational topics.

Despite the tremendous heterogeneity found in ASD, autism itself, the most severe form of ASD, is also considered the most clearly defined of all the ASDs and one of the most reliably defined psychiatric disorders emerging in childhood (Volkmar et al., 1997). Autism can be reliably diagnosed starting at age 2 by an experienced clinician, using standardized methods based on criteria in the *Diagnostic and Statistical Manual on Mental Disorders*–4th edition (DSM–IV; APA, 1994) and in the World Health Organization's *International Statistical Classification of Diseases and Related Health Problems*, 10th Revision (ICD–10; WHO, 1992). Through the use of multiple standard instruments targeting developmental history, cognitive and communicative functioning, and observation of the symptoms of autism, uniform standards for a comprehensive assessment of ASD have been created. Providing a comprehensive review of ASD diagnostic instruments is beyond the scope of this chapter; for this purpose, see Lord and Corsello (2004) or Worley and Matson (2011). In this chapter, changes recently made to two diagnostic tools for ASD, the Autism Diagnostic Observation Schedule (ADOS; Lord et al., 1999) and Autism Diagnostic Interview–Revised (ADI–R; Rutter Le Couteur & Lord, 1994) will be reviewed.

Diagnosis and classification of ASD

Standardized diagnostic instruments

Standardized diagnostic instruments based on criteria in the DSM–IV (American Psychiatric Association, 1994) and in the ICD–10 (WHO, 1990) have created uniform standards for a diagnosis of ASD. Past studies have consistently suggested that the diagnosis of ASD should be made based on a comprehensive assessment of developmental history, cognitive and communicative functioning, and observation of the symptoms of autism using multiple diagnostic and cognitive instruments (Corsello et al., 2007; Kim & Lord, 2011a; LeCouteur et al., 2008; Risi et al., 2006).

The Autism Diagnostic Observation Schedule (ADOS; Lord et al., 1999) is a semi-structured, standardized assessment of communication, social interaction, and play or imaginative use of materials for individuals who have been referred because of a possible autism spectrum disorder (ASD). As part of the schedule, planned social occasions, referred to as 'presses' (Lord et al., 1989) are created to elicit spontaneous behaviours in standardized contexts. Structured activities and materials, and less structured interactions, provide standard contexts within the ADOS in which social, communicative, and other behaviours relevant to the understanding of ASDs are observed.

The ADOS consists of four modules that are selected by the individual's age and language levels. The ADOS provides the diagnostic algorithms for the classifications of autism or ASDs. Original algorithms have been revised to improve diagnostic validity (Gotham et al., 2007). However, research has indicated that the algorithms showed lower diagnostic validity for toddlers, especially those with limited nonverbal mental age and language level, than for older children. Thus, a standardized diagnostic measure applicable for toddlers was needed for early identification; this prompted the development of Toddler Module of the ADOS applicable to very young children from 12 to 30 months' of age who are walking independently (Lord et al., 2012; Luyster et al., 2009). The ADOS–T consists of 11 activities with 41 accompanying ratings. Since differential diagnoses are not as stable in toddlers, the ADOS–T algorithms generate range of concern (little-or-no, mild-to-moderate, moderate-to-severe) that can be used to indicate whether the child needs to be recommended for follow-up assessments and services. Certain cutoff scores are also available for clinicians and researchers who wish to use the classification of ASD (rather than autism and ASD).

The Autism Diagnostic Interview–Revised (ADI–R; Lord et al., 1994) is a standardized, semi-structured, investigator-based interview for parents or caregivers of individuals referred for a possible ASD. The ADI–R includes 93 items in three domains of functioning, language, and communication, reciprocal social interactions, and restricted, repetitive, and stereotyped behaviours and interests, as well as other aspects of behaviours. Up to 42 of the interview items are systematically combined to produce a formal, diagnostic algorithm for autism based on the ICD–10 and DSM–IV criteria as specified by the authors. Other criteria, including using lower cutoffs with the same set of items, have been used to create an algorithm for broader classification of ASD as in several collaborative studies (Lainhart et al., 2006; Risi et al., 2006). A 'Toddler' version of the ADI–R was also developed several years ago to provide descriptive data to be used for research purposes with children under 4 years of age.

Previous analyses have suggested that the diagnostic algorithm for the ADI–R was useful for children with a nonverbal mental age above 2 years, but lower sensitivities and specificities were obtained for children under 3 years of age and/or nonverbal mental age below 2 years (Le Couteur et al., 1989; Lord et al., 1994; Risi et al., 2006; Rutter et al., 2003). For this reason, new ADI–R algorithms specific for toddlers and young preschoolers have been developed, which showed improved predictive validity for young children from 12 to 47 months of age compared to results obtained with the preexisting algorithm forms (Kim & Lord, 2011b). The new algorithms include items that overlap between the toddler and standard versions of the ADI–R such that the algorithms can be used for either version, expanding the lowest age of application to 12 months with a lowest nonverbal developmental level of 10 months.

As mentioned above, past studies have shown that combining information from both the ADOS and ADI–R better reflected the clinical best estimate diagnosis of ASD than when a single instrument was used for a diagnosis of ASD in populations across toddlers to adolescents (Kim & Lord, 2011a; Le Couteur et al., 2008; Risi et al., 2006). Therefore, ADOS and ADI–R make independent, additive contributions to more accurate diagnostic decisions for clinicians evaluating individuals with ASD. Combinations of the other alternative instruments, such as the Social Responsiveness Scale (SRS; Constantino et al., 2005), the Social Communication Questionnaire (SCQ; Rutter et al., 2003), and the Children's Communication Checklist (CCC; Bishop, 2005), with or without ADOS and/or ADI–R, may work equally to provide the most reliable, best-estimate diagnoses.

Classification of ASD

The newly proposed criteria for the DSM–5 (American Psychiatric Association, 2010) include one category, ASD, unlike the case in the DSM–IV (which included separate criteria for differential diagnoses, such as autistic disorder, Asperger's syndrome, childhood disintegrative disorder, and pervasive developmental disorders–not otherwise specified [PDD–NOS]). This decision was based on different factors. First, the diagnoses of autism *versus* PDD–NOS have been found to be relatively unstable, variable across sites, and often associated with severity, language level or intelligence rather than features of the disorder (Kleinman *et al.*, 2008; Lord *et al.*, 2006, 2012; Turner & Stone, 2006) in contrast to overall diagnoses of ASD *versus* other non-ASD developmental disorders that are consistent over time. This is also in line with recently developed ADOS and ADI–R algorithms and criteria for toddlers and young preschoolers, which include classifications of ASD *vs.* non-ASD rather than autism, ASD *vs.* non-ASD (Kim & Lord, 2011b; Luyster *et al.*, 2009).

In the past, the criteria for an autistic disorder in the DSM–IV were determined based on three domains, including communication, social interaction, and restricted and repetitive patterns of behaviour and interests. However, the most recent proposal for DSM–5 (American Psychiatric Association, 2010) has defined ASD symptoms according to two domains: reciprocal social communication and a broad domain of restricted, repetitive interests and behaviours. This change reflects the recent findings that social and communication impairments are highly associated with each other (Gotham *et al.*, 2007; Kim & Lord, 2011b; Luyster *et al.*, 2009; Snow *et al.*, 2009). For instance, studies have shown the common symptoms that are shown in ASD, such as limited use of eye contact and gestures, a lack of engagement in social chat, difficulties in reciprocal conversation, and deficits in imitation and play, are as much a part of communication as social factors are (Snow *et al.*, 2009). Moreover, nonverbal communication items on the ADI–R have been found to correlate very highly with social behaviours (Snow *et al.*, 2009). For these reasons, recent studies have suggested that it is more valid and parsimonious to think of the social and communication domains as a single domain rather than separate entities (Gotham *et al.*, 2007; Kim & Lord, 2011b).

In addition, individuals are required to have at least two symptoms of RRBs in order to receive a diagnosis of ASD. The scope of the RRB domain has been expanded to include examples such as stereotyped or repetitive speech and hyper- or hyporeactivity to sensory input. This decision has been supported by different studies that suggested that even though RRBs are present in non-spectrum disorders, RRBs in children with ASD are significantly more prevalent and higher in severity than children with other developmental disorders (*e.g.*, Kim & Lord, 2010; Richler *et al.*, 2010; Watson *et al.*, 2007). It has been also found that when parent interviews and clinician observations are both used, all children with ASD show RRBs (*e.g.*, Kim & Lord, 2010), highlighting the importance of combining information from multiple sources for a diagnosis of ASD. Requiring two symptoms for RRBs has been also found to improve specificity of the criterion without significant decrements in sensitivity (APA, 2010).

Another major change made to the newly proposed DSM–5 criteria concerns the levels of severity that will be used to indicate the level of support the individuals need. These levels are: *Level 1*: requiring support; *Level 2*: requiring substantial support; and *Level 3*: requiring very substantial support. These levels are based on the levels of impairment in social communication skills and the degree to which RRBs interfere with the individual's daily functioning.

Conclusions

ASD is one of the most reliably, if not the most reliably, defined psychiatric disorder emerging in childhood (Volkmar & Rutter, 1997). The diagnosis of ASD is based on standardized assessments of both observable behaviour and developmental history since there is not yet a valid genetic or biological marker of ASD. New diagnostic tools have been developed and refined recently, especially for very young children with ASD, with an increase in demand for valid instruments for diagnosing ASD in these young children. Major changes have also been proposed for the classification of ASD based on recent research findings. These newly developed and refined methods can help to contribute to more reliable and valid diagnosis of ASD.

Conflicts of interest: The author declares no conflicts of interest.

References

American Psychiatric Association (1994): *Diagnostic and Statistical Manual of Mental Disorders*, 4th ed. Washington, DC: APA.

American Psychiatric Association (2010): Autism spectrum disorder. Retrieved August 15, 2011 from <http://www.dsm5.org/proposedrevision/pages/proposedrevision.aspx?rid=94>

Bishop, D. (2005): *The Children's Communication Checklist–2*. London: Psychological Corporation.

Constantino, J. & Gruber, C. (2005): *Social Responsiveness Scale*. Los Angeles, CA: Western Psychological Services.

Corsello, C., Hus, V., Pickles, A., Risi, S., Cook, E., Leventhal, B. & Lord, C. (2007): Between a ROC and a hard place: decision making and making decisions about using the SCQ. *J. Child Psychol. Psychiatry* **48,** 932–940.

Gotham, K., Risi, S., Pickles, A. & Lord, C. (2007): The Autism Diagnostic Observation Schedule: revised algorithms for improved diagnostic validity. *J. Autism Dev. Disord.* **37,** 613–627.

Kim, S.H. & Lord, C. (2010): Restricted and repetitive behaviors in toddlers and preschoolers with autism spectrum disorders based on the autism diagnostic observation schedule (ADOS). *Autism Res.* **3,** 162–173.

Kim, S. & Lord, C. (2011a): Combining information from multiple sources in the diagnosis of autism spectrum disorders using the new ADI–R algorithms for toddlers from 12 to 47 months of age. *J. Child Psychol. Psychiatry* **53,** 143–151.

Kim, S. & Lord, C. (2011b): New Autism Diagnostic Interview-Revised (ADI–R) algorithms for toddlers and young preschoolers from 12 to 47 months of age. *J. Autism Dev. Disord.* **42,** 82–93.

Kim, S. & Lord, C. (in press): Behavioral manifestations of autism spectrum disorders. In: *The Neuroscience of Autism Spectrum Disorders*, eds. J.D. Buxbaum & P.R. Hofman. New York: Elsevier.

Kleinman, J.M., Ventola, P.E., Pandey, J., *et al.* (2008): Diagnostic stability in very young children with autism spectrum disorders. *J. Autism Dev. Disord.* **38,** 606–615.

Lainhart, J., Bigler, E., Bocain, M., *et al.* (2006): Head circumference and height in autism: a study by the collaborative program of excellence in autism. *Am. J. Med. Genet.*, A **140,** 2256–2274.

Le Couteur, A., Haden, G., Hammal, D. & McConachie, H. (2008): Diagnosing autism spectrum disorders in preschoolers using two standardised assessment instruments: the ADI–R and the ADOS. *J. Autism Dev. Disord.* **38,** 362–372.

Lord, C. & Corsello, C. (2005): Diagnostic instruments in autism spectrum disorders. In: *Handbook of Autism and Pervasive Developmental Disorders*, eds. F. Volkmar, A. Klin, R. Paul & D. Cohen. Hoboken, NJ: Wiley.

Lord, C., Rutter, M., Goode, S. & Heemsbergen, J. (1989): Autism Diagnostic Observation Schedule: a standardized observation of communicative and social behavior. *J. Autism Dev. Disord.* **19,** 185–212.

Lord, C., Rutter, M., DiLavore, P. & Risi, S. (1999): *Autism Diagnostic Observation Schedule: Manual*. Los Angeles, CA: Western Psychological Services.

Lord, C., Risi, S., DiLavore, P., Shulman, C., Thurm, A. & Pickles, A. (2006): Autism from 2 to 9 years of age. *Arch. Gen. Psychiatry* **63,** 694–701.

Lord, C.E., Luyster. R, Gotham, K. & Guthrie, W.J. (2012): Autism Diagnostic Observation Schedule – Toddler Module. Los Angeles, CA: Western Psychological Services.

Lord, C., Petkova, E., Hus, V., Gan W., Lu, F., Martin, D., et al. (2012): A multisite study of the clinical diagnosis of different autism spectrum disorders. *Arch. Gen. Psychiatry* **69**, 306–313.

Luyster, R., Gotham, K., Guthrie, W., Coffing, M., Petrak, R., Pierce, K., et al. (2009): The Autism Diagnostic Observation Schedule–Toddler Module: a new module of a standardized diagnostic measure for autism spectrum disorders. *J. Autism Dev. Disord.* **39**, 1305–1320.

Richler, J., Huerta, M., Bishop, S. & Lord, C. (2010): Developmental trajectories of restricted and repetitive behaviors and interests in children with autism spectrum disorders. *Dev. Psychopathol.* **22**, 55–69.

Risi, S., Lord, C., Gotham, K., et al. (2006): Combining information from multiple sources in the diagnosis of autism spectrum disorders. *J. Am. Acad. Child Adolesc. Psychiatry* **45**, 1094–1103.

Rutter, M., Le Couteur, A.L. & Lord, C. (1994): Autism Diagnostic Interview–Revised: a revised version of a diagnostic interview for caregivers of individuals with possible pervasive developmental disorders. *J. Autism Dev. Disord.* **24**, 659–685.

Rutter, M., Bailey, A. & Lord, C. (2003): *The Social Communication Questionnaire*. Los Angeles, CA: Western Psychological Services.

Snow, A.V., Lecavalier, L. & Houts, C. (2009): The structure of the Autism Diagnostic Interview-Revised: diagnostic and phenotypic implications. *J. Child Psychol. Psychiatry* **50**, 734–742.

Turner, L. & Stone, W. (2007): Variability in outcome for children with an ASD diagnosis at age 2. *J. Child Psychol. Psychiatry Allied Discipl.* **48**, 793–802.

Volkmar, F.R., Klin, A. & Cohen, D.J. (1997): Diagnosis and classification of autism and related conditions: consensus and issues. In: *Handbook of Autism and Pervasive Developmental Disorders*, 2nd ed., eds. D.J. Cohen & F.R. Volkmar, pp. 5–40. New York: Wiley.

Watson, L.R., Baranek, G.T., Crais, E.J., Reznick, J.S., Dykstra, J. & Perryman, T. (2007): The first year inventory: retrospective parent responses to a questionnaire designed to identify one year-olds at risk for autism. *J. Autism Dev. Disord.* **37**, 49–61.

World Health Organization (1992): *The ICD–10 Classification of Mental and Behavioral Disorders: Clinical Descriptions and Diagnostic Guidelines*. Geneva: WHO.

Worley, J.A. & Matson, J.L. (2011): Diagnostic instruments for the core features of autism. In: *International Handbook of Autism and Pervasive Developmental Disorders*, ed. J.L. Matson, pp. 215–231. New York: Springer.

Chapter 3

Conventional neuroimaging in autism

Alessandra Erbetta

Department of Neuroradiology, Fondazione IRCCS Istituto Neurologico 'C. Besta',
via Celoria 11, 20133 Milan, Italy
aerbetta@istituto-besta.it

Summary

Autism spectrum disorder (ASD) refers to a syndrome of social communication deficits, repetitive behaviours, and restricted interests. It remains a behaviourally defined syndrome with no reliable biological markers. Neuroimaging is increasingly involved in the diagnostic challenge of ASD forms. Its role is to exclude any gross pathology that can be identified by standard magnetic resonance imaging (MRI) such as neurocutaneous syndromes (*e.g.*, tuberous sclerosis), epileptic encephalopathies, neurometabolic diseases, and dystrophinopathies that might mimic or accompany ASD. Although a diagnostic imaging marker is lacking at present, a high rate of minor MRI abnormalities was found in a few series of conventional MRI investigations with respect to controls. These findings could contribute to research into the aetiology of autism and, in any case, complete the clinical assessment of children with ASD. The current literature on volumetric and voxel-based morphometry (VBM) studies shows a considerable variation of anatomic findings, within the broad construct of ASD. The goal of this review is to summarize the available conventional, volumetric, and VBM neuroimaging data and examine their implication for understanding of the neurobiology of ASD.

Introduction

Autism is clearly a disorder of neural development, but *when*, *where*, and *how* brain pathology occurs remain elusive. Typical brain development is composed of several stages, including proliferation and migration of neurons, creation of dendritic arbors and synaptic connections, and eventually dendritic pruning and programmed cell death. Any deviation at one or more of these stages could produce downstream effects. MRI studies of autism have provided important clues, describing an aberrant trajectory of growth during early childhood that is both present in the whole brain and marked in specific structures. Because MRI is safe and noninvasive, it can be used repeatedly in large numbers of living subjects. This allows MRI studies to provide a framework for when, where, and in whom there is a deviation from typical brain development. Common types of structural MRI images include T1-weighted images, which provide the greatest level of anatomic detail, and T2-weighted images, which highlight brain tissue signal abnormalities. Volumetric MRI studies typically utilize high-resolution T1-weighted images and can identify whether a particular region (*e.g.*, cerebral gray or white matter) or structure is larger or smaller in individuals with autism. Another important strength of MRI is its ability to acquire large enough samples of individuals to identify phenotype subgroups. Indeed, autism is increasingly recognized as an extremely heterogeneous disorder, with multiple phenotypes and aetiologies (Amaral *et al.*, 2008). A final major strength of MRI studies is that many analytic approaches can be applied to the same data set from the same case. These range from volumetric analyses of specific anatomically-defined structures to exploratory whole brain and VBM studies of gray and white matter alterations (Riva *et al.*, 2011). Other features that may be examined include cortical shape and cortical thickness (Ecker *et al.*, 2010). Despite the powerful advantages of MRI, there are several significant challenges as well. One challenge is that any movement during an MRI scan, whose duration is typically 30 min to an hour, adversely affects the quality of the image and makes the volume measurement of any brain region less reliable. For this reason, most MRI studies to date have focused on adults and adolescents with high-functioning autism despite the developmental nature of the disorder. Sedation or anesthesia has been utilized in some studies of young children and lower-functioning individuals with autism. Moreover, it is difficult to find neuroradiologic findings from healthy subjects to compare with those of very young patients. Another challenge is that careful advance planning is required to conduct multi-site MRI acquisition, which would be the most efficient way to acquire large sample sizes. MRI data from different scanners cannot be pooled together *post hoc*. Volumetric measurements of both total brain and subregions can differ significantly between acquisition locations. This may be attributed to differences in individual scanners, pulse sequences, and even scanning room environment, which produce differences in hardware-induced geometric distortions. MRI studies could explain some of the heterogeneity of autism by identifying different brain phenotypes or subgroups. Despite these contributions, it is important to keep in mind that the resolution of MRI is still so coarse that only gross, macroscopic changes can be detected. MRI researchers must look to postmortem research to understand the neurobiologic underpinnings of their findings. Postmortem brain tissue, acquired from individuals who had autism during life, is an important tool for understanding the underlying neurobiology and genetics of autism. Efforts to carry out postmortem brain studies of autism have historically been hindered by poor tissue quality and small sample sizes, with fewer than 150 autism cases studied to date and a mean sample size of 5 per study. Additionally, postmortem studies are obviously limited to observing the end result of each patient's neuropathologic course, which is influenced by their individualized exposure to environmental factors, medications, comorbid symptoms, cause of death, and particular type of autism (Schumann & Wu Nordahl, 2011).

Review of the topic

Neuropathologic findings

Despite the limitations of small sample sizes, bias in quantification techniques, and comorbidity that hamper neuropathologic investigation, some neuropathologic findings are available. Kemper and Bauman (1998) demonstrated an increased cell packing density and reduced cell size in hippocampus, subiculum, and amygdalae. Ritvo *et al.* (1986) and Fatemi *et al.* (2002) showed a decreased number of Purkinje cells in the cerebellar hemisphere and vermis of the autistic cases. Cortical dysgenesis with thickened cortices, high neuronal density, presence of neurons in the molecular layer, irregular laminar patterns and poor grey–white matter boundaries was reported by Bailey *et al.* (1998). Recently, Wegiel *et al.* (2010) detected changes within the subependymal cell layer with subependymal nodular dysplasia, subcortical and periventricular heterotopias, and neocortex, archicortex, dentate gyrus, cornu Ammonis, and cerebellar dysplasia. These findings reflect focal modification of neurogenesis, migration, and alterations of the cytoarchitecture of brain cortex, subcortical structures, and cerebellum in autism. Detection of the broad spectrum of focal developmental alterations in the brains of 92 per cent of the autistic subjects indicates that focal changes are a reflection of global developmental abnormalities and that regional changes may have their own contribution to the clinical heterogeneity of autism.

Conventional MR findings

At present, a diagnostic imaging marker is lacking and MRI is judged to be of little value in the clinical diagnosis of ASD. Computerized tomography and MRI demonstrated a very low prevalence of focal lesions or other structural abnormalities often incidental to coexisting anatomic disorders and probably unrelated to autism itself. Prevalence of lesions seen on MRI in children with autism was considered similar to that of normal control subjects and their inconsistent localization marked them as coincidental. For this reason, conventional MRI was judged to be of little value in the clinical diagnosis of autism according to the guidelines of the American Academy of Neurology and Child Neurology Society (Filipek *et al.*, 2000). Currently, MRI studies of autistic subjects screen to exclude those with disorders other than autism and confirm the absence of significant structural brain abnormalities. However, this statement was based on results obtained from small samples of patients and, more importantly, included mostly insufficient MRI sequences. Taber *et al.* (2004) demonstrated unusually large Virchow–Robin spaces in the centrum semiovale. More recently, Zeegers *et al.* (2006) demonstrated an abnormal rate of arachnoid cysts and Boddaert *et al.* (2009) reported an unexpected high rate of white matter signal abnormalities, and temporal lobe abnormalities in larger series of autistic patients using an appropriate set of sequences. In our series we detected enlargement of the cisterna magna, dilated Virchow–Robin spaces and white matter, and subcortical signal abnormalities (unpublished data).

Volumetric MR findings

Macrocephaly and increased brain volume in autism

Several epidemiologic studies of autism revealed an increased proportion (almost 15 per cent) of macrocephaly (defined as head circumference greater than the 97th percentile) in patients. Although macrocephaly is common in children and adults with autism, it is not common at birth. Macrocephaly appears to develop after birth in about 80 per cent of cases as an aberrant early postnatal brain overgrowth (Lainhart *et al.*, 1997; Courchesne *et al.*, 2001) Cross-sectional imaging studies that span toddlerhood through adulthood have provided valuable information for more than a decade about the neuropathology of autism at different ages (Courchesne *et al.*, 2001; Schumann *et al.*, 2010). These studies have revealed that there is brain enlargement during infancy and early childhood in the disorder, but normalization of volume in adolescence and adulthood (Amaral *et al.*, 2008; Courchesne *et al.*, 2007). Recently, longitudinal studies have confirmed the cross-sectional findings in young children (Mosconi *et al.*, 2009; Schumann *et al.*, 2010). Theoretically, brain enlargement in autism can occur as the result of three distinct developmental processes: increased neurogenesis, decreased neuronal death, and/or increased production of non-neuronal brain tissues such as glial cells or blood vessels.

Cerebellum

The cerebellum was extensively studied by different groups. In 1988 Kemper and Bauman reported a hypoplasia of the vermian lobules VI and VII in a group of autistic patients. This finding was consistent with earlier data from postmortem studies (*i.e.*, reduction in the number of Purkinje cells). These abnormalities could indirectly affect, through their connections to the brain stem, hypothalamus, and thalamus, the development and functioning of one or more systems involved in cognitive, sensory, autonomic, and motor activities (Courchesne *et al.*, 1988; Murakami *et al.*, 1989). Eventually, a meta-analysis done by Stanfield *et al.* (2007) confirmed the reduction in size of the lobules VI to VII of the vermis in autistic patients. About the role of the cerebellum in the aetiopathogenesis of autism, we recommend the reading of the consensus paper published by Fatemi *et al.* (2012).

Amigdalae

Amigdalae volumes have been examined in different small samples with inconsistent results. Some studies show increased and some decreased volume, whereas others revealed no significant group differences. The meta-analysis of Stanfield *et al.* (2007) indicated that age was an important factor in these conflicting results. Enlargement of amygdalae present in young autistic patients was not found in older subjects.

The cingulate gyrus

The cingulate gyrus was studied by Haznedar *et al.* (1997), who performed structural MRI and positron emission tomography (PET) scans on seven high-functioning autistic patients. The right anterior cingulate area in autistic subjects was significantly smaller in relative volume and was also metabolically less active in autistic subjects. These findings do not necessarily conflict with the neuropathologic findings.

Corpus callosum

Although various segments of the corpus callosum have been implicated in MRI studies of autism, there is consistency across studies in the finding that the corpus callosum is generally reduced in size. This reduction may diminish interhemispheric connectivity and may be involved in the pathophysiology of cognitive impairments and clinical features of autism (Cody *et al.*, 2002; Stanfield *et al.*, 2007).

Basal ganglia

At the level of the basal ganglia an enlargement of the caudate nucleus was shown. The caudate has connections to the prefrontal cortex and is known to play an inhibitory role in behaviour. A correlation was found between ritualistic and repetitive behaviours and increased volume of the caudate nucleus (Brambilla *et al.*, 2003).

Voxel-based morphometric studies

The development of new quantitative structural imaging studies like VBM analysis led to more standardized methods for data analysis. VBM analysis showed significant localized grey matter reductions within the fronto-striatal and parietal networks. Additional decreases were described in the ventral and superior temporal grey matter (Brambilla *et al.*, 2003; McAlonan *et al.*, 2005). Morphometric differences were also shown in key language regions. Boys with autism showed a significant asymmetric reversal in the inferior lateral frontal language cortex, which was 27 per cent larger on the right side The authors hypothesize that semantic encoding, normally performed by the inferior frontal gyrus, in autistic patients is performed via alternative pathways (Herbert *et al.*, 2005).

In our series of ASD patients, volume loss was found to affect the basal forebrain, nucleus accumbens, perisylvian regions, and other cortical brain regions functionally connected to the above-mentioned areas, as well as the putamen and cerebellum (Riva *et al.*, 2011). The volume reduction in the basal forebrain was not previously found in VBM studies of autistic children. This area and its extensive cholinergic multiple cortical connections are involved in social, communicative, and cognitive behaviour. The basal forebrain involvement may be also related to the contemporary presence of developmental delay in our autistic children.

Conclusions

As you can see, no characteristic is unique and uniform for all ASD patients. The autism phenotype comprises a spectrum of disorders varying in their presentation, course and outcome and in the quality and intensity of the symptoms. Conventional MRI demonstrated a high rate of MRI abnormalities which are not specific to ASD diagnosis. However, these findings may contribute to the aetiopathologic research and to complete the clinical assessment of ASD patients.

Regarding VBM abnormalities in individuals with ASD, many factors, such as inclusion and exclusion criteria, population age, MR acquisition parameters, details of the image processing, features of extraction procedures, analytic methods used to detect group differences, and sample sizes may have contributed to these disparities. Reviewing the present state of the art, we have to conclude that there are still a great number of incongruencies. However, because MRI is safe and noninvasive, it can be used repeatedly in large numbers of living subjects. This allows advanced MRI studies, such as functional MRI and DTI to provide a framework for when, where, and in whom there is a deviation from typical brain development. Neuroimaging can provide the framework by identifying different subgroups of ASD patients with distinct patterns of affected brain areas or the timing of aberrant development.

Conflicts of interest: The author declares no conflicts of interest.

References

Amaral, D.G., Schumann, C.M. & Nordahl, C.W. (2008): Neuroanatomy of autism. *Trends Neurosci.* **31,** 137–145.

Bailey, A., Luthert, P., Dean, A., *et al.* (1998): A clinicopathological study of autism. *Brain* **121,** 889–905.

Boddaert, N., Zilbovicius, M., Philipe, A., *et al.* (2009): MRI findings in 77 children with non-syndromic autistic disorder. *PLoS One* **4,** 1–7.

Brambilla, P., Hardan, A., di Nemi, S.U., Perez, J., Soares, J.C. & Barale, F. (2003): Brain anatomy and development in autism: review of structural MRI studies. *Brain Res Bull.* **61,** 557–569.

Cody, H., Pelphrey, K. & Piven, J. (2002): Structural and functional magnetic resonance imaging of autism. *Int. J. Dev. Neurosci.* **20,** 421–438.

Courchesne, E., Courchesne, R.Y., Press, G.A., Hesselink, J.R. & Jernigan T.L. (1988): Hypoplasia of cerebellar vermal lobules VI and VII in autism. *N. Engl. J. Med.* **318,** 1349–1354.

Courchesne, E., Karns, C., Davis, H.R., *et al.* (2001): Unusual brain growth patterns in early life in patients with autistic disorder: an MRI study. *Neurology* **57,** 245–254.

Courchesne, E., Pierce, K., Schumann, C.M., *et al.* (2007): Mapping early brain development in autism. *Neuron* **56**, 399–413.

Ecker, C., Marquand, A., Mourão-Miranda, J., *et al.* (2010): Describing the brain in autism in five dimensions: magnetic resonance imaging-assisted diagnosis of autism spectrum disorder using a multiparameter classification approach. *J. Neurosci.* **30**, 10612–10623.

Fatemi, S.H., Halt, A.R., Realmuto, G., *et al.* (2002): Purkinje cell size is reduced in cerebellum of patients with autism. *Cell Mol. Neurobiol.* **22**, 171–175.

Fatemi, S.H., Aldinger, K.A., Ashwood, P., *et al.* (2012): Consensus paper: pathological role of the cerebellum in autism. *Cerebellum* **11**, 777–807.

Filipek, P.A., Accardo, P.J., Ashwal, S., *et al.* (2000): Practice parameter: screening and diagnosis of autism: report of the Quality Standards Subcommittee of the American Academy of Neurology and the Child Neurology Society. *Neurology* **55**, 468–479.

Haznedar, M.M., Buchsbaum, M.S., Metzger, M., Solimando, A., Spiegel-Cohen, J. & Hollander, E. (1997): Anterior cingulate gyrus volume and glucose metabolism in autistic disorder. *Am. J. Psychiatry* **154**, 1047–1050.

Herbert, M.R., Ziegler, D.A., Deutsch, C.K., *et al.* (2005): Brain asymmetries in autism and developmental language disorder: a nested whole-brain analysis. *Brain* **128**, 213–226.

Kemper, T.L. & Bauman, M.L. (1998): Neuropathology of infantile autism. *J. Neuropath. Exp. Neurol.* **57**, 645–652.

Lainhart, J.E., Piven, J., Wzorek, M., *et al.* (1997): Macrocephaly in children and adults with autism. *J. Am. Acad. Child. Adolesc. Psychiatry* **36**, 282–290.

McAlonan, G.M., Cheung, V., Cheung, C., *et al.* (2005): Mapping the brain in autism: a voxel-based MRI study of volumetric differences and intercorrelations in autism. *Brain* **128**, 268–276.

Mosconi, M.W., Cody-Hazlett, H., Poe, M.D., Gerig, G., Gimpel-Smith, R. & Piven, J. (2009): Longitudinal study of amygdala volume and joint attention in 2- to 4-year-old children with autism. *Arch. Gen. Psychiatry* **66**, 509–516.

Murakami, J.W., Courchesne, E., Press, G.A., Yeung-Courchesne, R. & Hesselink, J.R. (1989): Reduced cerebellar hemisphere size and its relationship to vermal hypoplasia in autism. *Arch. Neurol.* **46**, 689–694.

Ritvo, E.R., Freeman, B.J., Scheibel, A.B., *et al.* (1986): Lower Purkinje cell counts in the cerebella of four autistic subjects: initial findings of the UCLA-NSAC Autopsy Research Report. *Am. J. Psychiatry* **143**, 862–866.

Riva, D., Bulgheroni, S., Aquino, D., Di Salle, F., Savoiardo, M. & Erbetta, A. (2011): Basal forebrain involvement in low functioning autistic children: a voxel-based morphometry study. *Am. J. Neuroradiol.* **32**, 1430–1435.

Schumann, C.M. & Wu Nordahl, C. (2011): Bridging the gap between MRI and postmortem research in autism. *Brain Res.* **380**, 175–186.

Schumann, C.M., Bloss, C., Barnes, C.C., *et al.* (2010): Longitudinal MRI study of cortical development through early childhood in autism. *J. Neurosci.* **30**, 4419–4427.

Stanfield, A.C., McIntosh, A.M., Spencer, M.D., Philip, R., Gaur, S. & Lawrie, S.M. (2007): Towards a neuroanatomy of autism: a systematic review and meta-analysis of structural magnetic resonance imaging studies. *Eur. Psychiatry* **23**, 289–299.

Taber, K.H., Shaw, J.B., Loveland, K.A., Pearson, D.A., Lane, D.M. & Hayman, L.A. (2004): Accentuated Virchow-Robin spaces in the centrum semiovale in children with autistic disorder. *J. Comput. Assist. Tomog.* **28**, 263–268.

Wegiel, J., Kuchna, I., Nowicki, K., *et al.* (2010): The neuropathology of autism: defects of neurogenesis and neuronal migration, and dysplastic changes. *Acta Neuropathol.* **119**, 755–770.

Zeegers, M., Van Der Grond, J., Durston, S., *et al.* (2006): Radiological findings in autistic and developmentally delayed children. *Brain Dev.* **28**, 495–499.

Chapter 4

Multimodal imaging of brain connectivity in autism spectrum disorders: an overview

Patrizia Chiesa and Ludovico Minati

U.O. Scientific Direction, Fondazione IRCCS Istituto Neurologico 'Carlo Besta',
via Celoria 11, 20133 Milan, Italy
lminati@ieee.org

Summary

While the aetiology of autism spectrum disorders is largely unknown, and clear pathologic hallmarks of disease are lacking, in recent years a remarkable body of literature has accumulated suggesting that anatomic connectivity (*i.e.*, axonal connections) as well as functional connectivity (*i.e.*, spatiotemporal coherencies of intrinsic or task-related neural activity) are significantly altered. There is solid evidence that long-range connectivity is impaired, mildly to severely, and recent data suggest that, on the contrary, short-range connectivity may be enhanced. This altered balance could be closely related to the presence of islands of spared or even excellent cognitive function, in the face of general impairment in associative reasoning, language, and social behaviour. Here, we provide a non exhaustive summary of results obtained in this area, and offer an introduction to two major investigational tools: diffusion tensor imaging (DTI) and resting-state functional MRI (rs-fMRI).

Introduction

While the aetiology of autism spectrum disorders (ASDs) remains for the most part not understood, and gross pathologic hallmarks are absent, a recurring observation is the altered development of brain connectivity, from the level of synaptic trees through to macroscopic fibre bundles (Casanova, 2007; Penzes *et al.*, 2011). One of the behavioural features of autistic individuals is the sheer difficulty in integrating information from multiple sensory domains into abstract representations: a paradigmatic example is the tendency to play with parts of toys, showing little or no interest in their functioning as a whole. This is in stark contrast with the occurrence of relatively preserved or even enhanced cognitive abilities in specific areas, *e.g.*, mathematical and logical reasoning. Such observations have been conceptualized in the *weak central coherence* theory, which postulates that the behavioural features of autism can be, at least in part, accounted for by inability to establish effective connectivity across sparse neocortical representations, leading to an imbalance in the integration of information, whereby there is excessive processing of details, but severely impaired representation of the whole. This theory is substantiated by observations that autistic individuals generally perform very poorly in tasks requiring multi-domain integration (Frith, 1989; Frith & Happe, 1994; López & Leekam, 2003; Mottron *et al.*, 2003).

A natural extension of this cognitive theory is the postulate that such situation will be directly reflected in structural as well as functional connectivity – either as a substrate, a consequence, or more likely both. On this basis, approximately a decade ago it was hypothesized that long-range connections would be weaker in autistic than neurotypical individuals and that short-range connectivity could be boosted. Such hypothesis has an obvious appeal given that the complex and variable behavioural phenotype of autism cannot be accounted for through localizationalist approaches, *i.e.*, in terms of maldevelopment of isolated regions or dysfunction of single neurotransmitter systems (Belmonte *et al.*, 2004; Just *et al.*, 2004; Wass, 2011).

The study of brain connectivity in autism is developing at a tremendous rate, also thanks to the widespread availability of high-field scanners and advanced computational tools. Here, we shall provide an overview of the main findings obtained to date. There is no presumption of completeness, the aim only being to exemplify the potential of such studies. A brief methodologic overview of diffusion-tensor imaging (DTI) and resting-state functional MRI (rs-fMRI) is also offered.

Microscopic and gross anatomic studies

There is growing consensus that altered connectivity is detectable through morphologic studies, particularly those exploring neocortical architecture in terms of 'minicolumns', *i.e.*, 30–60-µm cylindrical clusters comprising around 80–120 densely-interconnected neurons. Minicolumnar cytoarchitecture comparisons have shown that peripheral neuropil is reduced, but that there is increased spacing among neurons within each radial column, and that minicolumns are overall more abundant, but smaller in the prefrontal cortex (Brodmann area 9) and temporal lobe (BA 21 and 22). These features result in altered dendritic growth, with enhanced intra-columnar connectivity and fewer synapses across distant neurons; they may also imply a reduced proportion of interneurons, with consequences for local excitatory–inhibitory balance and large-scale regulation and stability of neurotransmitter systems (Casanova *et al.*, 2002, 2006; Casanova & Trippe, 2009; Rubenstein & Merzenich, 2003).

Altered connectivity can also be inferred through studies of gross anatomy, performed *ex vivo* by dissection or *in vivo* by structural MRI. The most widely studied bundle is the corpus callosum, which is the primary means of interhemispheric communication and harbours the majority of long-distance axonal projections in the brain. Given its anatomic conformation, inferences about the relative number of axons can be made simply through measurement of its cross-section on the mid-sagittal plane. On this premise, volumetric analyses have shown that marked reduction is detectable in all subregions (genu, body, and splenium) throughout the spectrum of severity of autism spectrum disorders. As the anterior-to-posterior organization of the corpus callosum closely matches the location of the somas of the projecting neurons, *i.e.*, frontal through to posterior parietal, these observations substantiate the hypothesis that there is pervasive interhemispheric underconnectivity affecting multiple lobes and systems (Casanova *et al.*, 2011; Just *et al.*, 2007; Vidal *et al.*, 2006).

Other gross anatomic observations are also relevant. Although some controversy remains, particularly because of sexual dimorphism and gender-selection biases, several studies have suggested that white matter volume may be reduced in autism, plausibly reflecting hypoplasia rather than atrophy (Beacher et al., 2012; Boger-Megiddo et al., 2006; Chung et al., 2004). On the other hand, there is fluctuating evidence of increased grey matter volume, which could by proxy signal greater density of intracortical, short-range connections, particularly in the prefrontal cortex (Carper et al., 2002; Herbert et al., 2005; McAlonan et al., 2005). Of note, increased total intracranial volume in autistic children has also been reported, fuelling the hypothesis that this could be causally related to long-range underconnectivity, i.e., that excessively rapid brain growth due to excessive neural proliferation or inadequate pruning in a critical phase could hamper the development of long-range axonal connections (Courchesne et al., 2007; Kates et al., 2004; Sparks et al., 2002). Yet some caution is needed when interpreting these results, as the heterogeneity of findings across studies remains substantial, probably because of sampling issues with respect to gender, age, and severity and because of methodologic differences.

Structural connectivity

Methodologic overview

DTI is an MR imaging modality that offers a window on the microstructure of tissues, utilizing the thermally-induced Brownian motion of water molecules as a sensitive probe for the density and orientational arrangement of biological membranes. The underlying concept is that both cellular membranes and myelin sheaths are largely impermeable to water, given sufficiently short diffusimetric time-windows, and that the study of their microstructural properties at a statistical level may thus provide information on the density of cells, irrespective of the presence of an orderly arrangement, and on the density of coherently-oriented axons, quantifying, through compound indices, the coherence of their alignment, their density, and their preferential orientation (Beaulieu, 2002; Minati & Weglarz, 2007). The physical basis of DTI is the ability to render the MR signal sensitive to water diffusion along a given direction, set by the orientation of a sensitizing gradient. Through measurements conducted using between 6 and hundreds of diffusion-weighting directions, it is possible to determine mathematical models of orientational microstructure within each image voxel: The simplest model is the rank-2 tensor, which captures only a single preferential orientation and is therefore inadequate in areas of complex axonal architecture, but much more sophisticated models, such as the q-ball, also exist, which can accurately represent the orientation of multiple fibre bundles within each voxel. Hence, DTI enables one to gather information on the microstructure of tissues at a scale (10–10 µm) much smaller than the spatial resolution (1–3 mm) directly attainable on a human scanner.

At its simplest, DTI provides a measurement of the directionally-averaged Apparent Diffusion Coefficient (ADC), also and more properly referred to as mean diffusivity (MD), which indicates the overall intensity of Brownian motion in a voxel: This parameter correlates negatively with the density of cells and myelin sheaths, and is by definition insensitive to orientational architecture (Hagmann et al., 2006; Minati & Weglarz, 2007). A more abstract parameter is Fractional Anisotropy (FA), which represents the orientational coherency of axonal fibres within a voxel: While this is a good proxy of axonal density for voxels within thick, highly-coherent fibre bundles, FA becomes meaningless in areas, such as subcortical white matter, where many heterogeneously-oriented axonal subpopulations are present within each voxel. More abstract parameters, such as Generalized Anisotropy (GA) propose to alleviate this issue

(Minati *et al.*, 2008). Importantly, the fields of tensors or other representations of orientation can serve as the basis for tractography, *i.e.*, iterative three-dimensional reconstruction of the path of given axonal bundles (Hagmann *et al.*, 2006).

Principal findings

Across studies, there is a general tendency for patients with autism spectrum disorders to exhibit reduced FA and increased MD in the white matter, suggesting reduced axonal density (Groen *et al.*, 2011; Shukla *et al.*, 2010).

The corpus callosum is a large, highly compact, and coherently-oriented fibre bundle, and hence many studies have naturally focused on this structure to search for indications of altered interhemispheric connectivity. There is good agreement across studies that such alterations are present (Keller *et al.* 2007; Noriuchi *et al.*, 2010) and high MD and low FA have been found to parametrically predict slowest integrative processing speeds (Alexander *et al.*, 2007).

Alterations are not confined to interhemispheric connectivity, and reduced FA has also been observed in the anterior, superior, and posterior thalamic radiations, substantiating the notion that altered thalamic connectivity may have a role in the pathophysiology of autism (Cheon *et al.*, 2011).

Further, reduced FA has also been found across the 'social cognition network' (*e.g.*, fusiform gyrus and superior temporal sulcus) and diffusely in the frontal lobe (ventromedial prefrontal and anterior cingulated cortex; see Barnea-Goraly *et al.*, 2004). Other reports indicate abnormally low FA in the dorsolateral prefrontal cortex, superior longitudinal fasciculus, occipito-frontal fasciculus, and anterior cingulate cortex (Noriuchi *et al.*, 2010), which are key constituents of circuits supporting inhibition, planning, cognitive flexibility and social cognition and which are closely related to the mirror neuron system.

There remains, however, some inconsistency across studies. For example, according to Sundaram *et al.* (2008), in ASD participants long-range association fibres in the frontal lobe are significantly longer than in controls. Other studies have demonstrated that in Asperger's syndrome the FA is reduced across the internal capsule, frontal, temporal, parietal and occipital lobes, cingulum, and corpus callosum (Bloemen *et al.*, 2010). Furthermore, by using diffusion tensor tractography Thomas *et al.* (2011) have found that the inferior longitudinal fasciculus, the inferior fronto-occipital fasciculus and the uncinate fasciculus are increased in volume and the corpus callosum is reduced, providing some evidence for the hypothesis of a local over-connectivity and a reduced long-range connectivity in the autistic brain. Even the variability in motor behaviour has been linked to overall white matter injury (Hadders-Algra, 2008).

Taken together, these studies clearly demonstrate that DTI is able to reveal profound, pervasive connectivity deficits and possibly even compensatory changes in autism spectrum disorders. There appears to be a general maldevelopment of white matter, reflected in reduced FA and increased MD across the principal association bundles. There is some evidence for increased intrahemispheric, short-range connectivity, but the topic remains controversial. Clearly, a significant proportion of the variability observed across studies may be down to mismatches in the populations under study (*e.g.*, age, gender, severity, specific behavioural phenotype) and to methodologic differences in the measurement and fibre reconstruction techniques. Of note, recent work demonstrates that the expression of autism in white matter integrity may significantly interact with sexual dimorphism, differentially affecting males and females and underscoring the need for detailed studies in both genders (Beacher *et al.*, 2012).

Functional connectivity

Methodologic overview

Abstract behaviours do not result from isolated regional activity, but rather emerge from complex, large-scale dynamics across networks of information flow that rapidly form and dissolve contingent on cognitive state and environmental demands (Mesulam, 1998; Sporns, 2009; Stephan, 2004). Hence it is hardly surprising that diffuse, highly-structured spatiotemporal coherencies in synaptic activity are found, both during wakeful rest and the performance of structured tasks. The *blood oxygen level–dependent* (BOLD) signal at the basis of fMRI closely tracks the intensity of postsynaptic activity and, in spite of contamination by systemic physiologic confounds (*e.g.*, cardiovascular activity), significant temporal smoothing due to the physiologic time-constant of the haemodynamic response (*e.g.*, 4–5 s), and temporal aliasing due to low sampling rate following instrumental limitations (*e.g.*, 0.2–1 Hz), powerfully reflects such activity coherencies. Functional connectivity is thus studied through fMRI by means of exploring correlations among BOLD signal time-series recorded from separated voxels (Buckner, 2010; Fox & Raichle, 2007; Logothetis & Pfeuffer, 2004; Rosazza & Minati, 2011).

Several data-analytic techniques are available, and a conceptual distinction is made between *functional connectivity*, also referred to as intrinsic connectivity, and *effective connectivity*: the former refers to the spatiotemporal coherencies observed in the awake 'idle', resting brain, whereas the latter refers to the *modulation* of such coherencies by the act of performing an active task or attending a stimulus (Friston *et al.*, 1997; Sporns, 2009; Stephan, 2004). Functional connectivity can be explored with *hypothesis-driven* or *data-driven* approaches: a notable example of the former is *seed-based analysis* (SBA) using pre-selected anatomic regions, whereas a common implementation of the latter is *independent-component analysis* (ICA), a decomposition technique that attempts to isolate a given small number of neural sources (*e.g.*, 20) by searching for un-mixing matrices that render the corresponding signals maximally independent. ICA and SBA share the same underlying approach, that is, calculating topographic maps that represent the correlation of each image voxel with respect to a reference time-course (Buckner, 2010; Fox & Raichle, 2007; Rosazza & Minati, 2011).

Effective connectivity, on the other hand, is generally studied through modelling how the activity of a 'target' region (which can be all brain voxels, one by one) is predicted by activity in a fixed 'seed' region *convoluted* with a function representing an external task: in other words, by answering the question of whether functional connectivity is significantly modulated by a psychological variable. This approach is termed *psycho-physiological interaction* (PPI) and provides invaluable insights into how connectivity encodes specific task features [which may not necessarily reflect on the intensity of activity in each region considered in isolation (Friston *et al.*, 1997; Stephan, 2004)]. A powerful abstraction of this concept is termed *dynamic causal modelling* (DCM) and involves setting up explicit, generative models of directed interactions among pre-determined cortical regions; a detailed account of haemodynamic coupling supports the generation of expected BOLD signal time-courses, which enables the comparison of competing models (or families of models) through Bayesian statistics (Friston *et al.*, 2003).

All these approaches, while very informative of their own, fail to capture one key element of connectivity: its large-scale topologic structure. In other words, ICA, SBA, and PPI explore the correlation between a seed signal and all brain voxels, hence providing *topographic* representations of connectivity, devoid of *topologic* information regarding how the connections across all possible combinations of regions are architected. DCM, on the other hand, does test explicit topologic models, but is limited by the need to pre-specify restricted networks, typically limited to less than 10 brain areas.

Brain networks, like many other self-organizing networks – biological as well as not – exhibit specific topologic features, most notably small-worldness, that is, a specific balance between the density of connections and the topologic distance (number of hops) between the network nodes, and scale-freeness, that is, a power-law distribution of the number of connections found for each node (Barabasi &Albert, 1999; Bassett & Bullmore, 2006; Park et al., 2005; Stam & de Bruin, 2004; Watts & Strogatz, 1998). The natural instrument to represent such features is a graph, i.e., a mathematical entity constituted by nodes (here corresponding to cortical regions) and edges (here corresponding to functional, or anatomic, connections). Recent studies of functional and effective connectivity are beginning to use graphs rather than topographic maps as standard, i.e., parcellating the cortex into a large set of regions and subsequently exploring all possible pair-wise associations, through linear regression, PPI, or other techniques (like Granger causality; see Bressler & Seth, 2011). Graph network models offer a substrate to quantify specific topologic features that complement the topographic information made available by ICA, SBA, and traditional PPI. Recent work has demonstrated that graph-based analysis of large-scale connectivity reveals intricate networks of startling complexity, wherein a small number of cortical regions feature as prominent 'hubs', representing information convergence–divergence zones (Buckner et al., 2009; Bullmore & Bassett, 2011; Mesulam, 1998; Minati et al., 2012; Salvador et al., 2005).

Principal findings

Most studies on functional connectivity in autism spectrum disorders have focused on the default-mode network, which is a prominent spatiotemporal coherency of activity across the precuneus, medial prefrontal cortex, and bilateral angular/supramarginal gyri, with ramifications to the superior frontal gyrus, medial temporal lobe, and insula. Although the exact nature of this finding remains unclear, there is converging evidence that is represents a functional network supporting introspection and memory consolidation, and predictive associations have been found between its integrity and the clinical outlook of early-dementia patients, for example (Buckner et al., 2008; Fox & Raichle, 2007; Greicius et al., 2004; Rosazza & Minati, 2011).

There is a certain variability of findings in autism: Cherkassky et al. (2006) and Weng et al. (2010) reported diffusely weakened connectivity, whereas other studies, such as that of Assaf et al. (2010), only detected reduced connectivity with the anterior node of the default-mode network, i.e., the medial prefrontal cortex/anterior cingulate cortex. Some studies have also demonstrated altered connectivity in regions that the default-mode network ramifies to, even though they are not deemed to be its main constituent nodes: For instance, Monk et al. (2009) found weaker connectivity between the precuneus and the superior frontal gyrus and stronger connectivity between the precuneus and both the right temporal lobe and right parahippocampal gyrus. Other investigations have explicitly focused on connectivity of the insula and amygdala, concluding that significant disconnection is present (von dem Hagen et al., 2012); because both regions are critically involved in emotion formation and emotional awareness of self and others, this might represent a correlate of the altered emotional experience and social reciprocity found in autism spectrum disorders (Craig, 2009; Ebisch et al., 2011). Notably, negative correlations between the Social Responsiveness scale and functional connectivity between the cingulate cortex and middle insula have been reported, even in neurotypical individuals (Di Martino et al., 2009).

Some resting-state studies also confirm the anatomic results of decreased interhemispheric functional connectivity in autism, specifically affecting the sensorimotor cortex, anterior insula, fusiform gyrus, superior temporal gyrus, and superior parietal lobe (Anderson et al., 2011).

In parallel, there is a growing body of work on effective connectivity during the performance of active tasks. In spite of the methodologic complexity, the approach has advantages in that it is less sensitive to physiologic contamination than resting-state fMRI and in that it allows the investigation of the neural correlates of specific tasks that are of particular relevance to the condition of interest. These studies are disparate and have investigated sensory association, language, and executive function as well as emotion.

An early, highly influential investigation on language comprehension demonstrated impaired synchronization between the left superior temporal area (Wernicke's area) and the left inferior frontal gyrus (Broca's area) in the autistic individuals, providing an explicit demonstration of dysfunctional information integration across language networks (Just et al., 2004). A later study extended these findings by showing reduced connectivity between frontal and parietal areas (Just et al., 2007).

A paradigmatic finding comes from the analysis of visuospatial tasks, in which autistic participants can exhibit boosted performance, which reveals weakened connectivity through frontal and parietal-occipital regions, corresponding to higher-order working memory/executive and visuospatial processing, in line with the notion of long-range cortical underconnectivity (Damarla et al., 2010). Visual processing has been particularly well-investigated on account of the relative ease of implementation of active tasks suitable for patients and because existing tools (PPI, DCM) are particularly well-suited to exploring associative sensory processing. One finding is that of reduced connectivity in the dorsal stream, involving the inferior frontal Brodmann area 44, which is part of the mirror neuron system (Villalobos et al. 2005), enhanced connectivity in the thalamocortical pathway, particularly left insula and postcentral and frontal regions, and increased but inefficiently organized functional connectivity between caudate and neocortex during visuomotor coordination (Mizuno et al., 2006). Though any interpretation remains necessarily speculative at this stage, enhanced subcortico-cortical connectivity is hypothesized to reflect a compensatory attempt after dysfunctional cortico-cortical connectivity, whereas the involvement of the caudate nuclei potentially accounts for stereotypic behaviours and executive deficits (Turner et al., 2006). Atypically increased connectivity during a searching task, which requires a huge attentional resource allocation, has also been shown in the occipital regions, both locally and with respect to long-distance connections with frontal regions (Keehn et al., 2012).

Other studies have targeted the connectivity correlates of impaired social reasoning and emotional behaviour. Abnormalities during functional integration of face processing have been found in amygdala and parahippocampal gyrus, and, though less saliently, in anterior cingulate, inferior occipital, and inferior frontal cortex (Welchew et al., 2005). Lower connectivity between the fusiform face area and both amygdalae and superior temporal sulcus has been found (Kleinhans et al., 2008). During the processing of emotional faces, impaired long-range connectivity was found between the amygdala and both V2 and the dorsolateral prefrontal cortex, and between the right pars opercularis of the inferior frontal gyrus and the ventromedial prefrontal cortex (Rudie et al., 2012). Further, during emotion processing, information flow from posterior to frontal association cortex, and the modulation of activation of posterior areas by frontal brain regions has been evaluated, revealing an abnormal pattern of effective connectivity in which the prefrontal cortex seems to be the key site of dysfunction (Wicker et al., 2008).

Summing up, these findings provide robust evidence for altered functional connectivity in autism, particularly affecting the default-mode network at rest and functional networks subserving emotional, language, and visuospatial processing during the performance of specific tasks. As with DTI studies, substantial challenges remain, in that heterogeneity of populations and investigational techniques across studies injects considerable discrepancy and fragmentation in the literature. Now that the available studies have proven the enormous potential of these techniques, it would be in the common interest to standardize upon consensus on a small number of tasks and associated data-analytic approaches, and share them across worldwide centres so that extensive investigations can be conducted to corroborate the existing results and establish credible, robust associations with clinical phenotype.

Conclusions

Diffusion-tensor imaging and resting-state functional MRI have radically extended the contribution of MRI to the study and, potentially, diagnostic work-up of autism, by providing new windows onto anatomic and functional connectivity. The field is developing rapidly, and there is good agreement across studies demonstrating impaired long-range connectivity; some evidence is also available for enhanced short-range connectivity, but findings are less clear-cut. Given the outstanding potential of these two techniques, researchers in large-scale, multi-centric studies are clearly motivated to characterize in detail the relationship between the observed effects and the clinical phenotype.

Conflicts of interest: The authors declare no conflicts of interest.

References

Alexander, A.L., Lee, J.E., Lazar, M., et al. (2007): Diffusion tensor imaging of the corpus callosum in autism. *NeuroImage* **34**, 61–73.

Anderson, J.S., Druzgal, T.J., Froehlich, A., et al. (2011): Decreased interhemispheric functional connectivity in autism. *Cereb. Cortex.* **21**, 1134–1146.

Assaf, M., Jagannathan, K., Calhoun V.D., et al. (2010): Abnormal functional connectivity of default mode subnetworks in autism spectrum disorder patients. *NeuroImage* **53**, 247–256.

Barabasi, A.L. & Albert, R. (1999): Emergence of scaling in random networks. *Science* **286**, 509–512.

Barnea-Goraly, N., Kwon, H., Menon, V., Eliez, S., Lotspeich, L. & Reiss, A.L. (2004): White matter structure in autism: preliminary evidence from diffusion tensor imaging. *Biol. Psychiatry* **55**, 323–326.

Bassett, D.S. & Bullmore, E. (2006): Small-world brain networks. *Neuroscientist* **12**, 512–523.

Beacher, F.D., Minati, L., Baron-Cohen, S., et al. (2012): Autism attenuates sex differences in brain structure: a combined voxel-based morphometry and diffusion tensor imaging study. *AJNR Am. J. Neuroradiol.* **33**, 83–98.

Beaulieu, C. (2002): The basis of anisotropic water diffusion in the nervous system: a technical review. *NMR Biomed.* **15**, 435–455.

Belmonte, M.K., Allen, G., Beckel-Mitchener, A., Boulanger, L.M., Carper, R.A. & Webb, S.J. (2004): Autism and abnormal development of brain connectivity. *J. Neurosci.* **24**, 9228–9231.

Bloemen, O.J., Deeley, Q., Sundram, F., et al. (2010): White matter integrity in Asperger syndrome: a preliminary diffusion tensor magnetic resonance imaging study in adults. *Autism Res.* **3**, 203–213.

Boger-Megiddo, I., Shaw, D.W., Friedman, S.D., *et al.* (2006): Corpus callosum morphometrics in young children with autism spectrum disorder. *J. Autism Dev. Disord.* **36**, 733–739.

Bressler, S.L. & Seth, A.K. (2011): Wiener–Granger causality: a well established methodology. *NeuroImage* **58**, 323–329.

Buckner, R.L. (2010): Human functional connectivity: new tools, unresolved questions. *Proc. Natl. Acad. Sci. USA* **107**, 10769–10770.

Buckner, R.L., Andrews-Hanna, J.R. & Schacter, D.L. (2008): The brain's default network: anatomy, function, and relevance to disease. *Ann. N.Y. Acad. Sci.* **1124**, 1–38.

Buckner, R.L., Sepulcre, J., Talukdar, T., *et al.* (2009): Cortical hubs revealed by intrinsic functional connectivity: mapping, assessment of stability, and relation to Alzheimer's disease. *J. Neurosci.* **29**, 1860–1873.

Bullmore, E.T. & Bassett, D.S. (2011): Brain graphs: graphical models of the human brain connectome. *Annu. Rev. Clin. Psychol.* **7**, 113–140.

Carper, R.A., Moses, P., Tigue, Z.D. & Courchesne, E. (2002): Cerebral lobes in autism: early hyperplasia and abnormal age effects. *NeuroImage* **16**, 1038–1051.

Casanova, M.F. (2006): Neuropathological and genetic findings in autism: the significance of a putative minicolumnopathy. *Neuroscientist.* **12**, 435–441.

Casanova, M.F. (2007): The neuropathology of autism. *Brain Pathol.* **17**, 422–433.

Casanova, M. & Trippe, J. (2009): Radial cytoarchitecture and patterns of cortical connectivity in autism. *Phil. Trans. Roy. Soc. (Lond.)* **364**, 1433–1236.

Casanova, M.F., Buxhoeveden, D.P., Switala, A.E. & Roy, E. (2002): Minicolumnar pathology in autism. *Neurology* **58**,428–432.

Casanova, M.F., El-Baz, A., Elnakib, A., *et al.* (2011): Quantitative analysis of the shape of the corpus callosum in patients with autism and comparison individuals. *Autism* **15**, 223–238.

Cheon, K., Kim, Y., Ohio, S., *et al.* (2011): Involvement of the anterior thalamic radiation in boys with high functioning autism spectrum disorders: a diffusion tensor imaging study. *Brain Res.* **1417**, 77–86.

Cherkassky, V.L., Kana, R.K., Keller, T.A. & Just, M.A. (2006): Functional connectivity in a baseline resting-state network in autism. *NeuroReport* **17**, 1687–1690.

Chung, M.K., Dalton, K.M., Alexander, A.L. & Davidson, R.J. (2004): Less white matter concentration in autism: 2D voxel-based morphometry. *NeuroImage* **23**, 242–251.

Courchesne, E., Pierce, K., Schumann, C.M., *et al.* (2007): Mapping early brain development in autism. *Neuron* **56**, 399–413.

Craig, A.D. (2009): How do you feel – now? The anterior insula and human awareness. *Nat. Rev. Neurosci.* **10**, 59–70.

Damarla, S.R., Keller, T.A., Kana, R.K., Cherkassky, V.L., Williams, D.L. & Minshew, N.J. (2010): Cortical underconnectivity coupled with preserved visuospatial cognition in autism: evidence from an fMRI study of an embedded figures task. *Autism Res.* **3**, 273–279.

Di Martino, A., Shehzad, Z., Kelly, C., *et al.* (2009): Relationship between cingulo-insular functional connectivity and autistic traits in neurotypical adults. *Am. J. Psychiatry.* **166**, 891–899.

Ebisch, S.J., Gallese, V., Willems, R.M., *et al.* (2011): Altered intrinsic functional connectivity of anterior and posterior insula regions in high-functioning participants with autism spectrum disorder. *Hum. Brain Mapp.* **32**, 1013–1028.

Fox, M.D. & Raichle, M.E. (2007): Spontaneous fluctuations in brain activity observed with functional magnetic resonance imaging. *Nat. Rev. Neurosci.* **8**, 700–711

Friston, K.J., Buechel, C., Fink, G.R., Morris, J., Rolls, E. & Dolan, R.J. (1997): Psychophysiological and modulatory interactions in neuroimaging. *NeuroImage* **6**, 218–229.

Friston, K.J., Harrison, L. & Penny, W. (2003): Dynamic causal modelling. *NeuroImage* **19**, 1273–1302.

Frith, U. (1989): *Autism: Explaining the Enigma.* Oxford: Blackwell.

Frith, U. & Happe, F. (1994): Autism: beyond 'theory of mind'. *Cognition* **50**, 115–132.

Greicius, M.D., Srivastava, G., Reiss, A.L. & Menon, V. (2004): Default-mode network activity distinguishes Alzheimer's disease from healthy aging: evidence from functional MRI. *Proc. Natl. Acad. Sci. USA* **101**, 4637–4642.

Groen, W.B., Buitelaar, J.K., van der Gaag, R.J. & Zwiers, M.P. (2011): Pervasive microstructural abnormalities in autism: a DTI study. *J. Psych. Neurosci.* **36**, 32-40.

Hadders-Algra, M. (2008): Reduced variability in motor behaviour: an indicator of impaired cerebral connectivity? *Early Hum. Dev.* **84**, 787–789.

Hagmann, P., Jonasson, L., Maeder, P., Thiran, J.P., Wedeen, V.J. & Meuli, R (2006): Understanding diffusion MR imaging techniques: from scalar diffusion-weighted imaging to diffusion tensor imaging and beyond. *Radiographics* **26**, 205–223.

Herbert, M.R., Ziegler, D.A., Deutsch, C.K., *et al.* (2005): Brain asymmetries in autism and developmental language disorder: a nested whole-brain analysis. *Brain* **28**, 213–226.

Just, M.A., Cherkassky, V.L., Keller, T.A. & Minshew, N.J. (2004): Cortical activation and synchronization during sentence comprehension in high-functioning autism: evidence of underconnectivity. *Brain* **127**, 1811–1821.

Just, M.A., Cherkassky, V.L., Keller, T.A., Kana, R.K & Minshew, N.J. (2007): Functional and anatomical cortical underconnectivity in autism: evidence from an FMRI study of an executive function task and corpus callosum morphometry. *Cereb. Cortex* **17**, 951–961.

Kates, W.R., Burnette, C.P., Eliez, S., *et al.* (2004): Neuroanatomic variation in monozygotic twin pairs discordant for the narrow phenotype for autism. *Am. J. Psychiatry* **161**, 539–546.

Keehn, B., Shih, P., Brenner, L.A., Townsend, J. & Müller, R.A. (2012): Functional connectivity for an 'island of sparing' in autism spectrum disorder: an fMRI study of visual search. *Hum. Brain Mapp.* doi: 10.1002/hbm.22084 [E-pub ahead of print].

Keller, T.A., Kana, R.K. & Just, M.A. (2007): A developmental study of the structural integrity of white matter in autism. *NeuroReport* **18**, 23–27.

Kleinhans, N.M., Richards, T., Sterling, L., *et al.* (2008): Abnormal functional connectivity in autism spectrum disorders during face processing. *Brain* **131**, 1000–1012.

Logothetis, N.K. & Pfeuffer, J. (2004): On the nature of the BOLD fMRI contrast mechanism. *Magn. Reson. Imag.* **22**, 1517–1531.

López, B. & Leekam, S.R. (2003): Do children with autism fail to process information in context? *J. Child Psychol. Psychiatry* **44**, 285–300.

McAlonan, G.M., Cheung, V., Cheung, C., *et al.* (2005): Mapping the brain in autism: a voxel-based MRI study of volumetric differences and intercorrelations in autism. *Brain* **128**, 268–276.

Mesulam, M.M. (1998): From sensation to cognition. *Brain* **121**, 1013–1052.

Minati, L. & Weglarz, W.P. (2007): Physical foundations, models, and methods of diffusion magnetic resonance imaging of the brain: a review. *Conc. Magn. Reson.* **30**, 278–307.

Minati, L., Banasik, T., Brzezinski, J., *et al.* (2008): Elevating tensor rank increases anisotropy in brain areas associated with intra-voxel orientational heterogeneity (IVOH): a generalised DTI (GDTI) study. *NMR Biomed.* **21**, 2–14.

Minati, L., Grisoli, M., Seth, A.K. & Critchley, H.D. (2012): Decision-making under risk: a graph-based network analysis using functional MRI. *NeuroImage* **60**, 2191–2205.

Mizuno, A., Villalobos, M.E., Davies, M.M., Dahl, B.C. & Müller, R.A. (2006): Partially enhanced thalamocortical functional connectivity in autism. *Brain Res.* **1104**, 160–174.

Monk, C.S., Peltier, S.J., Wiggins, J.L., Weng, S.J., Carrasco, M., Risi, S. & Lord, C. (2009): Abnormalities of intrinsic functional connectivity in autism spectrum disorders. *NeuroImage* **47**, 764–724.

Mottron, L., Burack, J.A., Iarocci, G., Belleville, S. & Enns, J.T. (2003): Locally oriented perception with intact global processing among adolescents with high-functioning autism: evidence from multiple paradigms. *J. Child Psychol. Psychiatry* **44**, 904–913.

Noriuchi, M., Kikuchi, Y., Yoshiura, T., *et al.* (2010): Altered white matter fractional anisotropy and social impairment in children with autism spectrum disorder. *Brain Res.* **1362**, 141–149.

Park, K., Lai, Y.C. & Ye, N. (2005): Self-organized scale-free networks. *Phys. Rev. E Stat. Nonlin. Soft Matter Phys.* **72**, 026131.

Penzes, P., Cahill, M.E., Jones, K.A., VanLeeuwen, J.E. & Woolfrey, K.M. (2011): Dendritic spine pathology in neuropsychiatric disorders. *Nat. Neurosci.* **14**, 285–293.

Rosazza, C. & Minati, L. (2011): Resting-state brain networks: literature review and clinical applications. *Neurol. Sci.* **32**, 773–850.

Rubenstein, J.L. & Merzenich, M.M. (2003): Model of autism: increased ratio of excitation/inhibition in key neural systems. *Genes Brain Behav.* **2**, 255–267.

Rudie, J.D., Shehzad, Z., Hernandez, L.M., *et al.* (2012): Reduced functional integration and segregation of distributed neural systems underlying social and emotional information processing in autism spectrum disorders. *Cereb. Cortex* **22**, 1025–1037.

Salvador, R., Suckling, J., Coleman, M.R., Pickard, J.D., Menon, D. & Bullmore, E. (2005): Neurophysiological architecture of functional magnetic resonance images of human brain. *Cereb. Cortex* **15**, 1332–1342.

Shukla, D.K., Keehn, B., Lincoln, A.J. & Müller, R.A. (2010): White matter compromise of callosal and subcortical fiber tracts in children with autism spectrum disorder: a diffusion tensor imaging study. *J. Am. Acad. Child Adolesc. Psychiatry* **12**, 1269–1278.

Sparks, B.F., Friedman, S.D., Shaw, D.W., *et al.* (2002): Brain structural abnormalities in young children with autism spectrum disorder. *Neurology* **59**, 184–192.

Sporns, O. (2009): *Networks of the Brain*. Cambridge, MA: The MIT Press.

Stam, C.J. & de Bruin, E.A. (2004): Scale-free dynamics of global functional connectivity in the human brain. *Hum. Brain Mapp.* **22**, 97–109.

Stephan, K.E. (2004): On the role of general system theory for functional neuroimaging. *J. Anat.* **205**, 443–470.

Sundaram, S.K., Kumar, A., Makki, M.I., Behen. M.E., Chugani, H.T. & Chugani, D.C. (2008): Diffusion tensor imaging of frontal lobe in autism spectrum disorder. *Cereb. Cortex* **18**, 2659–2665.

Thomas, C., Humphreys, K., Jung, K.J., Minshew, N. & Behrmann, M. (2011): The anatomy of the callosal and visual-association pathways in high-functioning autism: a DTI tractography study. *Cortex* **47**, 863–873.

Turner, K.C., Frost, L., Linsenbardt, D., McIlroy, J.R. & Müller, R.A. (2006): Atypically diffuse functional connectivity between caudate nuclei and cerebral cortex in autism. *Behav. Brain Funct.* **2**, 34.

Vidal, C.N., Nicolson, R., Devito, T.J., *et al.* (2006): Mapping corpus callosum deficits in autism: an index of aberrant cortical connectivity. *Biol. Psychiatry* **60**, 218–225.

Villalobos, M.E., Mizuno, A., Dahl, B.C., Kemmotsu, N. & Müller, R.A. (2005): Reduced functional connectivity between V1 and inferior frontal cortex associated with visuomotor performance in autism. *NeuroImage* **25**, 916–925.

von dem Hagen, E.A., Stoyanova, R.S., Baron-Cohen, S. & Calder, A.J. (2012): Reduced functional connectivity within and between 'social' resting state networks in autism spectrum conditions. *Soc. Cogn. Affect Neurosci.* [E-pub ahead of print].

Wass, S. (2011): Distortions and disconnections: disrupted brain connectivity in autism. *Brain Cogn.* **75**, 18–28.

Watts, D.J. & Strogatz, S.H. (1998): Collective dynamics of 'small-world' networks. *Nature* **393**, 440–442.

Welchew, D.E., Ashwin, C., Berkouk, K., *et al.* (2005): Functional disconnectivity of the medial temporal lobe in Asperger's syndrome. *Biol. Psychiatry* **57**, 991–998.

Weng, S.J., Wiggins. J.L., Peltier, S.J., Carrasco, M., Risi, S., Lord, C. & Monk, C.S. (2010): Alterations of resting state functional connectivity in the default network in adolescents with autism spectrum disorders. *Brain Res.* **1313**, 202–214.

Wicker, B., Fonlupt, P., Hubert, B., Tardif, C., Gepner, B. & Deruelle, C. (2008): Abnormal cerebral effective connectivity during explicit emotional processing in adults with autism spectrum disorder. *Soc. Cogn. Affect. Neurosci.* **3**, 135–143.

Chapter 5

Autism: the genetic viewpoint

Orsetta Zuffardi

Department of Molecular Medicine, University of Pavia, Pavia, Italy
IRCCS 'C. Mondino' Foundation, National Institute of Neurology, Pavia, Italy
zuffardi@unipv.it

Summary

Autism is a condition with a strong genetic basis, as demonstrated by the correlation of the condition in monozygotic and dizygotic twins, and among brothers, respectively, of 50–90 per cent, 0–30 per cent and 3–26 per cent, and by the presence of syndromic forms of autism such as fragile X syndrome. Only recently, however, has it been possible to identify at least some of the genetic components of the disorder, although most of them are still unknown. In the last decade, new approaches to a genome-wide analysis have identified several submicroscopic chromosomal imbalances (not detectable by conventional chromosome analysis because smaller than the resolution power of chromosome preparations analyzed by microscope) significantly associated with this condition. These new technologies–including the array-comparative genomic hybridization (CGH) and SNP (single nucleotide polymorphisms) arrays–are now dramatically part of the diagnostic routine under the name of chromosomal microarray (CMA) and should in theory be required by paediatricians and psychiatrists in place of the conventional chromosome investigation. In addition, CMA has now become imperative for a number of conditions for which chromosomal analysis was not usually required, such as isolated intellectual disabilities, autism, epilepsy and schizophrenia. Altogether syndromes associated with chromosomal imbalances identified by CMA are known as genomic disorders. Here the changes in copy number of genomic portions that are consistently associated with autism will be reviewed.

Introduction

A change in the copy number (CNV) is as a deletion or a duplication of a portion of DNA, in comparison to the reference genome. Such changes can vary in size from a kilobase (kb) to several megabases (Mbs) and may involve one or more genes. Deletions may be heterozygous, with only one copy missing, or more rarely homozygous, with both copies missing. X chromosome deletions in males are hemizygous deletions. Duplications result in three copies instead of the usual two. Some regions of the DNA may be present in more than three copies. Studies on a large number of controls have shown that some regions of the genome are tolerant to changes in the number of copies and that each normal person presents numerous CNVs, seemingly benign. As a result of this variability, two normal people may differ in DNA content for different megabases. The CNVs discussed here are associated with specific conditions such as autism and are generally not present in the control population. It should be emphasized, however, that some CNVs, largely recurrent (that is, characterized by identical breakpoints), have been considered as risk factors not only for autism but also for intellectual disability, epilepsy, schizophrenia and of deficits such as attention/hyperactivity disorder (ADHD) (Mefford, 2012). For example, microdeletions of 15q13.3 and 16p13.11 have been associated with all of these conditions, including autism, while the duplication of 16p13.11 is related to intellectual disability, ADHD, and autism. Another example of a CNV associated with significant phenotypic variability is a deletion in the proximal region of 16p11.2. This deletion may be associated with autism spectrum disorders as well as with intellectual disability without autism. The duplication of the same region is associated with schizophrenia. Even more surprising is the fact that many of these deletions/duplications can be inherited from a normal or nearly normal parent. For example, the recurrent deletion of 520 kb in 16p12.1 was significantly associated with psychomotor development delay, although it may also be present in control samples. In most cases the deletion 16p12.1 is inherited from a parent who often presents some slight neuropsychiatric disorder that is nevertheless compatible with a normal life. Although a remarkable phenotypic variability has long been known in subjects suffering from the same genomic disorder–think of the 22q11.2 deletion associated with the DiGeorge syndrome, which is inherited from one almost-normal parent in at least 10 per cent of cases–the deletion 16p12.1 is inherited in about 70 per cent of cases. It is therefore not obvious: (i) why some of these CNVs are often inherited from a normal or nearly normal parent; (ii) why the same CNV may be associated with so many different neuropsychiatric disorders; and (iii) why some CNVs, even in a different chromosomal location and with a different gene content are associated with similar phenotypes. With regard to (i), it has been shown that children with developmental delay or other neuropsychiatric problems, including autism, generally have a second large (greater than 500 kb) CNV not present in normal/near-normal controls. In other words, the clinical features of the subjects with two genomic imbalances are more severe than in those with a single one. With regard to (ii) and (iii), the most accredited hypothesis is that different CNVs may interfere with brain development in order to give minimal behavioural alterations, below the threshold of clinical diagnosis, while a second alteration of the genome is responsible for intellective disabilities, autism, epilepsy, or schizophrenia, depending on the genes it contains. In other words, the pathologic condition is the result of more imbalances according to the so-called 'two-hit' model (Girirajan *et al.*, 2012), where the clinical outcome of the destruction of a specific gene is determined by additional modifier factors.

Overall, studies using genomic arrays have definitely shown that rare CNVs, more than 500 kb in size, are more frequent (between 5 and 7 per cent) in individuals with autism than in controls (Pinto *et al.*, 2010). In addition, numerous studies of CNVs and autism have generated a list of candidate genes, destroyed by rare *de novo* CNVs: A2BP1, ANKRD11, C16orf72, CDH13, CDH18, DDX53, DLGAP2 [51.52], DPP6, DPYD, FHIT, FLJ16237, NLGN4, NRXN1, SHANK2, SHANK3, SLC4A10, SYNGAP1, and USP7 (Berg & Geschwind, 2012).

Currently, the major challenge is the search for genes associated with autism through new technologies of next-generation sequencing. Putting together genes with *de novo* variants identified by exome sequencing, genes of interest genes are: DYRK1A, POGZ, SCN2A, KATNAL2, and CHD8 (Berg & Geschwind, 2012). Although the molecular causes of this condition are far from being understood, there is convergence of opinion that autism is a disorder that involves proteins that modulate neuronal activity.

What tests may the clinician require when confronted with a patient with sporadic autism? Of course, the genomic array is presently a valuable tool even if the diagnostic probability does not exceed 10 per cent. Regarding familial cases, they should be considered for next-generation sequencing of the exome if not the whole genome.

Overall, the turning point for a molecular understanding of the disease, and therefore for the application of therapies aimed at bypassing the altered protein pathways, will only be achieved by a close collaboration between the clinician and the laboratory, who are called upon to interpret together the genomic profiles and to evaluate together every single alteration in respect to the endophenotype of that patient.

The clinician's role in interpreting an array analysis

The interpretation of the new genomic investigations requires a familiarity with specific databases that goes well beyond the expertise of the clinician, nor is it easily acquired through review of the scientific literature. Furthermore, our current knowledge of the genome is very poor, particularly with regard to the role of most of our genes and even more of their possible pathologic effects in cases of mutations, deletions, or duplications. As a result, the report of a potentially pathogenic CNV is based on well-established knowledge ('the genomic imbalance *xxxx* has been associated with the syndrome *xxxx*') and does not report deleted or duplicated genes whose possible pathogenic role is unknown ('current state of knowledge impairs establishing any association between the deleted or duplicated gene and the phenotype of the proband'). In an ideal practice of medicine, the report should be the result of a discussion between clinicians and geneticists in the laboratory, where each gene within the potentially pathologic CNV is examined with respect to its tissue expression and the role of the encoded protein in order to understand whether there could be a correlation between the genomic imbalance and some phenotypic characteristics of the patient. This approach would yield a hypothesis that should be further consolidated with other experiments, but which would be a first step towards the long-awaited translational medicine, where the doctor does not just treat the acute symptoms, but also clarifies the molecular basis of the condition for a more precise outcome and, in the future, not only alleviating symptoms, but also overcoming the molecular alteration. The example of chronic myeloid leukemia, which is now treated with a molecular drug to suppress the negative effects of the altered tyrosine kinase receptor, demonstrates the importance of the molecular approach to medicine.

Case report

We present here a report of using an array to help the clinician to interpret the data by him- or herself, and allow for a more profitable relationship with those working in the laboratory. The patient was a 4-year-old male characterized by neonatal hypotonia, global psychomotor delay with practically absent speech, and autistic behaviour. The family history was negative and the parents were healthy and non-consanguineous. A chromosome array showed a causative CNV consisting in heterozygous deletion of 274.141 kb of the distal region of the long arm of chromosome 22, defined as: arr 22q13.3 (50,924,617-51,198,757)x1. An extension of the investigation to the parents indicates that the deletion is *de novo*.

How to interpret this situation?

The fact that the deletion is not present in the genome of the parents argues in favor of its pathogenicity. However, this is not the only criterion for the interpretation of the data, as the occurrence of *de novo* CNV is relatively common in the population (about 2.5 CNVs *de novo* in every 100 live births), as shown by studies that have used an average array resolution of about 150 kb (Conrad *et al.*, 2010). On the other hand, there is the opposite condition, that is, the presence of the same CNV in a healthy parent cannot exclude the pathogenicity of the genomic imbalance for a number of reasons: (i) A gene on the not-deleted chromosome, lying in the region corresponding to the deletion, could be mutated so that the condition afflicting the proband is autosomal recessive and the parent with the same CNV is healthy heterozygotic. (ii) The CNV may contain a gene subjected to genomic imprinting that has a pathogenic effect only if inherited from the mother and not the father or vice versa: the healthy parent of the proband with the same CNV in turn inherited the CNV by a parent of the opposite sex. (iii) The CNV is a risk factor for a given pathologic feature that is manifested only in the presence of a second genome variant which is possibly unknown. In other words, the disease has incomplete penetrance and the risk that the disease occurs may not be currently evaluated through genetic analysis: this point is to be kept in mind for many neurologic disorders in which the presence of the second variant (second hit) is considered necessary for the full manifestation of the syndrome (Girirajan *et al.*, 2012).

To correctly interpret the identified CNVs it is first necessary to investigate whether it is listed in the database of the variants detected in the normal population (Fig. 1). Even this first stage of the inquiry requires a certain critical piece of information, that is, whether the variant has been reported in a significant proportion of healthy individuals or in only a few subjects. In the latter case, we cannot classify the variant as permanently free of pathogenicity, partly for reasons already mentioned, such as imprinting. In addition, the pathogenicity of the CNV may be due to incomplete penetrance or the CNV, although autosomal, can only be pathogenic in the XX background but not in the XY one (Vetro *et al.*, 2011).

The second step is to assess whether the CNV has already been identified by other laboratories and to evaluate the phenotypic characteristics associated with it. To this end, it is essential that different centres organize online databases and then continuously update them. These include the DECIPHER, ISCA, and ECARUCA databases, which are crucial to understanding whether there is a link between the phenotype of the patient and the CNV identified.

The last step, which is essential for the interpretation of the CNV, is to clarify the role of genes therein contained, although, at present, for many genes it is not known whether their alterations are causative of specific pathologic conditions.

All these processes, illustrated in Fig. 1, require a certain degree of experience as well as close cooperation with the clinician, who knows the patient.

The last, but not least, point to consider in the illustrated case (*de novo* pathogenic copy number change) is whether it is necessary to conduct further investigations to determine the risk of recurrence in the parents. In fact, despite the fact that the CNV is *de novo*, it is possible that the genomic region deleted in the patient is transposed in one of the parents on another chromosome. As a result, the parent would have a balanced chromosomal rearrangement (insertional translocation) that, as such, cannot be highlighted by the chromosome array. In this case, the risk of recurrence of genomic imbalance is 50 per cent and subsequent pregnancies must therefore be monitored by array investigations (Nowakowska *et al.*, 2012). A FISH analysis in the parents is thus recommended for all the *novo* deletions and duplications, and even more so when, in the proband, distal deletions and duplications are detected in different chromosomes, suggesting an unbalanced translocation.

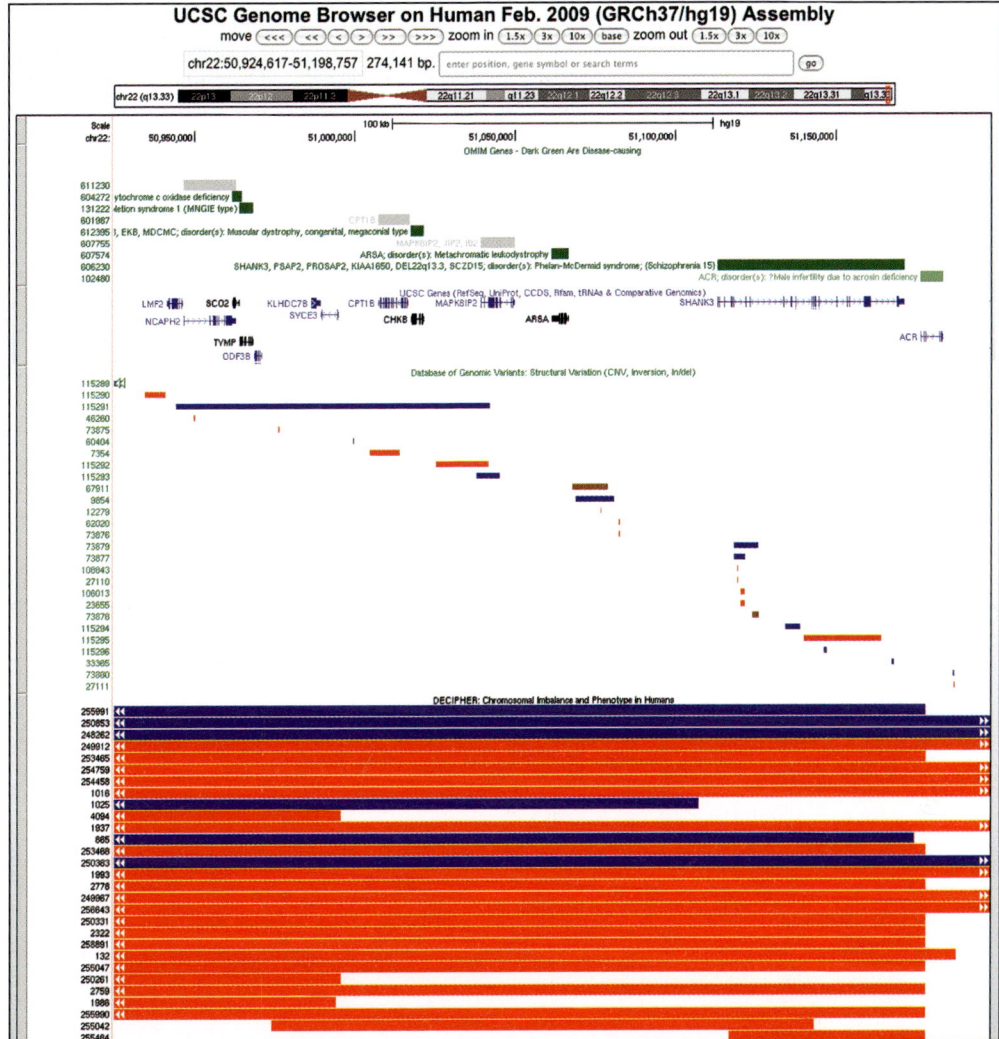

Fig. 1. This figure shows how any correlation between the identified CNV and the phenotype of the patient can be highlighted using the UCSC genome database. This example concerns the deletion of 22q13.3 discussed in the text. To obtain the necessary information, the UCSC browser is set as follows: First, set up the genomic assembly used in the array experiment, which is usually the most recent, here that of February 2009 (genome release hg19). The following items have to be turned on: Mapping and Sequencing Tracks: Base Position (dense or full), Chromosome Bands (pack or full); Phenotype and Disease Associations: DECIPHER (full), OMIM Genes (full); Genes and Gene Prediction Tracks: UCSC Gene (pack); Variation and Repeats: DGV Struct Var (full). In this figure, the OMIM genes appear below the image of chromosome 22. Those in green are 'disease-causing' while the gray ones are not currently known to have any established genotype-phenotype correlation. The analysis is limited to the green genes. Clicking the first four green ones from the left, it is possible to know that they all refer to autosomal recessive diseases. Therefore, they should not correlate to the disorder of the patient whose deletion is heterozygous,

while clicking the fifth green *gene, the information is obtained from* OMIM *that heterozygous deletions of SHANK3 are causative of the Phelan–McDermid syndrome, whose phenotype overlaps in fact with that of the patient under study. Proceeding downwards are the genes present in the deletion region, and by clicking each of them, a series of information on their function is obtained, if known. In the image, the gene products deriving from the various alternative splicings have been deleted. In principle, when the gene is represented multiple times, the information should be matched to the one with the more intense color (*blue *or* black*). By proceeding further, one can find the supposed benign CNV identified in the healthy population. These were selected by eliminating the CNVs identified by BAC array which may give false information. Finally, the DECIPHER information is provided:* red bars *refer to patients with deletion of the region and* blue bars *indicate patients with duplication. By clicking each of them, the information on the size of the CNV and the correlated phenotype is obtained (but, unfortunately, not for all cases).*

Conflicts of interest: The author declares no conflicts of interest.

References

Berg, J.M. & Geschwind, D.H. (2012): Autism genetics: searching for specificity and convergence. *Gen. Biol.* **13**, 247.

Conrad, D.F., Pinto, D., Redon, R., *et al.* (2010): Origins and functional impact of copy number, variation in the human genome. *Nature* **464**, 704–712.

Girirajan, S., Rosenfeld, J.A., Coe, B.P., *et al.* (2012): Phenotypic heterogeneity of rare disorders and genomic copy-number variants. *N. Engl. J. Med.* **367**, 1321–1331.

Mefford, H.C., Batshaw, M.L. & Hoffman, E.P. (2012): Genomics, intellectual disability, and autism. *N. Engl. J. Med.* **366**, 733–743.

Nowakowska, B.A., de Leeuw, N., Ruivenkamp, C.A., *et al.* (2012): Parental insertional balanced translocations are an important cause of apparently de novo CNVs in patients with developmental anomalies. *Eur. J. Hum. Genet.* **20**, 166–170.

Pinto, D., Pagnamenta, A.T., Klei, L., *et al.* (2010): Functional impact of global rare copy number variation in autism spectrum disorders. *Nature* **466**, 368–372.

Vetro, A., Ciccone, R., Giordano, R., *et al.* (2011): XX males SRY negative: a confirmed cause of infertility. *J. Med. Genet.* **48**, 710–712 [E-pub 7 Jun 2011].

Chapter 6

Gene–environment interactions in autism spectrum disorder

Antonio M. Persico

*Child & Adolescent Neuropsychiatry Unit & Laboratory of Molecular Psychiatry and Neurogenetics,
University Campus Bio-Medico, via Alvaro del Portillo 21, 00128 Rome, Italy;
and Department of Experimental Neurosciences, I.R.C.C.S. 'Fondazione Santa Lucia',
C.E.R.C., via del Fosso di Fiorano, 00143 Rome, Italy*
a.persico@unicampus.it

Summary

Autism spectrum disorder (ASD) encompasses a group of neurodevelopmental conditions characterized by deficits of variable severity in the areas of language, communication, and social interaction, as well as by the presence of stereotypic behaviours, restricted and unusual interests, and insistence on sameness. Post-mortem studies have unveiled neuropathologic abnormalities highly compatible with an early developmental origin of ASD (first and second trimester of pregnancy), despite behavioural onset typically occurring at 6–24 months of postnatal life. Genetic factors contribute strongly to ASD. However, twin studies performed two decades ago yielded heritability estimates above 90 per cent, whereas a recent study performed in California estimates heritability at 37 per cent and shared environmental factors at 55 per cent. Furthermore, the majority of patients do not carry mutations or copy number variants fully responsible for the disease. Finally, converging evidence supports frequent immune abnormalities in children with ASD, especially those affecting the innate immune system.

This surprising level of complexity has spurred interest into polygenic models of disease characterized by variable penetrance, labile genotype–phenotype correlations and gene–environment interactions. This chapter describes three evidence-based paradigms of gene–environment interaction relevant to autistic behaviours: (*a*) PON1 + RELN + prenatal exposure to organophosphate pesticides; (*b*) SLC25A12 + ATP2B2 + prenatal exposure to polychlorinated biphenyls; and (*c*) MET + prenatal exposure to polycyclic aromatic hydrocarbons. These three paradigms, which have received at least some experimental support, demonstrate that during critical periods in neurodevelopment specific environmental factors can play pathogenic roles when acting upon a vulnerable genetic background. In addition, pathoplastic roles (*i.e.*, significant influences on disease severity) by the postnatal exposure to toxicants can be exemplified by *p*-cresol, a compound primarily produced by the gut flora and seemingly associated with more severe forms of autism.

Introduction

Autism spectrum disorder (ASD) is a severe neuropsychiatric disorder characterized by deficits in social interaction and communication, as well as by stereotyped behaviours and insistence on sameness (*e.g.*, restricted patterns of interest and activities), with onset in early childhood, prior to 3 years of age (American Psychiatric Association, 1994). Its incidence has dramatically risen during the last two decades from 2–5/10,000 to approximately 1–2/1,000 children: broader diagnostic criteria and increased awareness in the medical community have contributed to this trend (Fombonne, 2005), but a real increase in incidence possibly due to gene–environment interactions is also likely (Landrigan, 2010; Persico & Bourgeron, 2006). Brain imaging and especially neuropathologic studies involving postmortem brains have uncovered important neuroanatomic abnormalities in the central nervous system (CNS) of ASD patients, generally resulting from reduced programmed cell death and/or increased cell proliferation, altered cell migration, and abnormal cell differentiation with reduced neuronal size and abnormal wiring (Bauman & Kemper, 2005; Persico & Bourgeron, 2006). Physiologically these neurodevelopmental processes occur during the first and second trimester of pregnancy, strongly supporting a prenatal origin for autism (Bauman & Kemper, 2005; Rice & Barone, 2000; Scott *et al.*, 2009), although postnatal exposure to toxicants can likely modulate the behavioral phenotype, as may occur with *p*-cresol (see below) (Altieri *et al.*, 2011).

Genetics is believed to strongly contribute to the pathogenesis of ASD (Persico, 2012). According to initial twin studies performed in the United Kingdom and in Sweden (Bailey *et al.*, 1995; Steffenburg *et al.*, 1989), ASD displayed the highest heritability (> 90 per cent) among all neuropsychiatric disorders, as well as a relevant sibling recurrence risk (5–6 per cent for severe non-syndromic autism and 15 per cent for broad spectrum) (Persico, 2012; Persico & Bourgeron, 2006). However, these heritability estimates have not been confirmed by a more recent twin study performed in California, which supports a larger proportion of variance explained by shared environmental factors as opposed to genetic heritability (55 per cent *vs.* 37 per cent for strict autism, respectively) (Hallmayer *et al.*, 2011). Furthermore, many patients reveal no causal mutations or pathogenic copy number variants. The vast majority of ASD patients conform to a 'multiple hit' model, encompassing gene–gene and gene–environment interactions, as well as epigenetic contributions related to several factors, such as increasing parental age at the time of conception (Leblond *et al.*, 2012; Persico, 2012; Persico & Bourgeron, 2006).

This unexpected complexity has spurred interest into polygenic models allowing for gene–environment interactions to produce large inter-individual phenotypic variability.

Review of the topic

Three gene–environment interaction paradigms relevant to ASD will now be presented. These three models have been selected because they have received experimental support, albeit to a variable degree.

RELN-PON1-prenatal exposure to organophosphate pesticides or excessive oxidative stress

The *RELN* gene encodes for reelin, a stop signal critical to neuronal migration in several regions of the CNS, including neocortex, cerebellum, and hindbrain; at the cellular level, reelin acts by binding to a variety of receptors, including the VLDL receptors and APOE-R2 (Förster *et al.*, 2010). In addition, it exerts a proteolytic activity on extracellular matrix proteins, which is inhibited by organophosphate (OP) pesticides (Quattrocchi *et al.*, 2002).

The *PON1* gene encodes for an enzyme usually denoted 'paraoxonase', which exerts several enzymatic activities including the inactivation of OPs, the degradation of lipid peroxides preventing atherosclerosis and vascular disease, the breakdown of bacterial endotoxins, and the prevention of protein lactonation (Gaita *et al.*, 2010).

Autistic individuals display a significant reduction in reelin protein levels both in plasma and in post-mortem brains compared to controls, as well as reduced serum *PON1* enzymatic activity measured as 'arylesterase' (Fatemi *et al.*, 2005; Gaita *et al.*, 2010; Lugli *et al.*, 2003; Paşca *et al.*, 2006). *RELN* gene polymorphisms yielding lower reelin gene expression both *in vitro* and *in vivo*, are significantly associated with autism, as occurs with *PON1* gene variants responsible for lower gene expression and reduced OP detoxification (D'Amelio *et al.*, 2005; Persico *et al.*, 2001, 2006). Therefore, individuals carrying genetic variants producing lower amounts of reelin and PON1 enzyme, if exposed to developmental neurotoxicants like OPs during critical periods in prenatal neurodevelopment, could be especially vulnerable to having abnormal neuronal migration, yielding altered neural networks and behavioral autism (Persico & Bourgeron, 2006). Recently, this model has received experimental and epidemiologic support by two important data sets, one showing an association between prenatal exposure to OPs, *PON1* genotypes, and poorer neurobehavioral development in humans (Eskenazi *et al.*, 2010), the other showing abnormal behavior and CNS lamination in the neocortex, hippocampus, and cerebellum of heterozygous *reeler* mice (expressing 50 per cent lower amounts of reelin compared to wild-type mice) prenatally exposed to the OP chlorpyrifos (Mullen *et al.*, 2010). As briefly outlined above, these results have been interpreted in reference to the capacity of OPs to inhibit cholinesterase activity, but alternative mechanisms are also possible. In particular, excessive prenatal and early postnatal oxidative stress may also play a prominent role, since our sample encompassing 174 autistic patients, 175 first-degree relatives, and 144 controls, unveiled a significant decrease in arylesterase, but not in diazoxonase PON1 activities (Gaita *et al.*, 2010). Interestingly, excessive oxidative stress has been documented in various tissues of ASD patients (Chauhan & Chauhan, 2006), and OP exposure further increases oxidative stress both *in vitro* and *in vivo* (Qiao *et al.*, 2005).

ATP2B2–SLC25A12–polychlorinated biphenyls (PCBs)

Intracellular Ca^{2+} spikes, when excessive either in extent or duration, have been convincingly shown to play a relevant role in the pathophysiology of autism (Krey & Dolmetsch, 2007). The *ATP2B2* gene encodes for the plasma membrane calcium ATPase 2 (PMCA2), which removes Ca^{2+} from the cytoplasm into the extracellular space with faster kinetics and broader affinity as compared to the other three PMCAs. For this reason, PMCA2 is especially critical to the function and plasticity of critical synaptic sites in the CNS, such as the parallel fibre-to-Purkinje cell synapse in the cerebellar cortex and in parvalbumin-positive GABAergic interneurons (Burette *et al.*, 2009; Empson *et al.*, 2007; Garside *et al.*, 2009). We have recently described an association of *ATP2B2* gene variants with autism in males (Carayol *et al.*, 2011). On the basis of preliminary data indicating reduced *ATP2B2* expression patterns in post-mortem brains of ASD patients, the autism-associated genetic variant is expected to yield reduced gene expression, leading to slower Ca^{2+} clearance from the cytoplasm in excitable cells. This genetic vulnerability could be exacerbated by environmental exposure to PCBs, important endocrine disruptors also able to promote Ca^{2+} entry from the extracellular space and Ca^{2+} release from the endoplasmic reticulum (Pessah *et al.*, 2010). Therefore, prenatal exposure to PCBs could lead to intracellular Ca^{2+} spikes of greater duration and/or amplitude in genetically vulnerable individuals carrying ATP2B2 gene variants possibly associated with reduced gene expression and Ca^{2+} clearance capacity. Excessive intracellular Ca^{2+} spikes can in turn interfere with neuronal migration, dendritic spine formation, and synaptogenesis by modulating numerous intracellular molecules and pathways. Especially important in this regard could be the role played by a Ca^{2+}-mediated activation of the exchange of aspartate for glutamate mediated by the mitochondrial carrier AGC1, resulting in abnormal energy metabolism and enhanced oxidative stress (Palmieri *et al.*, 2010; Palmieri & Persico, 2010). Interestingly, the *SLC25A12* gene, which encodes for AGC1, may encompass genetic variants able to influence disease risk in autism (Ramoz *et al.*, 2004).

MET–polycyclic aromatic hydrocarbons (PAHs)

The *MET* proto-oncogene encodes for the MET receptor tyrosine kinase, a key modulator of cell proliferation and migration, as well as neurite outgrowth and synaptogenesis in the development of the CNS, gut, and immune system (Campbell *et al.*, 2006). The *MET* gene promoter contains the single nucleotide polymorphism (SNP) rs1858830, whose C allele is significantly associated with autism and with lower *MET* transcription both *in vitro* and in post-mortem brains (Campbell *et al.*, 2006, 2007). Furthermore, ASD brains display profound 50 per cent decreases in *MET* mRNA and protein on average, compared to matched controls (Campbell *et al.*, 2007). Therefore, on the one hand, reduced *MET* gene expression confers autism risk. On the other hand, prenatal exposure of mice to the PAH benzo(*a*)pyrene blunts postnatal *MET* gene expression and yields behavioural deficits in a novelty test (Sheng *et al.*, 2010). Therefore, prenatal exposure to PAHs may either act in conjunction with the C allele at SNP rs1858830, further enhancing autism risk, or may more likely reduce the protection conferred by the G allele.

In addition to gene–environment interactions, where 'environment' is represented by man-made toxicants, the potential relevance of nongenetic factors in ASD is further underscored by gut-derived toxicants, which seemingly play at least pathoplastic, if not pathogenetic roles in ASD. In particular, experimental evidence provides initial support for two compounds, namely *p*-cresol (4-methylphenol) and propionic acid (PPA). *P*-cresol can essentially originate either from the gut or from environmental exposure. The largest source of this compound is represented by specific gut bacteria, such as *Clostridium difficile*, which express *p*-cresol-synthesizing enzymes not found in human cells. Environmental exposure is relatively common and occurs through the skin, as well as the gastrointestinal and respiratory systems. Propionic acid (PPA) is also produced in the gut by anaerobic bacteria, including Clostridia and Propionibacteria, through fermentation of dietary carbohydrates and several amino acids (Al-Lahham *et al.*, 2010). Also PPA can derive from environmental exposure, since it is used as a food preservative in many wheat and dairy products, but, differently from *p*-cresol, it is also an endogenous compound, namely an intermediate of human fatty acid metabolism (Al-Lahham *et al.*, 2010). Evidence supporting *p*-cresol and PPA roles in ASD is still growing and comes at this stage primarily from human and animal studies, respectively.

Urinary *p*-cresol and its conjugated derivative *p*-cresylsulfate have been found elevated in an initial sample and recently in a replica sample of autistic children below 8 years of age. In particular, we assessed urinary levels of *p*-cresol in 59 non-syndromic autistic children and in 59 tightly age- and sex-matched controls (Altieri *et al.*, 2011). Urinary concentrations of *p*-cresol were significantly higher in autistic children compared to controls (123.5 ± 12.8 *vs*. 91.2 + 8.7 µg/ml, $P < 0.05$). This elevation was surprisingly age-dependent, as it was clearly detectable only up until and including age 7 (134.1 ± 20.1 *vs*. 70.3 ± 6.7 µg/ml, $P = 0.005$), with urinary *p*-cresol levels normalizing at age 8 and beyond. Levels of *p*-cresol were correlated neither with body mass index nor with urinary cotinine levels, excluding spurious contamination from passive smoking. Instead, *p*-cresol levels were significantly higher among *female* autistic children compared to males ($P < 0.05$), *more severely affected* autistic children, regardless of sex ($P < 0.05$), and in children who underwent *regression at autism onset*, based on parents' reporting loss of language skills after acquisition of more than 5 spoken words and loss of social abilities after initial acquisition ($P < 0.05$).

A replication study was then undertaken on an independent sample of ASD children and controls recruited at the Center for Child and Adolescent Psychiatry of the Hôpital Bretonneau in Tours (France). Preliminary analyses run on 34 French children already replicate significantly higher urinary *p*-cresol levels in 17 ASD cases compared to 17 matched controls ($P < 0.05$). This significant increase occurs only in 8 case–control pairs aged 7 or below ($P < 0.01$), with no significant difference beyond 7 years of age. Urinary *p*-cresol is again significantly correlated with clinical severity, as documented using several clinical scales (Antonio Persico, Andrea Urbani, Sonia Cerullo, Catherine Barthélémy, Frédérique Bonnet-Brilhault and Gabriele Tripi, unpublished observation). In addition to measuring total *p*-cresol, as in our initial study (Altieri *et al.*, 2011), here we separately measured its three fractions, namely free *p*-cresol, *p*-cresylsulfate and *p*-cresylglucuronate. These compounds account for 0.06 per cent, 95.26 per cent, and 4.68 per cent, respectively, of total urinary *p*-cresol in controls. Statistically significant elevations in ASD children compared to controls were found for urinary *p*-cresylsulfate and *p*-cresylglucuronate ($P < 0.05$), whereas free *p*-cresol displays at this stage a nonsignificant trend ($P = 0.086$). Conceivably *p*-cresol, or its metabolite *p*-cresylsulfate, could thus exert negative pathoplastic effects on autistic behaviours and associated cognitive deficits.

Evidence for PPA comes primarily from animal studies. Intracerebroventricular administration of PPA in young rats yields behavioural abnormalities reminiscent of those of ASDs, including perseverance in object-directed behaviour, impaired reversal learning in the T-maze, and reduced interaction with a novel rat compared to a novel object (MacFabe *et al.*, 2011). The hippocampus and white matter of these same animals display neuroinflammation in the form of activated microglia and reactive astrogliosis (MacFabe *et al.*, 2011), similar to those detected in post-mortem autistic brains (Vargas *et al.*, 2005). Also, developmental delay and cognitive deficits have been documented in rodents prenatally exposed to PPA (Brusque *et al.*, 1999).

Once ongoing animal and cellular studies will have unveiled the mechanism of action of *p*-cresol, and human studies verified whether PPA plays concrete roles in human autism, it will be extremely interesting to study whether gene × *p*-cresol/PPA interactions may underlie interindividual differences in sensitivity to these compounds. It will also be very interesting to assess in baby–sibling studies whether elevated levels of these compounds derived from the maternal gut may play pathogenetic roles during early pregnancy.

Conclusions

The gene–environment interaction models and the possible roles of gut-derived compounds briefly presented above, stem from growing genetic, neurobiologic, and epidemiologic evidence, and are not mere hypotheses solely based on theoretical grounds. They are in no way exhaustive, as prenatal exposure to many other chemicals could favour the development of autism by interfering with the intracellular pathways best shown to underlie this disease (excessive Ca^{2+} signalling, PI3K/mTOR/ERK, oxidative stress, decreased synaptogenesis, epigenetic abnormalities, decreased oxidative phosphorylation). Nonetheless, these paradigms do stress the need to consider the encounter between environmental toxicants and an individual, or perhaps even more a feto-maternal unit, even when studying a behavioural disorder with prominent heritability. The validity of such models is strongly supported even by known prenatal teratologic agents, such as rubella or cytomegalovirus infection, and drugs like thalidomide, misoprostol, and valproic acid, which cause autism only in a subset of presumably vulnerable individuals (Landrigan, 2010; Persico & Bourgeron, 2006; Persico, 2012). Finally, this avenue of investigation holds promise to yield therapies able to at least ameliorate the clinical severity and co-morbidities commonly seen in many autistic children.

Acknowledgments: I gratefully acknowledge my collaborators (Roberto Sacco, Carla Lintas, Valerio Napolioni, Stefano Gabriele, Ignazio Stefano Piras, and Sarah Hastings) and all the patients and families who participated in our studies. We are also grateful for financial support from the Italian Ministry for University, Scientific Research and Technology; the Italian Ministry of Health; the Fondazione Gaetano e Mafalda Luce (Milan, Italy); Autism Aid ONLUS (Naples, Italy); Autism Speaks (Princeton, NJ); the Autism Research Institute (San Diego, CA); and the European Union (IMI project EU-AIMS).

Conflicts of interest: The author declares no conflicts of interest.

References

Al-Lahham, S.H., Peppelenbosch, M.P., Roelofsen, H., Vonk, R.J. & Venema, K. (2010): Biological effects of propionic acid in humans; metabolism, potential applications and underlying mechanisms. *Biochim. Biophys. Acta* **180**, 1175–1183.

Altieri, L., Neri, C., Sacco, R., *et al.* (2011): Urinary p-cresol is elevated in small children with severe autism spectrum disorder. *Biomarkers* **16**, 252–260.

American Psychiatric Association (1994): *Diagnostic and Statistical Manual of Mental Disorders* (4th ed). Washington DC: American Psychiatric Association.

Bauman, M.L. & Kemper, T.L. (2005): Neuroanatomic observations of the brain in autism: a review and future directions. *Int. J. Dev. Neurosci.* **23**, 183–187.

Bailey, A., Le Couteur, A., Gottesman, I., *et al.* (1995): Autism as a strongly genetic disorder: evidence from a British twin study. *Psychol. Med.* **25**, 63–77.

Brusque, A.M., Mello, C.F., Buchanan, D.N., *et al.* (1999): Effect of chemically induced propionic acidemia on neurobehavioral development of rats. *Pharmacol. Biochem. Behav.* **64**, 529–534.

Burette, A.C., Strehler, E.E. & Weinberg, R.J. (2009): 'Fast' plasma membrane calcium pump PMCA2a concentrates in GABAergic terminals in the adult rat brain. *J. Comp. Neurol.* **512**, 500–513.

Campbell, D.B., Sutcliffe, J.S., Ebert, P.J., *et al.* (2006): A genetic variant that disrupts *MET* transcription is associated with autism. *Proc. Natl. Acad. Sci. USA* **103**, 16834–16839.

Campbell, D.B., D'Oronzio, R., Garbett, K., *et al.* (2007): Disruption of cerebral cortex MET signaling in autism spectrum disorder. *Ann. Neurol.* **62**, 243–250.

Carayol, J., Sacco, R., Tores, F., *et al.* (2011): Converging evidence for an association of *ATP2B2* allelic variants with autism in males. *Biol. Psychiatry* **70**, 880–887.

Chauhan, A. & Chauhan, V. (2006): Oxidative stress in autism. Pathophysiology **13**, 171–181.

D'Amelio, M., Ricci, I., Sacco, R., *et al.* (2005): Paraoxonase gene variants are associated with autism in North America, but not in Italy: possible regional specificity in gene-environment interactions. *Mol. Psychiatry* **10**, 1006–1016.

Empson, R.M., Garside, M.L. & Knöpfel, T. (2007): Plasma membrane Ca2+ ATPase 2 contributes to short-term synapse plasticity at the parallel fiber to Purkinje neuron synapse. *J. Neurosci.* **27**, 3753–3758.

Eskenazi, B., Huen, K., Marks, A., *et al.* (2010): PON1 and neurodevelopment in children from the CHAMACOS study exposed to organophosphate pesticides in utero. *Environ. Health Perspect.* **118**, 1775–1781.

Fatemi, S.H., Snow, A.V., Stary, J.M., *et al.* (2005): Reelin signaling is impaired in autism. *Biol. Psychiatry* **57**, 777–787.

Fombonne, E. (2005): Epidemiology of autistic disorder and other pervasive developmental disorders. *J. Clin. Psychiatry* **66**, 3–8.

Förster, E., Bock, H.H., Herz, J., Chai, X., Frotscher, M. & Zhao, S. (2010): Emerging topics in Reelin function. *Eur. J. Neurosci.* **31,** 1511–1518.

Gaita, L., Manzi, B., Sacco, R., *et al.* (2010): Decreased serum arylesterase activity in autism spectrum disorders. *Psychiatry Res.* **180,** 105–113.

Garside, M.L., Turner, P.R., Austen, B., Strehler, E.E., Beesley, P.W. & Empson, R.M. (2009): Molecular interactions of the plasma membrane calcium ATPase 2 at pre- and post-synaptic sites in rat cerebellum. *Neuroscience* **162,** 383–395.

Hallmayer, J., Cleveland, S., Torres, A., *et al.* (2011): Genetic heritability and shared environmental factors among twin pairs with autism. *Arch. Gen. Psychiatry* **68,** 1095–1102.

Krey, J. & Dolmetsch, R. (2007): Molecular mechanisms of autism: a possible role for Ca^{2+} signaling. *Curr. Opin. Neurobiol.* **17,** 112–119.

Landrigan, P.J. (2010): What causes autism? Exploring the environmental contribution. *Curr. Opin. Pediatr.* **22,** 219–225.

Leblond, C.S., Heinrich, J., Delorme, R., *et al.* (2012): Genetic and functional analyses of SHANK2 mutations suggest a multiple hit model of autism spectrum disorders. *PLoS Genet.* **8,** e1002521.

Lugli, G., Krueger, J.M., Davis, J.M., Persico, A.M., Keller, F. & Smalheiser, N.R. (2003): Methodological factors influencing measurement and processing of plasma reelin in humans. *BMC Biochem.* **4,** 9.

MacFabe, D.F., Cain, N.E., Boon, F., Ossenkopp, K.P. & Cain, D.P. (2011): Effects of the entericbacterial metabolic product propionic acid on object-directed behavior, social behavior, cognition, and neuroinflammation in adolescent rats: relevance to autism spectrum disorder. *Behav. Brain Res.* **217,** 47–54.

Mullen, B., Khialeeva, E. & Carpenter, E.M. (2010): A Dab1-lacZ reporter reveals CNS lamination defects in a mouse model for autism. Program No. 147.12, 40th Annual Meeting of Neuroscience. Society for Neuroscience 2010 Daily Books, ed. Coe-Truman Technologies, San Diego, CA.

Palmieri, L. & Persico, A.M. (2010): Mitochondrial dysfunction in autism spectrum disorders: cause or effect? *Biochim. Biophys. Acta* **1797,** 1130–1137.

Palmieri, L., Papaleo, V., Porcelli, V., *et al.* (2010): Altered calcium homeostasis in autism-spectrum disorders: evidence from biochemical and genetic studies of the mitochondrial aspartate/glutamate carrier AGC1. *Mol. Psychiatry* **15,** 38–52.

Paşca, S.P., Nemeş, B., Vlase, L., *et al.* (2006): High levels of homocysteine and low serum paraoxonase 1 arylesterase activity in children with autism. *Life Sci.* **78,** 2244–2248.

Persico, A.M., D'Agruma, L., Maiorano, N., *et al.* (2001): Reelin gene alleles and haplotypes as a factor predisposing to autistic disorder. *Mol. Psychiatry* **6,** 150–159.

Persico, A.M. & Bourgeron, T. (2006): Searching for ways out of the autism maze: genetic, epigenetic and environmental clues. *Trends Neurosci.* **29,** 349–358.

Persico, A.M., Levitt, P. & Pimenta, A.F. (2006): Polymorphic GGC repeat differentially regulates human reelin gene expression levels. *J. Neural. Transm.* **113,** 1373–1382.

Persico, A.M. (2013): Autisms. In: *Neural Circuit Development and Function in the Brain: Comprehensive Developmental Neuroscience, Vol. 3*, eds. P. Rakic & J. Rubenstein, chapt. 45. San Diego, CA: Academic Press.

Pessah, I.N., Cherednichenko, G. & Lein, P.J. (2010): Minding the calcium store: ryanodine receptor activation as a convergent mechanism of PCB toxicity. *Pharmacol. Ther.* **125,** 260–285.

Qiao, D., Seidler, F.J. & Slotkin, T.A. (2005): Oxidative mechanisms contributing to the developmental neurotoxicity of nicotine and chlorpyrifos. *Toxicol. Appl. Pharmacol.* **206,** 17–26.

Quattrocchi, C.C., Wannenes, F., Persico, A.M., *et al.* (2002): Reelin is a serine protease of the extracellular matrix. *J. Biol. Chem.* **277,** 303–309.

Ramoz, N., Reichert, J.G., Smith, C.J., *et al.* (2004): Linkage and association of the mitochondrial aspartate/glutamate carrier *SLC25A12* gene with autism. *Am. J. Psychiatry* **161,** 662–669.

Rice, D. & Barone, S., Jr (2000): Critical periods of vulnerability for the developing nervous system: evidence from humans and animal models. *Environ. Health Perspect.* **108,** 511–533.

Scott, J.A., Schumann, C.M., Goodlin-Jones, B.L. & Amaral, D.G. (2009): A comprehensive volumetric analysis of the cerebellum in children and adolescents with autism spectrum disorder. *Autism Res.* **2,** 246–257.

Sheng, L., Ding, X., Ferguson, M., *et al.* (2010): Prenatal polycyclic aromatic hydrocarbon exposure leads to behavioural deficits and downregulation of receptor tyrosine kinase, MET. *Toxicol. Sci.* **118,** 625–634.

Steffenburg, S., Gillberg, C., Hellgren, L., *et al.* (1989): A twin study of autism in Denmark, Finland, Iceland, Norway and Sweden. *J. Child Psychol. Psychiatry* **30,** 405–416.

Vargas, D.L., Nascimbene, C., Krishnan, C., Zimmerman, A.W. & Pardo, C.A. (2005): Neuroglial activation and neuroinflammation in the brain of patients with autism. *Ann. Neurol.* **57,** 67–81.

Chapter 7

GABA is essential for the construction of neuronal circuits early in development: dysfunction in autism spectrum disorders

Rocco Pizzarelli and Enrico Cherubini

Department of Neuroscience, Scuola Internazionale Superiore di Studi Avanzati (SISSA),
via Bonomea 265, 34136 Trieste, Italy
cher@sissa.it

Summary

Autism spectrum disorders (ASDs) comprise a heterogeneous group of neuro-developmental disorders characterized by impaired social interaction, communication deficits, stereotyped and repetitive behaviours, and restricted interests. In a few cases, ASDs are associated with enhanced cognitive abilities (Garber, 2007) and in about 30 per cent of cases with epilepsy. ASDs affect one of every 150 children. The incidence of ASDs has risen dramatically over the past two decades, mainly because of the improvement of diagnostic means (Rutter, 2005).
ASDs are caused by genetic as well as environmental and epigenetic factors (Geschwind & Levitt, 2007; Persico & Bourgeron, 2006). Interestingly, in a small number of subjects with idiopathic ASD, a single mutation in genes involved in synaptic function has been identified, pointing to the synapse as one possible site of origin of autism (Südhof, 2008). Synapses are specialized intercellular junctions which ensure communication between neurons and therefore ASDs can be considered as disorders of synapses or synaptopathies.
Some gene mutations involved in ASD have been introduced in animal models in order to elucidate the underlying pathophysiologic mechanisms and to develop new appropriately targeted therapeutic tools. Although the behavioural deficits found in animals and humans may be substantially different because of the high complexity of the human brain, basic disruption of elementary neuronal functions may be very similar.
Neuronal wiring, which is established very early in development, involves cell migration and differentiation, synapse formation, and stabilization and refinement following experience-dependent processes. Several lines of evidence suggest that GABA plays a key role in these processes and in maintaining an appropriate excitatory/inhibitory (E/I) balance necessary for the correct operation of neuronal networks. In this review we will focus on GABA, the neurotransmitter required for the proper assembly and construction of neuronal networks in the perinatal period. In particular we highlight how a dysfunction of GABAergic signaling during brain maturation leads to the impairment of the E/I balance, which may account for several behavioural deficits found in neurodevelopmental disorders.
Of interest, as illustrated in Fig. 1, the peak of the incidence of ASDs coincides with the period of maximal experience-dependent synapse formation.

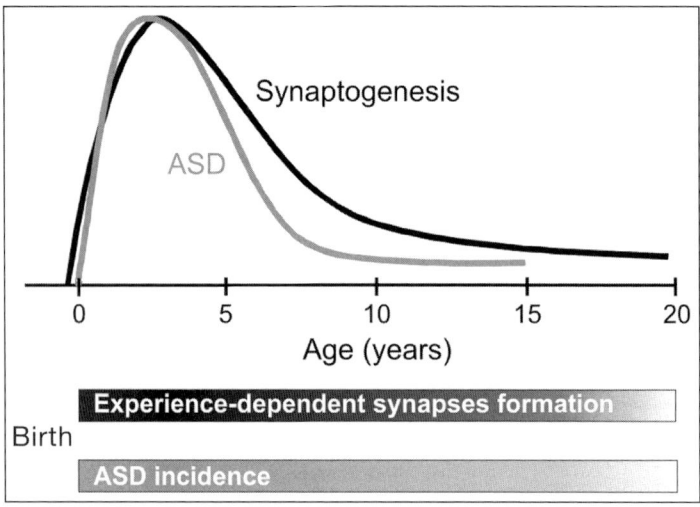

Fig. 1. The peak of the incidence of ASDs (in grey) coincides with the period of maximal experience-dependent synapse formation (in black).

GABA, a key player in the development of neuronal circuits

GABA (γ-aminobutyric acid), the major inhibitory transmitter in the adult brain, plays a crucial role in controlling neuronal excitability and in generating oscillatory activity crucial for information processing. GABA acts by activating two different classes of receptors: $GABA_A$ and $GABA_B$. $GABA_A$ receptors are ligand-gated ion channels, permeable mainly to Cl^- and HCO_3^- (Cherubini & Conti, 2001). The opening of $GABA_A$ receptor channels causes a net flux of chloride inside the cells with consequent membrane hyperpolarization and reduction of cell firing. The $GABA_B$ receptors do not contain an integral ion channel, but are coupled with cationic channels (usually inwardly rectifying potassium channels) via G_i and G_o proteins (Bettler et al., 2004). Activation of $GABA_B$ receptors causes a membrane hyperpolarization and a reduction of cell firing (Luscher et al., 1997).

One peculiarity of the GABAergic signaling is that the polarity of its action is closely related to the intracellular concentration of chloride $[Cl^-]_i$, which is highly labile, leading in certain conditions to depolarising and even excitatory actions.

In the immediate postnatal period, when glutamatergic synapses are still poorly developed (Hosokawa et al., 1994; Tyzio et al., 1999), GABA, via $GABA_A$ receptors, depolarizes the membrane through an outwardly-directed flux of chloride (Ben-Ari et al., 1989), which enables reaching spike threshold via amplification through non-inactivating sodium conductances (Valeeva et al., 2010). As the spike threshold differs in different types of immature neurons, GABA will depolarize some neurons and excite others (Banke & McBain, 2006). GABA-induced membrane depolarization triggers calcium currents and removes the voltage-dependent magnesium block from NMDA receptors (Ben-Ari et al., 1997; Leinekugel et al., 1997). Calcium entry leads to the activation of second messengers involved in a variety of developmental processes, including cell migration and differentiation and synaptogenesis (Garaschuk et al., 1998; Leinekugel et al., 1997; Yuste et al., 1991).

The construction of the cerebral cortex from a single sheet of neuroepithelium requires multiple tightly regulated developmental processes working in concert. In order to form this complex structure, neurons must be generated in the correct numbers, migrate to the proper position, and form intricate connections with neighbours and targets. Of the many cell-intrinsic and -extrinsic signals involved in neocortical development, GABA has been proved to be an important regulator (Wang & Kriegstein, 2009).

Interestingly, the majority of GABAergic interneurons are derived from an extracortical source, the ganglionic eminences (GEs) of the ventral telencephalon (Faux et al., 2012). In the mouse, GEs, which appear around embryonic (E) day 11, can be structurally divided into three separate areas: lateral (LGE), medial (MGE), and caudal (CGE), depending on the rostrocaudal and mediolateral position. MGE-derived interneurons are mainly parvalbumin-positive (PV+), fast-spiking basket cells and somatostatin-positive intrinsic bursting Martinotti cells, while CGE-derived cells exhibit a wide range of firing patterns and are divided in vasoactive intestinal peptide (VIP)-, calretinin (CR)-, and neuropeptide-Y-positive cells (Faux et al., 2012). The majority of interneurons derived from the MGE and CGE undergo their final mitosis in these regions prior to their tangential migration into the cortical plate. Once there, they adopt various radial migration modes to settle into specific cortical layers in an inside-out manner according to their birth order (Faux et al., 2012). The migration process, supposed to be calcium dependent, is regulated by a sequence of well-orchestrated processes involving guidance cues, neurotransmitter receptors (NMDA, $GABA_A$ receptors), and voltage-dependent calcium channels (Komuro & Rakic, 1998; Spitzer, 2002).

In contrast to GABAergic interneurons, principal cells, generated locally in the neuroepithelium, migrate radially from progenitors in the ventricular/subventricular zone towards the cortical plate. Migrating neurons as well as radial glial cells express $GABA_A$ receptors (LoTurco et al., 1995; Owens et al., 1996, 1999) that, during corticogenesis, bind GABA with higher affinity than do mature neurons (Owens et al., 1999). In addition, at early developmental stages, $GABA_A$ receptors can be activated in a paracrine fashion by GABA released from growth cones and astrocytes in a calcium- and SNARE-independent way (Demarque et al., 2002). The absence of an efficient uptake system enables GABA to accumulate in the extracellular space and reach a concentration that is sufficient to exert its depolarizing and excitatory effects on distal neurons.

Blocking the depolarizing action of GABA *in utero* has a heavy impact on migration and circuit formation, indicating that GABA modulates these and many other functions (Cancedda et al., 2007; Manent et al., 2006; Wang & Kriegstein, 2010). The premature expression of the cation-chloride extruder KCC2, by *in utero* electroporation, eliminates the excitatory action of endogenous GABA in a subpopulation of newly-born cortical neurons and severely alters the structure of cortical cells (Cancedda et al., 2007) (Fig. 2).

This effect can be mimicked by over-expressing the inwardly rectifying K^+ channel, which lowers the membrane potential and reduces cell excitability, strongly suggesting that membrane depolarization caused by the early GABA excitation is essential for the functional maturation of cortical circuits *in vivo*.

Immediately after birth, GABAergic signals mature and operate before glutamatergic ones and this correlates with the level of dendritic arborization (Ben Ari et al., 2007; Khazipov et al., 2001; Tyzio et al., 1999). Three stages of development can be identified: (1) silent neurons with no apical dendrites without functional synapses; (2) GABA-only neurons with small apical and not basal dendrites that express GABA but not glutamate-mediated postsynaptic

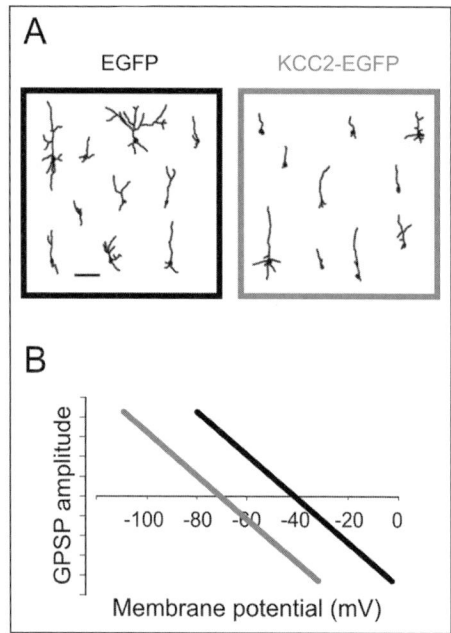

Fig. 2. The depolarizing and excitatory action of GABA early in postnatal development is essential for the morphologic maturation of principal cells. (A) EGFP-(black) or KCC2/EGFP (grey)-expressing neurons in layer II–III of the cerebral cortex at postnatal day 6. Note that in comparison with EGFP, EGFP/KCC2-expressing cells exhibit fewer and shorter dendritic processes; bar = 100 µm. (Modified from Cancedda et al., 2007). (B) EGFP/KCC2-expressing cells (grey) exhibit, compared to those expressing only EGFP (black), a more hyperpolarized reversal of $GABA_A$-mediated postsynaptic potentials (GPSPs).

currents; and (3) GABA- and glutamate neurons with extensive apical and basal dendrites that generate both GABA and glutamate PSCs. This sequence is also respected in GABAergic interneurons, albeit earlier. The vast majority of interneurons have already fully operative synapses at a time when most pyramidal cells are silent (Ben Ari et al., 2007). Therefore, GABAergic neurons provide the early source of activity in otherwise silent networks.

Giant depolarizing potentials (GDPs), a hallmark of developmental networks

Correlated neuronal activity occurring at late embryonic, early postnatal stages of development represents a hallmark of developmental circuits, well preserved during evolution (Ben-Ari et al., 2007). In the hippocampus, during the first week of postnatal life, the so-called *giant depolarizing potentials* or GDPs (Ben-Ari et al., 1989) constitute a primordial form of synchrony between neurons, preceding more organized forms of activity such as theta and gamma rhythms (Buzsáki & Draguhn, 2004). GDPs are characterized by recurrent membrane depolarizations (lasting several hundred of milliseconds) that give rise to bursts of action potentials, separated by quiescent periods. This network activity, thought to be the *in vitro* counterpart of 'sharp waves' recorded in pups during immobility periods, sleep, and feeding (Leinekugel et al., 2002), is reminiscent of the *tracé discontinu* first described by Dreyfus-Brisac in the electroencephalogram of immature babies and characterized by intermittent bursts separated by periods of virtually complete suppression of activity (Stockard-Pope et al., 1992).

The appearance of GDPs is preceded by a well-defined sequence of events consisting in calcium action potentials followed by spontaneous plateau assemblies (SPAs). SPAs involve small groups of neurons coupled by gap-junctions and consist in non-synaptic membrane oscillations generated by the activation of intrinsic membrane conductances (Crepel et al., 2007). SPAs are modulated by oxytocin, a maternal hormone essential for induction of labor, known to transiently convert GABA action from excitatory to inhibitory during parturition (Tyzio et al., 2006). In addition, SPAs are facilitated by the depolarizing action of GABA, which activates voltage-dependent calcium channels and facilitates the relief of the voltage-dependent magnesium block from NMDA receptors, thus allowing calcium entry and activation of second messengers.

In rodents, GDPs are already present at birth and disappear towards the end of the second postnatal week, in concomitance with the shift of GABA from the depolarizing to the hyperpolarizing direction (Ben-Ari et al., 1989, 2012). GDPs are generated by the activation of both principal cells and interneurons (Bonifazi et al., 2009; Garaschuk et al., 1998; Leinekugel et al., 1997), which, by releasing glutamate and GABA, activate $GABA_A$ and AMPA receptors, respectively. The GABAergic and glutamatergic components of GDPs can be unveiled by holding two neighbouring pyramidal neurons at E_{GABA} (− 70 mV) and E_{AMPA} (0 mV), respectively. With this procedure it appears that the GABAergic component always precedes the glutamatergic one by several milliseconds, suggesting that principal cells are driven by GABAergic interneurons (Cherubini et al., 2011; Mohajerani & Cherubini, 2005). Furthermore, using network dynamics, imaging, online reconstruction of functional connectivity, and targeted whole-cell recordings from immature hippocampal slices, it was recently demonstrated that functional hubs composed of subpopulations of GABAergic interneurons with large axonal arborizations are able to synchronize large ensembles of cells (Fig. 3; Bonifazi et al., 2009).

In analogy with the synchronized activity generated in the disinhibited hippocampus by $GABA_A$ receptor antagonists (De la Prida et al., 2006), it seems likely that GDPs emerge when a sufficient number of cells fire and the excitability of the network attains a certain threshold within a restricted window of time (De la Prida & Sanchez-Andres, 1999). Although the entire hippocampal network possesses the capacity to generate GDPs, for its anatomic characteristics, including extensive glutamatergic connections via recurrent collaterals, the CA3 area is particularly well equipped to generate synchronized oscillations. Furthermore, this area is able to initiate, upon membrane depolarization, intrinsic bursts which, by virtue of their spontaneous discharges and large spike output, can drive other neurons to fire (Safiulina et al., 2008; Sipila et al., 2005). Burst firing is facilitated by a persistent slow sodium current (Sipila et al., 2006) and by a tonic $GABA_A$-mediated conductance generated by the activation of extrasynaptic $GABA_A$ receptors by 'ambient' GABA, accumulated in the extracellular space by spillover from neighbouring synapses or by release from nonconventional release sites (Marchionni et al., 2007). This would bring the membrane to the voltage window for activation of voltage-dependent sodium and calcium channels. Intrinsic bursting activity is boosted by the low expression, of Kv7.2 and Kv7.3 channels responsible for the non-inactivating, low-threshold M current, which in adulthood controls spike after-depolarization and burst generation (Yue & Yaari, 2004). The low density of I_M at birth contributes to produce intrinsic bursts that, in comparison with those observed in adults, are more robust, last longer and recur more regularly (Safiulina et al., 2008).

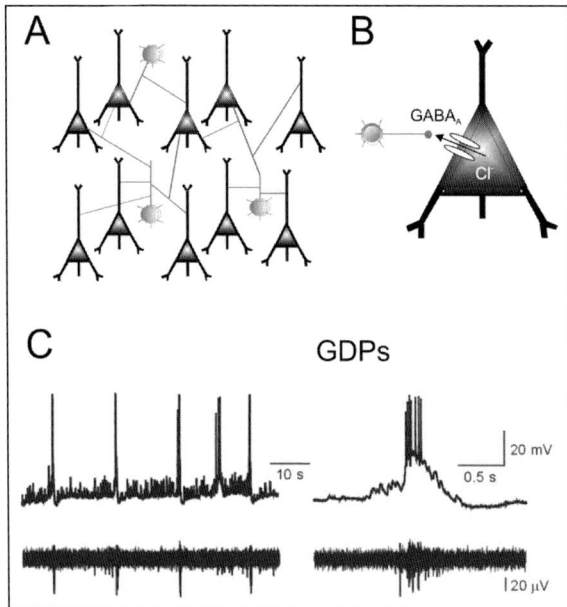

Fig. 3. Giant depolarizing potentials (GDPs) are generated within a local network by the interplay between GABAergic and glutamatergic neurons. (A) Schematic drawing showing interconnected pyramidal cells (triangular shapes) and GABAergic interneurons (circular shapes). (B) GABA, released from GABAergic interneurons, binds and opens $GABA_A$ receptor channels (white), leading to an outwardly directed flux of chloride (arrow), which depolarizes principal cells. (C) Patch clamp (upper trace) and field potentials recordings (lower trace) from an immature CA3 pyramidal cell. On the right, a GDP is shown on an expanded time scale.

Network synchronization may be facilitated by the slow hyperpolarization-activated cation current I_h, carried by HCN channels. The role of I_h on network-driven oscillations was suggested by the observations that extracellular cesium or the selective I_h blocker ZD 7288 (Bender et al., 2005; Strata et al., 1997) were able to disrupt GDPs in principal cells and interneurons, endowed since birth with the HCN1 isoform of HCN channels. However, the role of I_h is not essential, since synchronous oscillations may occur also in neurons lacking HCN channels (Bender et al., 2005). GDPs can be also facilitated by cell-coupling *via* gap junctions, whose expression early in development has been well documented (Rozental et al., 2000). This type of signaling, which plays a crucial role in SPA generation, may persist at later developmental stages when SPAs are replaced by GDPs (Strata et al., 1997).

In previous studies, the hypothesis that GDPs may act as coincidence detectors for enhancing synaptic efficacy in an associative and activity-dependent manner was tested (Kasyanov et al., 2004; Mohajerani et al., 2007). Activity-dependent modifications in synaptic strength such as long-term-potentiation (LTP) or long-term depression (LTD) are critical for information storage in the brain and for the development of neuronal circuits. These processes are particularly important in the developing brain, characterized by an elevated number of 'silent' synapses (Durand et al., 1996). These are synapses that do not conduct at rest because the neurotransmitter is not released when the presynaptic terminal is invaded by an action potential (presynaptically silent) or because they are unable to detect the release of the neurotransmitter due to the lack of the respective receptors on the subsynaptic membrane (postsynaptically silent). Silent synapses can be converted into active ones by activity-dependent processes and this represents the most common mechanism for LTP induction, particularly during development (Voronin & Cherubini, 2004). Using a pairing procedure, consisting in triggering MF stimulation with the rising phase of GDPs, in such a way that calcium transients associated with GDPs occurred simultaneously with MF-evoked GABAergic currents (MF-GPSCs), GDPs were found to act as coincident detector signals for enhancing, in a persistent way, synaptic efficacy at emerging glutamatergic Schaffer collateral-CA1 synapses (Mohajerani et al., 2007) and mossy fiber-CA3 synapses (Kasyanov et al., 2004), which are GABAergic immediately after birth (Safiulina et al., 2006). The pairing protocol was also able to switch presynaptically silent neurons into conductive ones.

In both Schaffer collateral-CA1 and mossy fibers-CA3 synapses, induction of LTP was clearly postsynaptic (dependent on the postsynaptic rise of calcium through GDPs), while its expression was presynaptic, suggesting a retrograde signal. One attractive candidate is BDNF, which can be released in a calcium-dependent way by depolarization of the postsynaptic cell and plays a crucial role in synaptic plasticity. BDNF acts on tropomyosin-related kinase receptor B (TrkB), and this interaction activates different signaling pathways. Indeed, at glutamatergic synapses, BDNF was able to mimic the effects of pairing on synaptic transmission and BDNF scavengers or tropomyosin-related kinase receptor B (TrkB) antagonists were able to block pairing-induced synaptic potentiation. Blocking TrkB receptors in the postsynaptic cell did not prevent the effects of pairing, suggesting that BDNF, possibly secreted from the postsynaptic cell during GDPs, acts on TrkB receptors localized on presynaptic neurons. Pairing-induced synaptic potentiation was blocked by ERK inhibitors, suggesting that BDNF activates the MAPK/ERK cascade, which may lead to transcriptional regulation and new protein synthesis in the postsynaptic neuron. Therefore, BDNF can act not only presynaptically to alter the probability of glutamate release, but also postsynaptically to produce structural modifications necessary for the formation of new synapses.

Overall, these results support the hypothesis that, during a critical period of postnatal development, GDPs act as coincidence detectors to establish the appropriate GABAergic and glutamatergic connections necessary for the construction of the adult neuronal circuit.

Is synaptic transmission unidirectional?

In contrast to electrical synapses, which conduct information in both directions, chemical synapses are considered unidirectional. According to the classical view, an action potential travelling along the axon invades the presynaptic terminal and induces calcium entry through voltage-dependent calcium channels, thus increasing the intracellular calcium concentration. Calcium binds to presynaptic calcium sensors and causes exocytosis of synaptic vesicles and neurotransmitter release. Once released, the neurotransmitter diffuses across the synaptic cleft and binds to postsynaptic receptors leading to channel opening. In this way, a voltage change in the presynaptic neuron is converted into a chemical signal in the postsynaptic one. However, to be highly efficient, synaptic transmission needs the coordinated activity of pre- and postsynaptic elements. In particular, the postsynaptic cell should exert a backward control on presynaptic signaling. This may occur *via* retrograde messengers or specialized adhesion molecules such as neuroligins (NLGs) and neurexins (NRXs), which, by bridging the cleft, provide a direct link between the pre- and the postsynaptic sites (Lisé & El-Husseini, 2006). NLGs, which are localized postsynaptically, bind to NRXs, which are localized presynaptically. The NLG–NRX complexes possess a potent 'synaptogenic' activity, as demonstrated by their ability, when expressed in heterologous non-neuronal cells, to induce presynaptic differentiation of contacting neuritis (Fu et al., 2003; Graf et al., 2004; Sara et al., 2005; Scheiffele et al., 2000). Postsynaptic NLGs promote the assembly of functional presynaptic specializations in axons, while presynaptic NRXs recruit postsynaptic scaffolding proteins and neurotransmitter receptors in dendrites *via* their interaction with NLGs (Huang & Scheiffele, 2008). By functionally coupling synaptic calcium channels with the release machinery, NRXs play an essential role in calcium-triggered neurotransmitter release (Missler *et al.*, 2003).

The NLG family comprises five different molecules, NLG1–NLG5, with various splice variants (encoded by five different genes), which form homodimers through the extracellular domain. Among these, NLG2 is preferentially associated with GABAergic synapses, while NLG1 is associated with glutamatergic synapses (Song *et al.*, 1999; Varoqueaux *et al.*, 2004). NLG3 is associated with both excitatory and inhibitory synapses (Budreck & Scheiffele, 2007). The NRX family includes α-NRX and β-NRX. Initially, α-NRXN was considered the main partner for NLGs, but recently α-NRX was also found to bind NLGs (Boucard *et al.*, 2005). Unlike β-NRX, which participates in the formation of both glutamatergic and GABAergic synapses, α-NRX seems to be specific for GABAergic synapses (Kang *et al.*, 2008). Therefore, it is clear that within a neuronal network, the NLG–NRX interaction controls the formation of both glutamatergic and GABAergic synapses (Craig & Kang, 2007).

At inhibitory synapses, $GABA_A$ receptors are first assembled in the endoplasmic reticulum from appropriate subunits and then delivered to the plasma membrane. Targeting and clustering $GABA_A$ receptors at synaptic and extrasynaptic sites is dynamically regulated by neuronal activity (Hanus *et al.*, 2006) and requires the precise interplay of various proteins and active transport processes along the cytoskeleton (Kneussel & Loebrich, 2007; Tretter *et al.*, 2008). In a recent study it was demonstrated that disrupting gephyrin function with selective recombinant antibodies led to a reduction of $GABA_A$ receptor clusters, an effect that was associated with a decrease in the density and size of NLG2 clusters and with a loss of GABAergic innervation (Varley *et al.*, 2011). Pair recordings from interconnected cells demonstrated that, with respect to controls, neurons transfected with recombinant antibodies against gephyrin, exhibited a lower probability of GABA release. This reduction involved NLG2 since it was possible, in gephyrin-deprived neurons, to rescue this effect by over-expressing NLG2, known to directly bind gephyrin through a conserved cytoplasmatic domain (Poulopoulos *et al.*, 2009; Varley *et al.*, 2011). Similarly, at glutamatergic synapses, the NLG–NRX complex has been shown to act as a coordinator between postsynaptic and presynaptic sites (Futai *et al.*, 2007). Hence, over-expressing the glutamatergic scaffold protein PSD-95 on the postsynaptic site enhanced the probability of glutamate release *via* a retrograde modulation of neurotransmitter release through the NLG–NRX complex.

From these studies it is clear how a dysfunction of synaptic proteins such as those belonging to the NLG–NRX families affects transynaptic signaling and severely alters the structural architecture of the synapses, resulting, at the network level, in a serious imbalance between excitation and inhibition (Fig. 4).

Therefore, it is not surprising that single mutations in genes encoding for adhesion molecules belonging to the NLG–NRX families have been found in some subjects with idiopathic forms of ASD (Südhof, 2008).

GABAergic dysfunction in autism spectrum disorders

ASD comprises a variety of neurodevelopmental disorders including the Fragile X, Rett, Asperger, Angelman or Prader-Willi syndromes as well as 'not otherwise specified' cases, showing many but not all the symptoms required for the diagnosis of autism (American

Chapter 7 GABA in early development of neuronal circuits

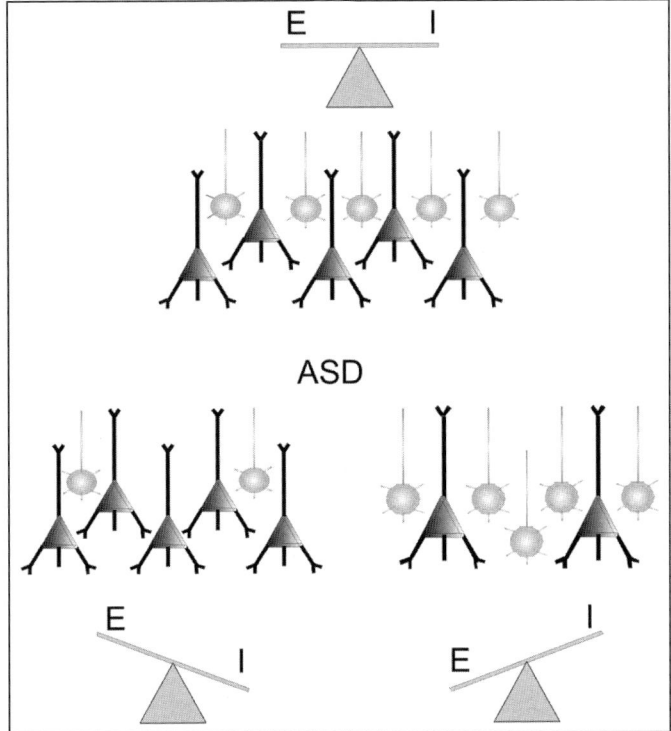

Fig. 4. A proper balance between excitation and inhibition is essential for the correct operation of neuronal networks. ASD may be associated with an increase of excitation (left) or inhibition (right). Excitatory neurons are triangle-shaped; inhibitory neurons are circular in shape.

Psychiatric Association, 2000). Although these disorders have a different aetiology, they share overlapping symptoms, suggesting a common deficit in some neurodevelopmental pathways. Among these, an impairment of the GABAergic function, seems to play a major role, as demonstrated by the high percentage of co-morbidity (~30 per cent) with epilepsy.

Evidence has been provided that many cases of ASD are caused by submicroscopic abnormalities known as 'copy-number variations' (CNVs) consisting in micro-deletions or micro-duplications. Interestingly, the most common chromosomal loci where CNVs have been found are 15q11–q13, which contains a number of genes coding for $GABA_A$ receptor subunits (Coghlan et al., 2012). This locus can be affected either directly by single point mutations or indirectly by epigenetic factors. Alterations may occur also up or downstream to $GABA_A$ receptor activation in genes encoding for scaffolding, adhesion, and signaling proteins, necessary for the proper function of GABAergic transmission. This may lead to the loss of GABAergic receptors, of some particular subtype of GABAergic interneuron, or to the inability of GABAergic interneurons to integrate local circuits and undergo activity-dependent plasticity processes.

Post-mortem studies from autistic patients have revealed alterations of glutamic acid decarboxylase (GAD_{65} and GAD_{67}), enzymes that catalyze the decarboxylation of glutamate to GABA, in the cerebellum and in the parietal cortex (Fatemi et al., 2002). In addition, changes in the vesicular GABA transporter (VGAT), of $GABA_A$ and $GABA_B$ receptors and a decreased expression of PV+ GABAergic interneurons have been reported (Lawrence et al., 2010).

A recent *in vivo* study using single photon emission computed tomography (SPECT) in ASD patients has demonstrated a reduced $GABA_A$–benzodiazepine ligand, liomazenil, suggesting a reduced expression of $GABA_A$ receptors (Mori et al., 2011).

New insights into the mechanisms of ASD come from animal studies in which gene-targeting introduction in mice of single gene mutations found in affected children have allowed linking cellular and network dysfunctions of particular brain areas with behaviour. The majority of animal models, so far examined, shows a loss of GABAergic function, involving phasic and sometimes tonic $GABA_A$-mediated conductances. Thus, relevant inhibitory synaptic abnormalities have been found in animal models of the Fragile X syndrome (*Fmr1* gene), tuberous sclerosis (*Tsc1* and *Tsc2* genes), and the Angelman (*Ube3a* gene) and Rett syndromes (*Mecp2* gene). They have been also detected in transgenic mice carrying mutations in homeobox genes *Dlx1* and *Dlx2*, involved in the development of most telencephalic GABAergic neurons or in the *Gabrb3* gene, encoding for the β3 subunit of $GABA_A$ receptors (highly expressed during brain development). Perturbations of GABAergic signals have been also found in pups from mothers chronically treated with valproic acid (VPA). This animal model has been developed on the basis of the observation that treatment of epilepsy or bipolar disorders in pregnant women with VPA, a histone deacetylase inhibitor, leads to an increased incidence of children with ASD (for a more detailed description of different animal models, see Pizzarelli & Cherubini, 2011).

It is worth noting that in a few cases GABAergic alterations lead to a gain of function, as in mice carrying the human R415C mutation of the *Nlgn3* gene. Single point mutations in *Nlgn3* and *Nlgn4* genes were among the first to be identified as causes of ASD. A missense mutation causing R451C substitution within a highly conserved region of *Nlgn3* gene was detected in two siblings: one with autism and the other with Asperger's syndrome. The first identified mutation in the *Nlgn4* gene occurred in a male with autism and in his brother with the Asperger syndrome. In both families, the mother was a carrier but did not manifest any phenotype as in many cases of X-linked disorders (Jamain et al., 2003; Laumonnier et al., 2004). $NLG3^{R451C}$ knock-in mice bear a striking phenotype which mimics in many aspects that found in ASD patients (Tabuchi et al., 2007). Functional characterization of these mice has revealed (in contrast with NLG3 knock-out mice) a loss of NLG3 in the forebrain associated with impaired social interactions and a 50 per cent increase in the frequency of spontaneous inhibitory events with apparently no effects on excitatory synaptic transmission. Of interest, in these mice, the gain of function was associated with a significant increase in the level of the vesicular transporter for GABA, VGAT, and gephyrin, the postsynaptic scaffolding protein. Moreover, these animals exhibited an asymmetric reduction of PV+ basket cells across the two hemispheres (Gogolla et al., 2009). These interneurons play an important role in the generation of high-frequency oscillations because of their fast-spiking characteristics and the short time constants of their synaptic interactions (Bartos et al., 2007). By *in vivo* inhibition of PV+ basket cells, γ-oscillations, thought to be associated with high cognitive functions, are suppressed (Sohal et al., 2009).

It is clear from the data reviewed here that a dysfunction of GABAergic transmission early in development may severely affect the E/I balance and the functionality of neuronal circuits, leading in some cases to ASD (Fig. 4). This may impair the connectivity between different brain regions, weakening their specialized functions. Interestingly, during brain maturation, disorders of the E/I balance may occur not only when the formation or maintenance of one class of synapses prevails over the others, but also when the shift in GABA action is altered or delayed beyond a critical period.

Concluding remarks

From the data reported here, it is clear that GABA is one of the major players in orchestrating the construction and refinement of neuronal circuits in the immature brain. A dysfunction of GABAergic signaling may contribute to the neurologic impairment found in several neuropsychiatric disorders, including ASDs. Although the causes of ASDs are multiple and still largely unknown, it is clear that a better understanding of the maturational processes by which GABAergic neurotransmission influences neuronal migration, differentiation, and synapse and circuit formation will allow identifying novel targets for therapeutic interventions. In this respect, it is worth mentioning that clinical trials for drugs that counter the E/I imbalance by selectively targeting glutamate and GABA pathways are now underway. In particular, selective GABA agonists have been shown to lessen clinical symptoms in a group of children affected by the Fragile X syndrome and idiopathic forms of ASD (Oberman, 2012). Furthermore, by reducing the intracellular chloride concentration and the excitatory drive of GABA, with chronic administration of bumetanide, a selective blocker of the cation–chloride importer NKCC1 (Dzhala *et al.*, 2008) has been shown to dramatically ameliorate the autistic behaviour in randomly selected autistic children with almost no side effects (Lemonnier & Ben-Ari, 2010; Lemonnier *et al.*, 2012). Although the mechanisms by which bumetanide acts are not clear, we cannot exclude the possibility that in some particular circumstances, pharmacologic manipulations might reactivate, as in the visual cortex (Castrén *et al.*, 2012), critical period-like plasticity. However, larger multicentre trials and more studies are warranted to better determine the population that will benefit from these novel therapeutic approaches as well as the underlying mechanisms of disorder.

Acknowledgments: This study was supported by Telethon (GGP11043) and by a grant from *Ministero Università e Ricerca* (PRIN 2012) to E.C.

Conflicts of interest: The authors declare no conflicts of interest.

References

American Psychiatric Association (2000): *Diagnostic and Statistical Manual of Mental Disorders* (DMS-IV-TR), Washington, DC: APA.

Bartos, M., Vida, I. & Jonas, P. (2007): Synaptic mechanisms of synchronized gamma oscillations in inhibitory interneuron networks. *Nat. Rev. Neurosci.* **8**, 45–56.

Ben-Ari, Y., Cherubini, E., Corradetti, R. & Gaiarsa, J.L. (1989): Giant synaptic potentials in immature rat CA3 hippocampal neurons. *J. Physiol. (Lond.)* **416**, 303–325.

Ben-Ari, Y., Khazipov, R., Leinekugel, X., Caillard, O. & Gaiarsa, J.L. (1997): GABAA, NMDA and AMPA receptors: a developmentally regulated 'ménage à trois'. *Trends Neurosci.* **20**, 523–529.

Ben-Ari, Y., Gaiarsa, J.L., Tyzio, R. & Khazipov, R. (2007): GABA: a pioneer transmitter that excites immature neurons and generates primitive oscillations. *Physiol. Rev.* **87**, 1215–1284.

Bender, R.A., Galindo, R., Mameli, M., Gonzalez-Vega, R., Valenzuela, C.F. & Baram, T.Z. (2005): Synchronized network activity in developing rat hippocampus involves regional hyperpolarization-activated cyclic nucleotide-gated (HCN) channel function. *Eur. J. Neurosci.* **22**, 2669–2674.

Bettler, B., Kaupmann, K., Mosbacher, J. & Gassmann, M. (2004): Molecular structure and physiological functions of GABA(B) receptors. *Physiol. Rev.* **84**, 835–867.

Bonifazi, P., Goldin, M., Picardo, M.A., *et al.* (2009): GABAergic hub neurons orchestrate synchrony in developing hippocampal networks. *Science* **326**, 1419–1424.

Boucard, A.A., Chubykin, A.A., Comoletti, D., Taylor, P. & Südhof, T.C. (2005): A splice code for trans-synaptic cell adhesion mediated by binding of neuroligin 1 to alpha- and beta-neurexins. *Neuron* **48**, 229–236.

Budreck, E.C. & Scheiffele, P. (2007): Neuroligin-3 is a neuronal adhesion protein at GABAergic and glutamatergic synapses. *Eur. J. Neurosci.* **26**, 1738–1748.

Buzsaki, G. & Draguhn, A. (2004): Neuronal oscillations in cortical networks. *Science* **304**, 1926–1929.

Cancedda, L., Fiumelli, H., Chen, K. & Poo, M.M. (2007): Excitatory GABA action is essential for morphological maturation of cortical neurons *in vivo*. *J. Neurosci.* **27**, 5224–5235.

Castrén, E., Elgersma, Y., Maffei, L. & Hagerman, R (2012): Treatment of neurodevelopmental disorders in adulthood. *J. Neurosci.* **32**, 14074–14079.

Cherubini, E. & Conti, F. (2001): Generating diversity at GABAergic synapses. *Trends Neurosci.* **24**, 155–162.

Cherubini, E., Griguoli, M., Safiulina, V. & Lagostena, L. (2011): The depolarizing action of GABA controls early network activity in the developing hippocampus. *Mol. Neurobiol.* **43**, 97–106.

Coghlan, S., Horder, J., Inkster, B., Mendez, M.A., Murphy, D.G. & Nutt, D.J. (2012): GABA system dysfunction in autism and related disorders: from synapse to symptoms. *Neurosci. Biobehav. Rev.* **36**, 2044–2055.

Craig, A.M. & Kang, Y. (2007): Neurexin-neuroligin signaling in synapse development. *Curr. Opin. Neurobiol.* **17**, 43–52.

Crepel, V., Aronov, D., Jorquera, I., Represa, A., Ben-Ari, Y. & Cossart, R. (2007): A parturition-associated nonsynaptic coherent activity pattern in the developing hippocampus. *Neuron* **54**, 105–120.

De la Prida, L.M. & Sanchez-Andres, J.V. (1999): Nonlinear transfer function encodes synchronization in a neural network from the mammalian brain. *Phys. Rev.* **60**, 3239–3243.

De la Prida, L.M., Huberfeld, G., Cohen, I. & Miles, R. (2006): Threshold behavior in the initiation of hippocampal population bursts. *Neuron* **49**, 131–142.

Demarque, M., Represa, A., Becq, H., Khalilov, I., Ben-Ari, Y. & Aniksztejn, L. (2002): Paracrine intercellular communication by a Ca2+- and SNARE-independent release of GABA and glutamate prior to synapse formation. *Neuron* **36**, 1051–1061.

Durand, G.M., Kovalchuk, Y. & Konnerth, A. (1996): Long-term potentiation and functional synapse induction in developing hippocampus. *Nature* **381**, 71–75.

Dzhala, V.I., Brumback, A.C. & Staley, K.J. (2008): Bumetanide enhances phenobarbital efficacy in a neonatal seizure model. *Ann. Neurol.* **63**, 222–235.

Fatemi, S.H., Halt, A.R., Stary, J.M., Kanodia, R., Schulz, S.C. & Realmuto, G.R. (2002): Glutamic acid decarboxylase 65 and 67 kDa proteins are reduced in autistic parietal and cerebellar cortices. *Biol. Psychiatry* **52**, 805–810.

Faux, C., Rakic, S., Andrews, W. & Britto, J.M. (2012): Neurons on the move: migration and lamination of cortical interneurons. *Neurosignals* **20**, 168–189.

Fu, Z., Washbourne, P., Ortinski, P. & Vicini, S. (2003): Functional excitatory synapses in HEK293 cells expressing neuroligin and glutamate receptors. *J. Neurophysiol.* **90**, 3950–3957.

Futai, K., Kim, M.J., Hashikawa, T., Scheiffele, P., Sheng, M. & Hayashi, Y. (2007): Retrograde modulation of presynaptic release probability through signaling mediated by PSD-95-neuroligin. *Nat. Neurosci.* **10**, 186–195.

Garaschuk, O., Hanse, E. & Konnerth, A. (1998): Developmental profile and synaptic origin of early network oscillations in the CA1 region of rat neonatal hippocampus. *J. Physiol. (Lond.)* **507**, 219–236.

Garber, K. (2007): Autism's cause may reside in abnormalities at the synapse. *Science* **317**, 190–191.

Geschwind, D.H. & Levitt, P. (2007): Autism spectrum disorders: developmental disconnection syndromes. *Curr. Opin. Neurobiol.* **17**, 103–111.

Gogolla, N., Leblanc, J.J., Quast, K.B., Südhof, T.C., Fagiolini, M. & Hensch, T.K. (2009): Common circuit defect of excitatory-inhibitory balance in mouse models of autism. *J. Neurodev. Disord.* **1**, 172–181.

Graf, E.R., Zhang, X., Jin, S.X., Linhoff, M.W. & Craig, A.M. (2004): Neurexins induce differentiation of GABA and glutamate postsynaptic specializations via neuroligins. *Cell* **119**, 1013–1026.

Hanus, C., Ehrensperger, M.V. & Triller, A. (2006): Activity-dependent movements of postsynaptic scaffolds at inhibitory synapses. *J. Neurosci.* **26**, 4586–4595.

Hosokawa, Y., Sciancalepore, M., Stratta, F., Martina, M. & Cherubini, E. (1994): Developmental changes in spontaneous $GABA_A$-mediated synaptic events in rat hippocampal CA3 neurons. *Eur. J. Neurosci.* **6**, 805–813.

Huang, Z.J. & Scheiffele, P. (2008): GABA and neuroligin signaling: linking synaptic activity and adhesion in inhibitory synapse development. *Curr. Opin. Neurobiol.* **18**, 77–83.

Jamain, S., Quach, H., Betancur, C., et al. & Paris Autism Research International Sibpair Study (2003): Mutations of the X-linked genes encoding neuroligins NLGN3 and NLGN4 are associated with autism. *Nat. Genet.* **34**, 27–29.

Kang, Y., Zhang, X., Dobie, F., Wu, H. & Craig, A.M. (2008): Induction of GABAergic postsynaptic differentiation by alpha-neurexins. *J. Biol. Chem.* **283**, 2323–2334.

Kasyanov, A.M., Safiulina, V.F., Voronin, L.L. & Cherubini, E. (2004): GABA-mediated giant depolarizing potentials as coincidence detectors for enhancing synaptic efficacy in the developing hippocampus. *Proc. Natl. Acad. Sci. USA* **101**, 3967–3972.

Khazipov, R., Esclapez, M., Caillard, O., *et al.* (2001): Early development of neuronal activity in the primate hippocampus in utero. *J. Neurosci.* **21**, 9770–9781.

Kneussel, M. & Loebrich, S. (2007): Trafficking and synaptic anchoring of ionotropic inhibitory neurotransmitter receptors. *Biol. Cell* **99**, 297–309.

Komuro, H. & Rakic, P. (1998): Orchestration of neuronal migration by activity of ion channels, neurotransmitter receptors, and intracellular Ca2+ fluctuations. *J. Neurobiol.* **37**, 110–130.

Laumonnier, F., Bonnet-Brilhault, F., Gomot, M., *et al.* (2004): X-linked mental retardation and autism are associated with a mutation in the *NLGN4* gene, a member of the neuroligin family. *Am. J. Hum. Genet.* **74**, 552–557.

Lawrence, Y.A., Kemper, T.L., Bauman, M.L. & Blatt, G.J. (2010): Parvalbumin-, calbindin- and calretinin-immunoreactive hippocampal interneuron density in autism. *Acta Neurol. Scand.* **121**, 99–108.

Leinekugel, X., Medina, I., Khalilov, I., Ben-Ari, Y. & Khazipov, R. (1997): Ca2+ oscillations mediated by the synergistic excitatory actions of GABA(A) and NMDA receptors in the neonatal hippocampus. *Neuron* **18**, 243–255.

Leinekugel, X., Khazipov, R., Cannon, R., Hirase, H., Ben-Ari, Y. & Buzsáki, G. (2002): Correlated bursts of activity in the neonatal hippocampus *in vivo*. *Science* **296**, 2049–2052.

Lemonnier, E. & Ben-Ari, Y. (2010): The diuretic bumetanide decreases autistic behaviour in five infants treated during 3 months with no side effects. *Acta Paediatr.* **99**, 1885–1888.

Lemonnier, E., Degrez, C., Phelep, M., *et al.* (2012): A randomized controlled trial of bumetanide in the treatment of autism in children. *Trans Psychiatry* **2**, e202; doi:10.1038/tp.2012.124 [E-pub 11 December 2012].

Lisé, M.F. & El-Husseini, A. (2006): The neuroligin and neurexin families: from structure to function at the synapse. *Cell Mol. Life Sci.* **63**, 1833–1849.

LoTurco, J.J., Owens, D.F., Heath, M.J., Davis, M.B., & Kriegstein, A.R. (1995): GABA and glutamate depolarize cortical progenitor cells and inhibit DNA synthesis. *Neuron* **15**, 1287–1298.

Luscher, C., Jan, L.Y., Stoffel, M., Malenka, R.C. & Nicoll, R.A. (1997): G protein-coupled inwardly rectifying K+ channels (GIRKs) mediate postsynaptic but not presynaptic transmitter actions in hippocampal neurons. *Neuron* **19**, 687–695.

Manent, J.B., Jorquera, I., Ben-Ari, Y., Aniksztejn, L. & Represa, A. (2006): Glutamate acting on AMPA but not NMDA receptors modulates the migration of hippocampal interneurons. *J. Neurosci.* **26**, 5901–5909.

Marchionni, I., Omrani, A. & Cherubini, E. (2007): In the developing rat hippocampus a tonic GABA(A)-mediated conductance selectively enhances the glutamatergic drive of principal cells. *J. Physiol. (Lond.)* **581**, 515–528.

Missler, M., Zhang, W., Rohlmann, A., *et al.* (2003): α-Neurexins couple Ca2+ channels to synaptic vesicle exocytosis. *Nature* **423**, 939–948.

Mohajerani, M.H. & Cherubini, E. (2005): Spontaneous recurrent network activity in organotypic rat hippocampal slices. *Eur. J. Neurosci.* **22**, 107–118.

Mohajerani, M.H., Sivakumaran, S., Zacchi, P., Aguilera, P. & Cherubini, E. (2007): Correlated network activity enhances synaptic efficacy via BDNF and the ERK pathway at immature CA3 CA1 connections in the hippocampus. *Proc. Natl. Acad. Sci. USA* **104**, 13176–13181.

Mori, T., Mori, K., Fujii, E., *et al.* (2011): Evaluation of the GABAergic nervous system in autistic brain: (123)I-iomazenil SPECT study. *Brain Dev.* **34**, 648–654.

Oberman, L.M. (2012): mGluR antagonists and GABA agonists as novel pharmacological agents for the treatment of autism spectrum disorders. *Exp. Opin. Invest.* **21**, 1819–1825.

Owens, D.F., Boyce, L.H., Davis, M.B. & Kriegstein, A.R. (1996): Excitatory GABA responses in embryonic and neonatal cortical slices demonstrated by gramicidin perforated-patch recordings and calcium imaging. *J. Neurosci.* **16**, 6414–6423.

Owens, D.F., Liu, X. & Kriegstein, A.R. (1999): Changing properties of GABA(A) receptor-mediated signaling during early neocortical development. *J. Neurophysiol.* **82**, 570–583.

Persico, A.M. & Bourgeron, T. (2006): Searching for ways out of the autism maze: genetic, epigenetic and environmental clues. *Trends Neurosci.* **29**, 349–358.

Pizzarelli, R. & Cherubini, E. (2011): Alterations of GABAergic signaling in autism spectrum disorders. *Neural Plast.* 297153 [E-pub 23 Jun 2011].

Poulopoulos, A., Aramuni, G., Meyer, G., *et al.* (2009): Neuroligin 2 drives postsynaptic assembly at perisomatic inhibitory synapses through gephyrin and collybistin. *Neuron* **63**, 628–642.

Rozental, R., Srinivas, M., Gökhan, S., et al. (2000): Temporal expression of neuronal connexins during hippocampal ontogeny. *Brain Res. Brain Res. Rev.* **32**, 57–71.

Rutter, M. (2005): Incidence of autism spectrum disorders: changes over time and their meaning. *Acta Paediatr.* **94**, 2–15.

Safiulina, V.F., Fattorini, G., Conti, F. & Cherubini, E. (2006): GABAergic signaling at mossy fiber synapses in neonatal rat hippocampus. *J. Neurosci.* **26**, 597–608.

Safiulina, V.F., Zacchi, P., Taglialatela, M., Yaari, Y. & Cherubini, E. (2008): Low expression of Kv7/M channels facilitates intrinsic and network bursting in the developing rat hippocampus. *J. Physiol.* **586**, 5437–5453.

Sara, Y., Biederer, T., Atasoy, D., et al. (2005): Selective capability of SynCAM and neuroligin for functional synapse assembly. *J. Neurosci.* **25**, 260–270.

Scheiffele, P., Fan, J., Choih, J., Fetter, R. & Serafini, T. (2000): Neuroligin expressed in nonneuronal cells triggers presynaptic development in contacting axons. *Cell* **101**, 657–669.

Sipila, S.T., Huttu, K., Soltesz, I., Voipio, J. & Kaila, K. (2005): Depolarizing GABA acts on intrinsically bursting pyramidal neurons to drive giant depolarizing potentials in the immature hippocampus. *J. Neurosci.* **25**, 5280–5289.

Sipila, S.T., Huttu, K., Voipio, J. & Kaila, K. (2006): Intrinsic bursting of immature CA3 pyramidal neurons and consequent giant depolarizing potentials are driven by a persistent Na current and terminated by a slow Ca-activated K current. *Eur. J. Neurosci.* **23**, 2330–2338.

Sohal, V.S., Zhang, F., Yizhar, O. & Deisseroth, K. (2009): Parvalbumin neurons and gamma rhythms enhance cortical circuit performance. *Nature* **459**, 698–702.

Song, J.Y., Ichtchenko, K., Südhof, T.C. & Brose, N. (1999): Neuroligin 1 is a postsynaptic cell-adhesion molecule of excitatory synapses. *Proc. Natl. Acad. Sci. USA* **96**, 1100–1105.

Spitzer, N.C. (2002): Activity-dependent neuronal differentiation prior to synapse formation: the functions of calcium transients. *J. Physiol. (Paris)* **96**, 73–80.

Stockard-Pope, J., Werner, S.S. & Bickford, R.G. (1992): *Atlas of Neonatal Electroencephalography.* New York: Raven Press.

Strata, F., Atzori, M., Molnar, M., Ugolini, G., Tempia, F. & Cherubini, E. (1997): A pacemaker current in dye-coupled hilar interneurons contributes to the generation of giant GABAergic potentials in developing hippocampus. *J. Neurosci.* **17**, 1435–1446.

Südhof, T.C. (2008): Neuroligins and neurexins link synaptic function to cognitive disease. *Nature* **455**, 903–911.

Tabuchi, K., Blundell, J., Etherton, et al. (2007): A neuroligin-3 mutation implicated in autism increases inhibitory synaptic transmission in mice. *Science* **318**, 71–76.

Tretter, V., Jacob, T.C., Mukherjee, J., Fritschy, J.M., Pangalos, M.N. & Moss, S.J. (2008): The clustering of GABA(A) receptor subtypes at inhibitory synapses is facilitated via the direct binding of receptor alpha 2 subunits to gephyrin. *J. Neurosci.* **28**, 1356–1365.

Tyzio, R., Represa, A., Jorquera, I., Ben-Ari, Y., Gozlan, H. & Aniksztejn, L. (1999): The establishment of GABAergic and glutamatergic synapses on CA1 pyramidal neurons is sequential and correlates with the development of the apical dendrite. *J. Neurosci.* **19**, 10372–10382.

Tyzio, R., Cossart, R., Khalilov, I., et al. (2006): Maternal oxytocin triggers a transient inhibitory switch in GABA signaling in the fetal brain during delivery. *Science* **314**, 1788–1792.

Valeeva, G., Abdullin, A., Tyzio, R., et al. (2010): Temporal coding at the immature depolarizing GABAergic synapse. *Front. Cell. Neurosci.* **4**, 17 (E-pub 14 Jul 2010).

Varley, Z.K., Pizzarelli, R., Antonelli, R., et al. (2011): Gephyrin regulates GABAergic and glutamatergic synaptic transmission in hippocampal cell cultures. *J. Biol. Chem.* **286**, 20942–20951.

Varoqueaux, F., Jamain, S. & Brose, N. (2004): Neuroligin 2 is exclusively localized to inhibitory synapses. *Eur. J. Cell Biol.* **83**, 449–456.

Voronin, L.L. & Cherubini, E. (2004): 'Deaf, mute and whispering' silent synapses: their role in synaptic plasticity. *J. Physiol.* **557**, 3–12.

Wang, D.D. & Kriegstein, A.R. (2009): Defining the role of GABA in cortical development. *J. Physiol.* **587**, 1873–1879.

Wang, D.D. & Kriegstein, A.R. (2010): Blocking early GABA depolarization with bumetanide results in permanent alterations in cortical circuits and sensorimotor gating deficits. *Cereb. Cortex* **21**, 574–587.

Yue, C. & Yaari, Y. (2004): KCNQ/M channels control spike afterdepolarization and burst generation in hippocampal neurons. *J. Neurosci.* **24**, 4614–4624.

Yuste, R. & Katz, L.C. (1991): Control of postsynaptic Ca2+ influx in developing neocortex by excitatory and inhibitory neurotransmitters. *Neuron* **6**, 333–644.

Chapter 8

The role of the immune response in autism spectrum disorders

Paul Ashwood and Milo Careaga

Department of Medical Microbiology and Immunology and the M.I.N.D. Institute, University of California at Davis, 2825 50th Street, Sacramento, California 95817, USA
pashwood@ucdavis.edu

Summary

Autism spectrum disorders (ASDs) are complex and heterogeneous with a spectrum of diverse symptoms and co-morbidities. Twenty years ago ASD was rare, with fewer than 1 in 1,000 children reported with the disorder. Current estimates, however, suggest that ASD affects approximately 1 per cent of all children, boys being more likely to be affected than girls. Despite decades of research, little is known about the factors that contribute to the pathogenesis of ASD, although both genetic and environmental factors have been implicated. A growing number of reports have linked ASD with immune dysfunction. A number of published findings have identified numerous immune abnormalities in subjects with ASD and their families, both at the systemic and cellular levels. These reports include altered immunogenetics, brain and CNS inflammation, systemic immune abnormalities, and animal models that show immune responses can cause 'autistic like' features. Collectively these findings point to a pivotal role for aberrant immune responses in the pathogenesis of ASD. A better understanding of how immune response can alter early brain development and how this is altered in ASD will have important mechanistic and therapeutic implications.

Introduction

The immune system is a complex and highly developed collection of cells, tissues, and molecules that combine to prevent and/or eradicate infections. The role of the immune response is important to provide protection to the host from the myriad of pathogens to which an individual can be exposed. For many years, because of the blood–brain barrier, the brain was considered to be 'immune restricted' or 'immune privileged' and largely separated from immune cells in the blood. The prevailing concept was that immune cells within the brain were a detrimental event linked with inflammation and either disease states such as multiple sclerosis or as a result of infection. However, over the last decade new data have emerged that suggest that there is extensive communication between cells of the immune and nervous systems and that immune cells play an important role in supporting and maintaining the health of the brain. In addition, immune tissue is highly innervated with 'hardwiring' of sympathetic and parasympathetic nerves. Bidirectional cross-communication mediated by signal molecules exists between the nervous and the immune systems. Neurons, microglia, and astrocytes produce immune molecules such as cytokines and have receptors to immune mediators that enable them to direct immune cells and respond to immunologic stimuli. Similarly, cells of the immune system secrete neurotransmitters and express their receptors and therefore can either influence neural processes or respond to neural stimuli. Products of immune cell activation have known effects on many behaviours including cognition, mood, appetite, and sleep. Activation of the immune response could potentially alter or modulate function of the peripheral nervous system, the central nervous system (CNS), or the expression of cellular messengers at the blood–brain barrier, and thus entry of immune cells into the brain may not be required. Finally, the immune and nervous systems have many similarities through shared molecules and receptors and shared transcriptional factors as both form synapses between cells that are structurally similar; they share guidance cues such as semaphorins, and, from a philosophical viewpoint, they are the only two systems in the body to be able to create memory or distinguish self from non-self.

Although, the aetiology of ASD has remained a mystery since Leo Kanner first described the syndrome in 1943 (Kanner, 1968), various immune system abnormalities have been reported in children and adults with ASD by a number of different laboratories around the world. Both autoimmunity and reduced immune function have been described in ASD. Additionally, a number of animal models with behaviours relevant to ASD have recently been developed with an immune basis. Overall the evidence for immune dysfunction in ASD highlights four areas: (1) immunogenetics; (2) brain and CNS inflammation; (3) skewing of systemic immune responses; and (4) immune activation in animal models that generates 'autistic-like' phenotypes. These four areas will be topics for discussion in the remainder of the chapter.

Immunogenetics in ASD

As early as 1971, a relationship between ASD and immune dysfunction or autoimmune diseases has been reported (Money *et al.*, 1971). Several epidemiologic studies have sought to determine whether a familial link exists between ASD and immune dysfunction. A number of immune disorders and autoimmune diseases have been repeatedly reported in families of subjects with ASD: these include asthma and allergy, coeliac disease, type-1 diabetes, autoimmune thyroid disease, rheumatoid arthritis, and rheumatic fever (Atladottir *et al.*, 2009; Valicenti-McDermott *et al.*, 2008). Together these studies point to abnormal immune function in the families of children with ASD, suggesting a probable role for immune dysfunction in the pathology of ASD. Many of the studies showed increased rates of immune dysfunction in both mothers and fathers of children with ASD (Atladottir *et al.*, 2009; Comi *et al.*, 1999; Keil *et al.*, 2010; Molloy *et al.*, 2006; Sweeten *et al.*, 2003a) and imply that immune dysfunction in parents may be related to shared genetic or physiologic pathways.

Many gene polymorphisms have been implicated in the development of ASD, with a number associated with the control of immune function. Among these, *HLA* genes have been implicated frequently (Daniels *et al.*, 1995; Lee *et al.*, 2006; Stubbs & Magenis, 1980; Torres *et al.*, 2002; Warren *et al.*, 1992). The *HLA* genes are located within a large genomic region found on chromosome 6 known as the major histocompatibility complex (MHC). The *HLA* genes are among the strongest predictors of risk for autoimmune conditions, and are associated with other neurodevelopmental disorders such as schizophrenia (Fernando *et al.*, 2008). A number of HLA haplotypes, in particular HLA-DR4, occur more often in children with ASD compared to the general population (Daniels *et al.*, 1995; Lee *et al.*, 2006; Torres *et al.*, 2002; Warren *et al.*, 1992). A study by Guerini *et al.* (2009) shows several microsatellite linkages within the MHC that are associated with ASD. This suggests that genetic abnormalities in the MHC are likely present in *HLA* genes or other genes in this genomic region consisting of a number of immune-related genes. For example, another gene associated with ASD in the MHC region codes for the complement protein C4. Complement is an important element of innate immunity, and is vital in protecting the host from a number of infectious agents. Deficiencies in the C4B allele, as well as its protein product, have been reported in ASD (Odell *et al.*, 2005; Warren *et al.*, 1994, 1995). Proteomic analyses of sera samples from children with ASD indicate that several complement proteins are differentially produced compared with age, gender, and geographically matched typically-developing control children (Corbett *et al.*, 2007).

Other genes with known effects on immune function have also been implicated in ASD. These include macrophage migration inhibitory factor (MIF) (Grigorenko *et al.*, 2008), MET tyrosine receptors (Campbell *et al.*, 2006; Correll *et al.*, 2004), serine and threonine kinase C gene *PRKCB1* (Lintas *et al.*, 2009), protein phosphatase and tensin homologue (PTEN) (Herman *et al.*, 2007), and reelin (Serajee *et al.*, 2006; Skaar *et al.*, 2005; Zhang *et al.*, 2002). Many products of these genes are important in key signaling pathways such as the mTOR/Akt pathway utilized by both the nervous and immune system (reviewed in Careaga *et al.*, 2010). However, it is currently unclear how dysregulation of these pathways contributes to the development of ASD, or to what level immune dysfunction is involved.

Brain and CNS immunity

A key finding in ASD research, and arguably the most important to an immunologist, has been the observations of pronounced ongoing neuroinflammation in postmortem brain specimens from individuals with ASD over a wide range of ages (4–45 years of age) (Li *et al.*, 2009b; Morgan *et al.*, 2010; Vargas *et al.*, 2005). These findings include astroglia and microglia activation and increased production of inflammatory cytokine and chemokines, including interferon (IFN)-γ, IL-1β, IL-6, IL-12p40, tumor necrosis factor (TNF)-α and chemokine C–C motif ligand (CCL)-2 in the brain tissue and cerebral spinal fluid (Li *et al.*, 2009b; Morgan *et al.*, 2010; Vargas *et al.*, 2005).

Microglia are the resident mononuclear phagocytic cells of the CNS and participate in immune surveillance of the CNS in normal neurodevelopment (Bessis *et al.*, 2007). Microglia are also activated in the postmortem brain specimens of individuals with other neurologic diseases including multiple sclerosis and Alzheimer's and Parkinson's diseases (Kim & de Vellis, 2005). Expression profiling of ASD postmortem brain tissue reveals increased messenger RNA transcript levels of several immune system–associated genes and altered transcriptome organization patterns in cortical patterning, further implicating neuroinflammatory processes in this disorder (Garbett *et al.*, 2008; Voineagu *et al.*, 2011).

Cytokines and chemokines are small molecules that are used as the messengers of the immune system and have been shown to interact with neurons, helping to shape their differentiation, proliferation, migration, and synaptic plasticity (Deverman & Patterson, 2009). The neurologic and immune systems maintain an intricate balance, and change in one system often results in change in the other (reviewed in Schwartz & Kipnis, 2010). Increased immune activation is associated with a number of neurodegenerative disorders and likely plays a role in psychiatric disorders such as schizophrenia (Strous & Shoenfeld, 2006), obsessive-compulsive disorder (Murphy *et al.*, 2010), depression (Dantzer *et al.*, 2008), bipolar disorder (Eaton *et al.*, 2010), Gilles de la Tourette syndrome (Murphy *et al.*, 2010) and ASD (Careaga *et al.*, 2010; Enstrom *et al.*, 2009c; Goines & Van de Water, 2010). Elevated levels of inflammatory cytokines in the CNS could reflect ongoing inflammatory processes affecting neuronal function. Increased levels of pro-inflammatory cytokines such as IL-6, TNF-α, and MCP-1 in brain specimens and cerebral spinal fluid (CSF) obtained from young and old individuals with ASD suggest that an active neuroinflammatory process is ongoing in ASD (Vargas *et al.*, 2005; Li *et al.*, 2009a).

Systemic immunity

Studies that determined cytokine levels in the circulation have shown increases in pro-inflammatory cytokines (Ashwood *et al.*, 2004; Jyonouchi *et al.*, 2001; Singh, 1996; Singh *et al.*, 1991) and decreases in anti-inflammatory or regulatory cytokines such as IL-10 and TGF-β1 (Ashwood & Wakefield, 2006; Ashwood *et al.*, 2004). These data suggest in ASD that a shift has occurred towards a more pro-inflammatory state. In a recent large population-based case-control study increased plasma cytokine levels were associated with more impaired communication and aberrant behaviours and the later onset of symptoms (Ashwood *et al.*, 2011). As a note of caution, the literature on cytokines and ASD has not always been consistent and likely reflects study design problems and a complexity in the patterns of immune activation among different subgroups of individuals with ASD. The data are further complicated by the use of siblings of children with ASD as controls in many studies, as it has been shown that siblings are themselves often on a broader autism phenotype (Constantino *et al.*, 2010), displaying both behavioural and immunologic aberrations more similar to children with ASD than to typically-developing controls (Saresella *et al.*, 2009).

The immune system is generally described as having two arms: the innate immune system, which uses genetically encoded receptors and nonspecific mechanisms to defend the host, and the adaptive immune system, which responds to a threat with great specificity and develops memory against future insults by the same threat. These two systems work together to protect the host and maintain proper homeostasis. A number of studies have demonstrated abnormalities in innate immune function in children and adults with ASD.

Several studies have reported differences in monocytes and macrophages in young children with ASD. As discussed earlier it is noteworthy that increased plasma cytokine levels (namely, IL-1β, IL-6, and IL-12) in children with ASD exhibit a profile that is produced predominantly by cells of the myeloid lineage, *i.e.*, monocytes and dendritic cells (Ashwood *et al.*, 2011). In keeping with this observation, Sweeten *et al.* (2003b) reported an increased number of monocytes in the peripheral blood of individuals with ASD. Furthermore, Jyonouchi and colleagues (2002) found that peripheral blood mononuclear cells (PBMCs) from individuals with ASD, when stimulated with the innate immune-activating TLR-4 agonist LPS, released more IL-1β, further suggesting involvement of monocytes and/or circulating dendritic cells in ASD. In a subset of ASD patients with recurrent infections, altered responses to a number of TLR ligands were also demonstrated (Jyonouchi *et al.*, 2008). These studies, however, used mixed cultures of peripheral cells and it is unclear whether the altered response was from monocytes alone, or from a more complex interaction between monocytes and other cells, including adaptive immune cells. By using isolated monocytes, Enstrom and colleagues found that IL-1β, IL-6, and TNF-α responses were increased following innate immune stimulation with TLR-2 agonists and that IL-1β production was increased following TLR-4 stimulation in children with ASD but not typically-developing controls (Enstrom *et al.*, 2010).

Other notable findings include alterations in natural killer (NK) cell activity. NK cells play an important role in viral defense, tumor surveillance, and help maintain the uterine environment during pregnancy. Early studies showed that NK cell-mediated lyses of the target cell K562 were decreased in some individuals with ASD (Warren et al., 1987). In a large multi-site study nearly half of the ASD subjects were found to have low NK cell cytotoxic activity against the target cell (Vojdani et al., 2008). A more in-depth investigation into NK cell function showed that baseline NK cells from subjects with ASD are in fact more activated in ASD, potentially reflecting their *in vivo* status, but when these cells are stimulated *in vitro* by culturing them with K562 cells, they fail to respond (Enstrom et al., 2009b). This feature has been described in several autoimmune diseases and may suggest that these innate immune cells are maximally stimulated *in vivo* and therefore are unable to respond further once challenged *in vitro*. Overall, these abnormal innate immune responses might, in part, help explain the increased rate of early childhood (first 30 days) infections seen in children with ASD compared with typically-developing controls (Rosen et al., 2007). During this critical early postnatal period, the adaptive immune system is immature and still being educated and the body is largely reliant on the innate immune system for host defense. Thus, inappropriate immune responses to pathogens at this stage might contribute to the symptoms or etiopathogenesis of ASD through direct interactions between immune mediators and neuronal targets, or indirectly by modulating the adaptive immune response.

Cellular studies in ASD have also demonstrated functional alterations in the adaptive immune response. Early work by Stubbs suggested that there were irregularities in cellular immune function in ASD (Stubbs, 1976). Further work by Warren et al. (1986) found T-cell abnormalities, including skewed CD4:CD8 T-cell frequencies and altered T-cell recall responses. More recent work has shown decreases in T-cell numbers in children with ASD who also have gastrointestinal (GI) problems (Ashwood et al., 2003); this may reflect efflux of T cells into the GI mucosa in this subset of ASD individuals. Cellular markers of activation show altered T-cell activation in children with ASD, suggesting an incomplete or altered activation profile (Ashwood et al., 2010; Ashwood & Wakefield, 2006; Plioplys et al., 1994). In a small study, there was an apparent skewing towards a T_H2 cytokine profile in some individuals with ASD (Gupta et al., 1998). However, the patterns of cytokines produced in T cells in ASD are complex and do not always fit easily into a traditional T_H2 classification. In a recent functional study, T cells from 63 children with ASD, following stimulation with phytohaemagglutinin (PHA), showed increases in levels of GM-CSF, TNF-α, and IL-13 and decreases in IL-12(p40) compared with 73 age-matched typically-developing controls. Furthermore, the increased cytokine production was associated with altered behaviours in children with ASD, such that increased pro-inflammatory cytokine production was associated with greater impairments in core features of ASD and more aberrant behaviours (Ashwood et al., 2011). In contrast, production of GM-CSF and T_H2 cytokines were associated with better cognitive and adaptive function (Ashwood et al., 2010). Overall, these findings suggest that altered T-cell function occurs in ASD and probably plays a role in the ongoing pathophysiologic process.

Currently there are no studies that have examined B-cell function directly in ASD; however, there are several lines of indirect evidence that suggest altered B-cell dysfunction in individuals with ASD. The primary role of B cells is the production of immunoglobulins against pathogens. In order to protect the host, B cells produce different immunoglobulins, each with a different role. IgA is present mainly in mucosal tissue, where it serves to bind pathogens within the lumen. Deficiencies in IgA are associated with increased infections (Aghamohammadi et al., 2009). Lower circulating levels of IgA have previously been reported in ASD (Warren et al., 1997), but more recent studies have not replicated this finding (Croonenberghs et al., 2002; Enstrom et al., 2009a; Heuer et al., 2008). However, reduced IgM and IgG production have been reported, with lower levels found to correlate with more aberrant behaviours (Heuer et *al.*, 2008). Analysis of specific IgG subclasses found that in spite of lower total levels for IgG, the IgG2 subtype (Croonenberghs *et al.*, 2002) and IgG4 subtype (Croonenberghs *et al.*, 2002; Enstrom *et al.*, 2009a) are elevated in ASD compared to controls. Interestingly, IgG2 is important for immune responses to carbohydrate antigens, whereas IgG4 functions as a blocking antibody and is associated with chronic infection. The IgG4 subtype has also been shown to function as a pathogenic antibody in certain autoimmune disorders (Qaqish *et al.*, 2009). In addition to altered immunoglobulin levels, a number of autoantibodies reactive to brain and CNS tissue have been identified in ASD (discussed later).

Reports of GI symptoms have been found in a significant number of individuals with ASD, with the more frequently reported GI symptoms being food insensitivities/food allergies. This has led several investigators to focus their research on cellular responses to dietary proteins such as gluten and casein. Jyonouchi *et al.* (2000) found that PBMCs responded to stimulation with gliadin, cow's milk protein, and soy by producing higher levels of inflammatory cytokines in children with ASD compared with typically-developing children. However, children in this study were selected on the basis of having previously seen behaviour improvements on a restricted diet, and may translate to a specific subgroup of ASD with GI symptoms. Other studies found increased pan-enteric infiltration of T-cells, monocytes, NK cells, and eosinophils in GI mucosa, suggesting a subtle but extensive mucosal immune activation in children with ASD who have GI symptoms (Ashwood *et al.*, 2003; Furlano *et al.*, 2001; Torrente *et al.*, 2000, 2004). T cells isolated from lamina propria mononuclear cells exhibited activation profiles with increased TNF-α, but lower IL-10 production in children with ASD and GI symptoms, compared with non-inflamed GI symptom controls, and children with coeliac disease or inflammatory bowel diseases (Ashwood *et al.*, 2003, 2004; Ashwood & Wakefield, 2006). Autoantibodies directed against gut epithelium were also observed in children with ASD, but not controls (Torrente *et al.*, 2002, 2004). These autoantibodies may represent nonspecific inflammation or an autoimmune response directed at the epithelial barrier that could lead to increased permeability. Other studies have suggested changes in the epithelial barrier function manifesting as increased gut permeability (de Magistris *et al.*, 2010; D'Eufemia *et al.*, 1996). Considerable controversy remains as to the prevalence of GI symptoms in individuals with ASD, with current estimates of GI symptoms in ASD ranging from 20–70 per cent. Moreover, whether these GI symptoms relate to a clinically defined GI pathology, or how GI symptoms relate to core features of ASD or associated behavioural symptoms is not clear. A number of small studies suggest that GI symptoms in ASD may be related to increased symptoms of aggression and hyperactivity and that some individuals with ASD may benefit from therapies targeting GI inflammation (Adams *et al.*, 2011; Buie *et al.*, 2010). In a case report of celiac disease that was mistaken for ASD, after removal of gluten from the patient's diet and implementation of a modified diet, behaviour improved (Genuis & Bouchard, 2009). Such studies suggest that an abnormal immune response and/or immune-mediated food insensitivity, in this case to a dietary protein, could contribute to behavioural abnormalities associated with ASD.

Autoantibodies in ASD

The presence of autoantibodies reactive against foetal brain or CNS tissue, but not adult brain tissue, has been repeatedly reported in young children with ASD (reviewed in Enstrom *et al.*, 2009c; Wills *et al.*, 2007). Several studies show that individuals with ASD display autoantibodies directed against a number of specific targets, including serotonin receptors (Todd & Ciaranello, 1985), brain-derived neurotrophic factor (BDNF) (Connolly *et al.*, 2006), myelin basic protein (MBP) (Connolly et al., 2006; Singh et al., 1993), neuron-axon acidic protein (NAFP) (Singh et al., 1997), glial fibrillary acidic protein (GFAP) (Singh et al., 1997), and gliadin (Vojdani et al., 2004). Other unidentified neuronal targets are also detected, and are associated with certain behavioural endophenotypes in ASD. Autoantibodies specific to a 45-kDa cerebellum protein were more frequent in children with ASD, and associated with worse adaptive and cognitive function, and increased aberrant behaviours (Goines et al., 2010; Wills et al., 2007). It is, however, unclear whether these autoantibodies have pathogenic relevance or are just biomarkers to previous cellular damage. It is known they are not present in all individuals with ASD (Morris et al., 2009) and their specificity to particular antigen targets such as MBP and GFAP has been difficult to replicate across studies (Kirkman et al., 2008; Libbey et al., 2008). This lack of specificity and the diverse array of antibody specificities may suggest that the antibodies are generated as a consequence of some previous indiscriminate damage, leading to the generation of different autoantibodies with different specificities, which can vary between individuals. It is plausible that the presence of these autoantibodies could denote a subgroup of children with ASD that are more prone to immune dysfunction.

Maternal immune activation

Pregnancy is a unique and complex process for the immune system, where protection of the mother from pathogens/infections is required, but complicated by the need to support and accept the foetal tissue that contains many 'non-self' paternal antigens. Uterine NK cells, macrophage and dendritic cells predominate in the human maternal–foetal interface and promote foetal development (Mor & Cardenas, 2010). Because of the complexity of regulating a balance between immune tolerance and protection from pathogens, pregnancy represents a period of vulnerability to immune insult not only for the mother, but also for the developing foetus. Both epidemiologic and animal studies suggest that immune dysregulation during this critical window can result in altered development and lead to neurodevelopmental and behavioural changes in the offspring.

One such risk factor of altered neurodevelopment is maternal infection during pregnancy. Early case reports and small comparative studies showed causal links between maternal infection and ASD (Chess, 1977; Libbey et al., 2005; Sweeten et al., 2004). In a more a recent population-based study using Denmark's medical registry from the period of 1980 to 2005 and consisting more than a million children, it was found that there was an increased rate of mothers with children with ASD who had been hospitalized for viral infections in the first trimester and bacterial infections in the second trimester compared with mothers of typically-developing children (Atladottir et al., 2010). Most maternal infections do not result in the development of ASD in offspring, suggesting that other factors such as a genetic susceptibility may be involved. Individuals with known genetic disorders that are associated with high rates of ASD, such as tuberous sclerosis (TCS), have a 25–50 per cent rate of ASD (Wiznitzer, 2004), and associations are found with season of birth and incidence of ASD, the peak occurring during flu season, during the later stages of pregnancy (Ehninger et al., 2010).

Animal models support this theory (Smith et al., 2010). Using both viral and bacterial analogues, researchers have shown that a generalized maternal immune activation, rather than a pathogen-specific response, results in behavioural changes in offspring (Borrell et al., 2002; Gilmore et al., 2005). It is not fully understood how immune activation affects foetal development, but it is hypothesized that activation of the maternal immune system leads to changes either in the placenta potentially affecting progenitor cells, or directly in the foetal brain (Hsiao & Patterson, 2010; Meyer et al., 2008). Although numerous cytokines are induced during maternal immune activation, IL-6 appears to be one of the major mediators in the animal models. This has been demonstrated by the use of either IL-6 knockout mice or blocking IL-6 with an antibody: both have proven to be protective in maternal immune activation models (Smith *et al.*, 2007). Genetic factors may further contribute to the neuropathology in offspring during maternal immune activation. Mice with disruptions to genes associated with altered neurodevelopment, such as DISC1 or TSC1, have more exaggerated behavioural phenotypes, with greater impairments in social interaction after maternal immune activation (Abazyan *et al.*, 2010; Ehninger *et al.*, 2010). The effects of maternal immune activation are not limited to neurodevelopment, and appear to result in ongoing immune dysfunction in the offspring (Hsiao *et al.*, 2012; Lasala & Zhou, 2007; Mandal *et al.*, 2010; Surriga *et al.*, 2009).

The maternal transfer of antibodies from the mother to child during pregnancy is well documented, and confers protection from a wide range of infectious agents to the foetus. However, along with antibodies that provide immunoprotection, antibodies that are potentially reactive to foetal 'self' proteins will also cross the placental barrier and can affect neonatal outcome (Tincani *et al.*, 2005). For example, the transfer to the foetus of maternal anti-Ro/SS-A and anti-La/SS-B antibodies in mothers with systemic lupus erythematosus (SLE) causes neonatal lupus syndrome, often leading to congenital heart block (Lee *et al.*, 2009; McAllister *et al.*, 1997; Neri *et al.*, 2004; Tincani *et al.*, 2006). Neurotoxic autoantibodies from patients with SLE transferred into pregnant mice result in altered brain development in offspring (Lee *et al.*, 2009). Abnormal thyroid function caused by placental transfer of maternal anti-thyroid antibodies is often seen in babies born to mothers with Hashimoto's thyroiditis or Graves' disease (Fu *et al.*, 2005), and some cases of neonatal anti-phospholipid syndrome (APS) are thought to occur on account of the transfer of maternal autoantibodies from mothers with primary APS (Rolim *et al.*, 2006). The presence of autoantibodies directed against critical neuronal components of foetal brain extracts in a subset of mothers of ASD children could suggest that a similar mechanism may occur in ASD (Braunschweig *et al.*, 2008; Silva *et al.*, 2004; Zimmerman *et al.*, 2007). The reactivity of these antibodies is to foetal brain proteins, and is observed in approximately 10 per cent of mothers who have children with ASD, but not mothers of children who are typically-developing or have developmental disorders other than ASD (Braunschweig *et al.*, 2008).

The ASD-specific nature of these antibodies warrants further study. One possibility is that they bind to neuronal targets during development, thereby interfering with or altering neurodevelopment. Although it is hard to recapitulate exactly the core features of ASD in animal models, certain behaviours associated with ASD, such as repetitive behaviours, difficulty in learning, and hyperactivity can be replicated (Klauck & Poustka, 2006). In one study IgG isolated from mothers of children with ASD that was transferred into rhesus macaque monkeys during midgestation resulted in increased stereotypical behaviour and hyperactivity in the offspring that were not observed in monkeys that received IgG from mothers of typically-developing children or monkeys from mothers that received only saline solution (Martin *et al.*, 2008). Evidence of a potential role for these autoantibodies and altered neurodevelopment are also seen in murine models (Singer *et al.*, 2009). Whether such behavioural changes are directly related to ASD or are themselves distinct phenomena is not clear. Future studies will need to fully characterize the ASD specific behavioural changes evoked by specific maternal antibodies, as well as the potential cellular targets of these antibodies. Although such antibodies are present in only a subset of mothers who have children with ASD, the significance of carrying these antibodies may be substantial (Braunschweig *et al.*, 2008) and presents an exciting avenue for screening and/or therapy.

Conclusion

Our understanding of ASD is still in its infancy; however, decades of research have provided many clues into the pathology of ASD. Current research into the role of the immune system in neuronal development and function suggest that findings of immune dysfunction in ASD, both in children and parents, indicate that there is a strong immune component to this disorder, at least in a subgroup of individuals. However, the exact role of the immune system in ASD remains to be defined. Epidemiologic and animal model studies suggest that maternal immune activation may be involved in the initiation of the disorder, and evidence of persistent immune dysregulation in children with ASD indicates a possible role for continued immune involvement in the pathology of ASD. Future studies will help clarify further the role of the immune response in ASD, as well as identifying potential targets for treatments.

Conflicts of interest: The authors declare no conflicts of interest.

References

Abazyan, B., Nomura, J., Kannan, G., *et al.* (2010): Prenatal interaction of mutant DISC1 and immune activation produces adult psychopathology. *Biol. Psychiatry* **68**, 1172–1181.

Adams, J., Johansen, L., Powell, L., Quiq, D. & Rubin, R. (2011): Gastrointestinal flora and gastrointestinal status in children with autism: comparisons to neurotypical children and correlation with autism severity. *BMC Gastroenterol.* **11**, 22.

Aghamohammadi, A., Cheraghi, T., Gharagozlou, *et al.* (2009): IgA deficiency: correlation between clinical and immunological phenotypes. *J. Clin. Immunol,* **29**, 130–136.

Ashwood, P. & Wakefield, A.J. (2006): Immune activation of peripheral blood and mucosal CD3+: lymphocyte cytokine profiles in children with autism and gastrointestinal symptoms. *J. Neuroimmunol.* **173**, 126–134.

Ashwood, P., Anthony, A., Pellicer, A.A., Torrente, F., Walker-Smith, J. & Wakefield, A.J. (2003): Intestinal lymphocyte populations in children with regressive autism: evidence for extensive mucosal immunopathology. *J. Clin. Immunol.* **23**, 504–517.

Ashwood, P., Anthony, A., Torrente, F. & Wakefield, A.J. (2004): Spontaneous mucosal lymphocyte cytokine profiles in children with autism and gastrointestinal symptoms: mucosal immune activation and reduced counter regulatory interleukin-10. *J. Clin. Immunol.* **24**, 664–673.

Ashwood, P., Krakowiak, P., Hertz-Picciotto, I., Hansen, R., Pessah, I.N. & Van De Water, J. (2010): Altered T cell responses in children with autism. *Brain Behav. Immun.* [E-pub, 15 September 2010].

Ashwood, P., Krakowiak, P., Hertz-Picciotto, I., Hansen, R., Pessah, I. & Van De Water, J. (2011): Elevated plasma cytokines in autism spectrum disorders provide evidence of immune dysfunction and are associated with impaired behavioural outcome. *Brain Behav. Immun.* **25**, 40–45.

Atladottir, H.O., Pedersen, M.G., Thorsen, P., *et al.* (2009): Association of family history of autoimmune diseases and autism spectrum disorders. *Pediatrics* **124**, 687–694.

Atladottir, H.O., Thorsen, P., Ostergaard, *et al.* (2010): Maternal infection requiring hospitalization during pregnancy and autism spectrum disorders. *J. Autism Dev. Disord.* **40**, 1423–1430.

Bessis, A., Bechade, C., Bernard, D. & Roumier, A. (2007): Microglial control of neuronal death and synaptic properties. *Glia* **55**, 233–238.

Borrell, J., Vela, J. M., Arevalo-Martin, A., Molina-Holgado, E. & Guaza, C. (2002): Prenatal immune challenge disrupts sensorimotor gating in adult rats: implications for the etiopathogenesis of schizophrenia. *Neuropsychopharmacology* **26**, 204–215.

Braunschweig, D., Ashwood, P., Krakowiak, P., *et al.* (2008): Autism: maternally derived antibodies specific for fetal brain proteins. *Neurotoxicology* **29**, 226–231.

Buie, T., Campbell, D.B., Fuchs, G.J., 3rd, *et al.* (2010): Evaluation, diagnosis, and treatment of gastrointestinal disorders in individuals with ASDs: a consensus report. *Pediatrics* **125** (Suppl. 1), S1–S18.

Campbell, D.B., Sutcliffe, J.S., Ebert, P.J., *et al.* (2006): A genetic variant that disrupts MET transcription is associated with autism. *Proc. Natl. Acad. Sci. USA* **103**, 16834–16839.

Careaga, M., Van De Water, J. & Ashwood, P. (2010): Immune dysfunction in autism: a pathway to treatment. *Neurotherapeutics* **7**, 283–292.

Chess, S. (1977): Follow-up report on autism in congenital rubella. *J. Autism Child Schizoph.* **7**, 69–81.

Comi, A.M., Zimmerman, A.W., Frye, V.H., Law, P.A. & Peeden, J.N. (1999): Familial clustering of autoimmune disorders and evaluation of medical risk factors in autism. *J. Child Neurol.* **14**, 388–394.

Connolly, A.M., Chez, M., Streif, E.M., *et al.* (2006): Brain-derived neurotrophic factor and autoantibodies to neural antigens in sera of children with autistic spectrum disorders, Landau-Kleffner syndrome, and epilepsy. *Biol. Psychiatry* **59**, 354–363.

Constantino, J.N., Zhang, Y., Frazier, T., Abbacchi, A.M. & Law, P. (2010): Sibling recurrence and the genetic epidemiology of autism. *Am. J. Psychiatry* **167**, 1349–1356.

Corbett, B.A., Kantor, A.B., Schulman, H., *et al.* (2007): A proteomic study of serum from children with autism showing differential expression of apolipoproteins and complement proteins. *Mol. Psychiatry* **12**, 292–306.

Correll, P.H., Morrison, A.C. & Lutz, M.A. (2004): Receptor tyrosine kinases and the regulation of macrophage activation. *J. Leukoc. Biol.* **75**, 731–737.

Croonenberghs, J., Wauters, A., Devreese, K., *et al.* (2002): Increased serum albumin, gamma globulin, immunoglobulin IgG, and IgG2 and IgG4 in autism. *Psychol. Med.* **32**, 1457–1463.

Daniels, W.W., Warren, R.P., Odell, J.D., *et al.* (1995): Increased frequency of the extended or ancestral haplotype B44-SC30-DR4 in autism. *Neuropsychobiology* **32**, 120–123.

Dantzer, R., O'Connor, J.C., Freund, G.G., Johnson, R.W. & Kelley, K.W. (2008): From inflammation to sickness and depression: when the immune system subjugates the brain. *Nat. Rev. Neurosci.* **9**, 46–56.

De Magistris, L., Familiari, V., Pascotto, A., *et al.* (2010): Alterations of the intestinal barrier in patients with autism spectrum disorders and in their first-degree relatives. *J. Pediat. Gastroenterol.Nutr.* **51**, 418–424.

D'Eufemia, P., Celli, M., Finocchiaro, R., *et al.* (1996): Abnormal intestinal permeability in children with autism. *Acta Paediatr.* **85**, 1076–1079.

Deverman, B.E. & Patterson, P.H. (2009): Cytokines and CNS development. *Neuron* **64**, 61–78.

Eaton, W.W., Pedersen, M.G., Nielsen, P.R. & Mortensen, P.B. (2010): Autoimmune diseases, bipolar disorder, and non-affective psychosis. *Bipolar Disord.* **12**, 638–646.

Ehninger, D., Sano, Y., De Vries, P.J., *et al.* (2010): Gestational immune activation and Tsc2 haploinsufficiency cooperate to disrupt fetal survival and may perturb social behaviour in adult mice. *Mol. Psychiatry* **17**, 62–70; erratum, **17**, 469.

Enstrom, A., Krakowiak, P., Onore, C., *et al.* (2009a): Increased IgG4 levels in children with autism disorder. *Brain Behav. Immun.* **23**, 389–395.

Enstrom, A.M., Lit, L., Onore, C.E., *et al.* (2009b): Altered gene expression and function of peripheral blood natural killer cells in children with autism. *Brain Behav Immun.* **23**, 124–133.

Enstrom, A.M., Van De Water, J.A. & Ashwood, P. (2009c): Autoimmunity in autism. *Curr. Opin. Investig. Drugs* **10**, 463–473.

Enstrom, A.M., Onore, C.E., Van De Water, J.A. & Ashwood, P. (2010): Differential monocyte responses to Tlr ligands in children with autism spectrum disorders. *Brain Behav. Immun.* **24**, 64–71.

Fernando, M.M., Stevens, C.R., Walsh, E.C., *et al.* (2008): Defining the role of the MHC in autoimmunity: a review and pooled analysis. *PLoS Genet.* **4**, e1000024.

Fu, J., Jiang, Y., Liang, L. & Zhu, H. (2005): Risk factors of primary thyroid dysfunction in early infants born to mothers with autoimmune thyroid disease. *Acta Paediatrica* **94**, 1043–1048.

Furlano, R.I., Anthony, A., Day, R., *et al.* (2001): Colonic CD8 and gamma delta T-cell infiltration with epithelial damage in children with autism. *J. Pediatr.* **138**, 366–372.

Garbett, K., Ebert, P.J., Mitchell, A., *et al.* (2008): Immune transcriptome alterations in the temporal cortex of subjects with autism. *Neurobiol. Dis.* **30**, 303–311.

Genuis, S.J. & Bouchard, T.P. (2010): Celiac disease presenting as autism. *J. Child Neurol.* **25**, 114–119.

Gilmore, J.H., Jarskog, L.F. & Vadlamudi, S. (2005): Maternal poly I:C exposure during pregnancy regulates TNF alpha, BDNF, and NGF expression in neonatal brain and the maternal-fetal unit of the rat. *J. Neuroimmunol.* **159**, 106–112.

Goines, P. & Van De Water, J. (2010): The immune system's role in the biology of autism. *Curr. Opin. Neurol.* **23**, 111–117. 10.1097/WCO.0b013e3283373514.

Goines, P., Haapanen, L., Boyce, R., *et al.* (2011): Autoantibodies to cerebellum in children with autism associate with behaviour. *Brain Behav. Immun.* **25**, 514–523.

Grigorenko, E.L., Han, S.S., Yrigollen, C.M., *et al.* (2008): Macrophage migration inhibitory factor and autism spectrum disorders. *Pediatrics* **122** e438–445.

Guerini, F.R., Bolognesi, E., Manca, S., *et al.* (2009): Family-based transmission analysis of HLA genetic markers in Sardinian children with autistic spectrum disorders. *Hum. Immunol.* **70**, 184–190.

Gupta, S., Aggarwal, S., Rashanravan, B. & Lee, T. (1998): Th1- and Th2-like cytokines in CD4+ and CD8+ T cells in autism. *J. Neuroimmunol.* **85**, 106–109.

Herman, G.E., Butter, E., Enrile, B., Pastore, M., Prior, T.W. & Sommer, A. (2007): Increasing knowledge of PTEN germline mutations: two additional patients with autism and macrocephaly. *Am. J. Med. Genet. A.* **143**, 589–593.

Heuer, L., Ashwood, P., Schauer, J., *et al.* (2008): Reduced levels of immunoglobulin in children with autism correlates with behavioural symptoms. *Autism Res.* **1**, 275–283.

Hsiao, E.Y. & Patterson, P.H. (2011): Activation of the maternal immune system induces endocrine changes in the placenta via IL-6. *Brain Behav Immun.* **25**, 604–615.

Hsiao, E.Y., McBride, S.W., Chow, J., Mazmanian, S.K. & Patterson, P.H. (2012): Modeling an autism risk factor in mice leads to permanent immune dysregulation. *Proc. Natl. Acad. Sci. USA* **109**, 12776–12781.

Jyonouchi, H., Sun, S. & Le, H. (2001): Proinflammatory and regulatory cytokine production associated with innate and adaptive immune responses in children with autism spectrum disorders and developmental regression. *J. Neuroimmunol.* **120**, 170–179.

Jyonouchi, H., Sun, S. & Itokazu, N. (2002): Innate immunity associated with inflammatory responses and cytokine production against common dietary proteins in patients with autism spectrum disorder. *Neuropsychobiology* **46**, 76–84.

Jyonouchi, H., Geng, L., Cushing-Ruby, A. & Quraishi, H. (2008): Impact of innate immunity in a subset of children with autism spectrum disorders: a case control study. *J. Neuroinflam.* **5**, 52.

Kanner, L. (1968): Autistic disturbances of affective contact. *Acta Paedopsychiatry* **35**, 100–136.

Keil, A., Daniels, J.L., Forssen, U., *et al.* (2010): Parental autoimmune diseases associated with autism spectrum disorders in offspring. *Epidemiology* **21**, 805–808.

Kim, S.U. & De Vellis, J. (2005): Microglia in health and disease. *J. Neurosci. Res.* **81**, 302–313.

Kirkman, N.J., Libbey, J.E., Sweeten, T.L., *et al.* (2008): How relevant are GFAP autoantibodies in autism and Tourette syndrome? *J. Autism Dev. Disord.* **38**, 333–341.

Klauck, S.M. & Poustka, A. (2006): Animal models of autism. *Drug Disc. Today: Dis. Models* **3**, 313–318.

Lasala, N. & Zhou, H. (2007): Effects of maternal exposure to LPS on the inflammatory response in the offspring. *J. Neuroimmunol.* **189**, 95–101.

Lee, L.C., Zachary, A.A., Leffell, M.S., *et al.* (2006): HLA-DR4 in families with autism. *Pediatr. Neurol.* **35**, 303–307.

Lee, J.Y., Huerta, P.T., Zhang, J., *et al.* (2009): Neurotoxic autoantibodies mediate congenital cortical impairment of offspring in maternal lupus. *Nat. Med.* **15**, 91–96.

Li, X., Chauhan, A., Sheikh, A.M., *et al.* (2009a): Elevated immune response in the brain of autistic patients. *J. Neuroimmunol.* **207**, 111–116.

Li, X., Chauhan, A., Sheikh, A.M., *et al.* (2009b): Elevated immune response in the brain of autistic patients. *J. Neuroimmunol.* **207**, 111–116.

Libbey, J.E., Sweeten, T.L., McMahon, W.M. & Fujinami, R.S. (2005): Autistic disorder and viral infections. *J. Neurovirol.* **11**, 1–10.

Libbey, J.E., Coon, H.H., Kirkman, N.J., *et al.* (2008): Are there enhanced MBP autoantibodies in autism? *J. Autism Dev. Disord.* **38**, 324–332.

Lintas, C., Sacco, R., Garbett, K., *et al.* (2009): Involvement of the *PRKCB1* gene in autistic disorder: significant genetic association and reduced neocortical gene expression. *Mol. Psychiatry* **14**, 705–718.

Mandal, M., Marzouk, A.C., Donnelly, R. & Ponzio, N.M. (2010): Preferential development of Th17 cells in offspring of immunostimulated pregnant mice. *J. Reprod. Immunol.* **87**, 97–100.

Martin, L.A., Ashwood, P., Braunschweig, D., Cabanlit, M., Van De Water, J. & Amaral, D.G. (2008): Stereotypies and hyperactivity in rhesus monkeys exposed to IgG from mothers of children with autism. *Brain Behav. Immun.* **22**, 806–816.

McAllister, D.L., Kaplan, B.J., Edworthy, S.M., *et al.* (1997): The influence of systemic lupus erythematosus on fetal development: cognitive, behavioural, and health trends. *J. Int. Neuropsychol. Soc.* **3**, 370–376.

Meyer, U., Nyffeler, M., Yee, B.K., Knuesel, I. & Feldon, J. (2008): Adult brain and behavioural pathological markers of prenatal immune challenge during early/middle and late fetal development in mice. *Brain Behav. Immun.* **22**, 469–486.

Molloy, C.A., Morrow, A.L., Meinzen-Derr, J., *et al.* (2006): Familial autoimmune thyroid disease as a risk factor for regression in children with autism spectrum disorder: a CPEA study. *J. Autism Dev. Disord.* **36**, 317–324.

Money, J., Bobrow, N.A. & Clarke, F.C. (1971): Autism and autoimmune disease: a family study. *J. Autism Child Schizophr.* **1**, 146–160.

Mor, G. & Cardenas, I. (2010): The immune system in pregnancy: a unique complexity. *Am. J. Reprod. Immunol.* **63**, 425–433.

Morgan, J.T., Chana, G., Pardo, C.A., *et al.* (2010): Microglial activation and increased microglial density observed in the dorsolateral prefrontal cortex in autism. *Biol. Psychiatry* **68**, 368–376.

Morris, C.M., Zimmerman, A.W. & Singer, H.S. (2009): Childhood serum anti-fetal brain antibodies do not predict autism. *Pediatr. Neurol.* **41**, 288–290.

Murphy, T.K., Kurlan, R. & Leckman, J. (2010): The immunobiology of Tourette's disorder, pediatric autoimmune neuropsychiatric disorders associated with Streptococcus, and related disorders: a way forward. *J. Child Adolesc. Psychopharmacol.* **20**, 317–331.

Neri, F., Chimini, L., Bonomi, F., *et al.* (2004): Neuropsychological development of children born to patients with systemic lupus erythematosus. *Lupus* **13**, 805–811.

Odell, D., Maciulis, A., Cutler, A., *et al.* (2005): Confirmation of the association of the C4B null allelle in autism. *Hum. Immunol.* **66**, 140–145.

Plioplys, A.V., Greaves, A., Kazemi, K. & Silverman, E. (1994): Lymphocyte function in autism and Rett syndrome. *Neuropsychobiology* **29**, 12–16.

Qaqish, B.F., Prisayanh, P., Qian, Y., *et al.* (2009): Development of an IgG4-based predictor of endemic pemphigus foliaceus (fogo selvagem). *J. Invest. Dermatol.* **129**, 110–118.

Rolim, A., Castro, M. & Santiago, M. (2006): Neonatal antiphospholipid syndrome. *Lupus* **15**, 301.

Rosen, N.J., Yoshida, C.K. & Croen, L.A. (2007): Infection in the first 2 years of life and autism spectrum disorders. *Pediatrics* **119**, e61–69.

Saresella, M., Marventano, I., Guerini, F.R., *et al.* (2009): An autistic endophenotype results in complex immune dysfunction in healthy siblings of autistic children. *Biol. Psychiatry* **66**, 978–984.

Schwartz, M. & Kipnis, J. (2011): A conceptual revolution in the relationships between the brain and immunity. *Brain Behav. Immun.* **25**, 817–819.

Serajee, F.J., Zhong, H. & Mahbubul Huq, A.H. (2006): Association of reelin gene polymorphisms with autism. *Genomics* **87**, 75–83.

Silva, S.C., Correia, C., Fesel, C., *et al.* (2004): Autoantibody repertoires to brain tissue in autism nuclear families. *J. Neuroimmunol.* **152**, 176–182.

Singer, H.S., Morris, C., Gause, C., Pollard, M., Zimmerman, A.W. & Pletniko, V.M. (2009): Prenatal exposure to antibodies from mothers of children with autism produces neurobehavioural alterations: a pregnant dam mouse model. *J. Neuroimmunol.* **211**, 39–48.

Singh, V.K. (1996): Plasma increase of interleukin-12 and interferon-gamma: pathological significance in autism. *J. Neuroimmunol.* **66**, 143–145.

Singh, V.K., Warren, R.P., Odell, J.D. & Cole, P. (1991): Changes of soluble interleukin-2, interleukin-2 receptor, T8 antigen, and interleukin-1 in the serum of autistic children. *Clin. Immunol. Immunopathol.* **61**, 448–455.

Singh, V.K., Warren, R.P., Odell, J.D., Warren, W.L. & Cole, P. (1993): Antibodies to myelin basic protein in children with autistic behaviour. *Brain Behav. Immun.* **7**, 97–103.

Singh, V.K., Warren, R., Averett, R. & Ghaziuddin, M. (1997): Circulating autoantibodies to neuronal and glial filament proteins in autism. *Pediatr. Neurol.* **17**, 88–90.

Skaar, D.A., Shao, Y., Haines, J.L., *et al.* (2005): Analysis of the RELN gene as a genetic risk factor for autism. *Mol. Psychiatry* **10**, 563–571.

Smith, S.E., Li, J., Garbett, K., Mirnics, K. & Patterson, P.H. (2007): Maternal immune activation alters fetal brain development through interleukin-6. *J. Neurosci.* **27**, 10695–10702.

Smith, S.E.P., Hsiao, E. & Patterson, P.H. (2010): Activation of the maternal immune system as a risk factor for neuropsychiatric disorders. In: *Maternal Influences on Foetal Neurodevelopment*, eds. A.W. Zimmerman & S.L. Connors. New York: Springer.

Strous, R.D. & Shoenfeld, Y. (2006): Schizophrenia, autoimmunity and immune system dysregulation: a comprehensive model updated and revisited. *J. Autoimmun.* **27**, 71–80.

Stubbs, E.G. (1976): Autistic children exhibit undetectable hemagglutination-inhibition antibody titers despite previous rubella vaccination. *J. Autism Child Schizophr.* **6**, 269–274.

Stubbs, E.G. & Magenis, R.E. (1980): HLA and autism. *J. Autism Dev. Disord.* **10**, 15–19.

Surriga, O., Ortega, A., Jadeja, V., Bellafronte, A., Lasala, N. & Zhou, H. (2009): Altered hepatic inflammatory response in the offspring following prenatal LPS exposure. *Immunol. Lett.* **123,** 88–95.

Sweeten, T.L., Bowyer, S.L., Posey, D.J., Halberstadt, G.M. & McDougle, C.J. (2003a): Increased prevalence of familial autoimmunity in probands with pervasive developmental disorders. *Pediatrics* **112,** e420.

Sweeten, T.L., Posey, D.J. & McDougle, C.J. (2003b): High blood monocyte counts and neopterin levels in children with autistic disorder. *Am. J. Psychiatry* **160,** 1691–1693.

Sweeten, T.L., Posey, D.J. & McDougle, C.J. (2004): Brief report: autistic disorder in three children with cytomegalovirus infection. *J. Autism Dev. Disord.* **34,** 583–586.

Tincani, A., Rebaioli, C.B., Frassi, M., et al. (2005): Pregnancy and autoimmunity: maternal treatment and maternal disease influence on pregnancy outcome. *Autoimmun. Rev.* **4,** 423–428.

Tincani, A., Danieli, E., Nuzzo, M., et al. (2006): Impact of in utero environment on the offspring of lupus patients. *Lupus* **15,** 801–807.

Todd, R.D. & Ciaranello, R.D. (1985): Demonstration of inter- and intraspecies differences in serotonin binding sites by antibodies from an autistic child. *Proc. Natl. Acad. Sci. USA* **82,** 612–616.

Torrente, F., Ashwood, P., Day, R., et al. (2002): Small intestinal enteropathy with epithelial IgG and complement deposition in children with regressive autism. *Mol. Psychiatry* **7,** 334, 375–382.

Torrente, F., Anthony, A., Heuschkel, R.B., Thomson, M.A., Ashwood, P. & Murch, S.H. (2004): Focal-enhanced gastritis in regressive autism with features distinct from Crohn's and *Helicobacter pylori* gastritis. *Am. J. Gastroenterol.* **99,** 598–605.

Torres, A.R., Maciulis, A., Stubbs, E.G., Cutler, A. & Odell, D. (2002): The transmission disequilibrium test suggests that HLA-DR4 and DR13 are linked to autism spectrum disorder. *Hum. Immunol.* **63,** 311–316.

Valicenti-McDermott, M.D., McVicar, K., Cohen, H.J., Wershil, B.K. & Shinnar, S. (2008): Gastrointestinal symptoms in children with an autism spectrum disorder and language regression. *Paediatr. Neurol.* **39,** 392–398.

Vargas, D.L., Nascimbene, C., Krishnan, C., Zimmerman, A.W. & Pardo, C.A. (2005): Neuroglial activation and neuroinflammation in the brain of patients with autism. *Ann. Neurol.* **57,** 67–81.

Voineagu, I., Wang, X., Johnston, P., et al. (2011): Transcriptomic analysis of autistic brain reveals convergent molecular pathology. *Nature* **474,** 380–384.

Vojdani, A., O'Bryan, T., Green, J.A., et al. (2004): Immune response to dietary proteins, gliadin and cerebellar peptides in children with autism. *Nutr. Neurosci.* **7,** 151–161.

Vojdani, A., Mumper, E., Granpeesheh, D., et al. (2008): Low natural killer cell cytotoxic activity in autism: the role of glutathione, IL-2 and IL-15. *J. Neuroimmunol.* **205,** 148–154.

Warren, R.P., Margaretten, N.C., Pace, N.C. & Foster, A. (1986): Immune abnormalities in patients with autism. *J. Autism Dev. Disord.* **16,** 189–197.

Warren, R. P., Foster, A. & Margaretten, N.C. (1987): Reduced natural killer cell activity in autism. *J. Am. Acad. Child Adolesc. Psychiatry* **26,** 333–335.

Warren, R.P., Singh, V.K., Cole, P., et al. (1992): Possible association of the extended MHC haplotype B44-SC30-DR4 with autism. *Immunogenetics* **36,** 203–207.

Warren, R.P., Burger, R.A., Odell, D., Torres, A.R. & Warren, W.L. (1994): Decreased plasma concentrations of the C4B complement protein in autism. *Arch. Pediatr. Adolesc. Med,* **148,** 180–183.

Warren, R.P., Yonk, J., Burger, R.W., Odell, D. & Warren, W.L. (1995): DR-positive T cells in autism: association with decreased plasma levels of the complement C4B protein. *Neuropsychobiology* **31,** 53–57.

Warren, R.P., Odell, J.D., Warren, W.L., et al. (1997): Brief report: immunoglobulin A deficiency in a subset of autistic subjects. *J. Autism Dev. Disord.* **27,** 187–192.

Wills, S., Cabanlit, M., Bennett, J., Ashwood, P., Amaral, D. & Van De Water, J. (2007): Autoantibodies in autism spectrum disorders (ASD). *Ann. N.Y. Acad. Sci.* **1107,** 79–91.

Wiznitzer, M. (2004): Autism and tuberous sclerosis. *J. Child Neurol.* **19,** 675–679.

Zhang, H., Liu, X., Zhang, C., et al. (2002): Reelin gene alleles and susceptibility to autism spectrum disorders. *Mol. Psychiatry* **7,** 1012–1017.

Zimmerman, A.W., Connors, S.L., Matteson, K.J., et al. (2007): Maternal antibrain antibodies in autism. *Brain Behav. Immun.* **21,** 351–357.

Psychopharmacology

Chapter 9

New prospects towards more effective medication for ASDs

Roberta Zanni, Silvia Petza and Alessandro Zuddas

*Unit of Child and Adolescent Neuropsychiatry, Section of Neuroscience
and Clinical Pharmacology, Department of Biomedical Science, University of Cagliari, 09124 Cagliari, Italy
azuddas.unica@gmail.com*

Summary

Despite considerable progress in understanding the neurobiology of autism spectrum disorders (ASDs), currently available treatments for these disorders are inadequate. Specific educational and behavioural interventions still remain the main therapeutic strategy. When behavioural symptoms significantly interfere with daily activities and quality of life, making the therapeutic education program impossible or extremely difficult to carry out, pharmacologic intervention is then considered. In fact, stimulants and second-generation-antipsychotic drugs have shown some benefit for comorbid symptoms (hyperactivity, impulsivity, irritability, agitation, aggression) in the person with ASD, seldom mitigating the core symptom domain. The identification of new effective treatments for the core symptoms of ASDs is thus considered a primary unmet therapeutic need. Recently, the focus of this research has changed from behavioural observation of ASD to translating findings from animal models, genomic manipulation studies, and basic science studies to pharmacologic agents with the aim of lessening or reversing the core of the autistic symptoms. Understanding the pathophysiology of single-gene disorders associated with ASD may establish a molecular logic for development of novel therapeutic interventions. New insight from old medications such as SSRIs, from single-gene disorders as tuberous sclerosis and fragile X syndrome as well as from allosteric manipulation of specific glutamatergic receptor, will be briefly described in this chapter.

Introduction

Autism spectrum disorders (ASDs) are severe childhood disorders presenting in the first 3 years of life with a prevalence of 0.6 to 1.1 per cent in European and US children and adolescents, respectively (CDC, 2011; Wittchen *et al.* 2011), corresponding to 0.6 million European children and adolescents at a reported annual cost of about 50,000 euros per year per patient (Gustavsson *et al.*, 2011). ASD is characterized by deficits in social interaction, in verbal and nonverbal communication, imagination, and restricted and repetitive behaviours and/or interests. Symptomatic expression and severity are broad and many individuals also experience unusual sensory responses and motor patterns, anxiety, depression, sleep disturbances, attention problems, and aggression or self-injury (Levy *et al.*, 2009).

Youth with autism spectrum disorders are at increased risk of developing co-occurring mental health conditions. Symptoms of anxiety are among those most commonly reported (Brereton *et al.*, 2006; Skokauskas & Gallagher, 2012). High rates of comorbid psychopathology have been found in a population-derived sample (Simonoff *et al.*, 2012) as well as in community and clinic-based samples of youth with ASD (de Bruin *et al.*, 2007; Leyfer *et al.*, 2006). A majority of children in these samples met diagnostic criteria for at one least additional DSM Axis I diagnosis (American Psychiatric Association, 2000), and anxiety disorders were among the most commonly reported concurrent diagnoses.

Current therapeutic options

Despite considerable progress in understanding the neurobiology of ASD, currently available treatments for ASDs are inadequate (McPheeters *et al.*, 2011; Warren *et al.*, 2011). Specific educational and behavioural interventions still remain the main therapeutic strategy. When behavioural symptoms significantly interfere with daily activities and quality of life, making it impossible or extremely difficult to employ a therapeutic educational program, pharmacologic intervention may be needed: in fact pharmacologic intervention has shown some benefit for comorbid symptoms in ASD rather than on the core symptom domain (McPheeters *et al.*, 2011). Stimulants and second-generation antipsychotics have been shown to be effective in reducing hyperactivity and impulsivity or irritability, agitation and aggression, respectively (McCracken *et al.*, 2002; RUPP, 2005; Zuddas *et al.*, 2000, 2011).

Risperidone and aripirazole are most extensively studied medications for associated symptoms in ASD: efficacy of both medications has been shown by randomized placebo-controlled studies (Marcus *et al.*, 2009; McCracken *et al.*, 2002; McDougle *et al.*, 2005; Owen *et al.*, 2009); both drugs are registered for this indication in the United States, but only risperidone is indicated in Europe. A key obstacle to the use of pharmacotherapy in ASDs management includes the deeply entrenched position of behavioural interventions in treatment guidelines and the negative perceptions surrounding the use of antipsychotic agents. Because there are no disease-modifying drugs for ASDs, treatment guidelines state that pharmacologic approaches should only be initiated for the management of disruptive symptoms, in order to aid compliance and outcomes of behavioural interventions (Nightingale, 2012). Data on 5-HT reuptake inhibitors (SRIs) are inconsistent, showing some benefit in mitigating repetitive behaviours in some patients, while others drugs show a lack of efficacy, and significant side effects in other SRIs.

People with ASD share behaviour that is similar to that in persons affected by ADHD. Pharmacologic treatments for ADHD, such as methylphenidate, decreased hyperactivity and inattention and improved social communication in children with ASD. The most commonly reported side effects in these children include irritability, lethargy, tics, sadness, and social withdrawal [Di Martino *et al.*, 2004; Jahromi *et al.*, 2009; Posey *et al.*, 2007; Research Units on Paediatric Psychopharmacology (RUPP), 2005].

SSRIs as a putative innovative approach

Existing approaches to developing pharmacotherapeutic targets include observing for phenotypic similarities between ASD core symptoms and other known neuropsychiatric disease. One example is the case of selective serotonin reuptake inhibitors (SSRIs), with their dramatic effects on decreasing the repetitive behaviours and intrusive thoughts of obsessive-compulsive disorder.

Converging evidence from genetic, imaging, and drug treatment studies has implicated serotonin dysregulation in ASD (Hanley et al., 1977; Cook & Leventhal, 1996; Di Martino et al., 2007; Nakamura et al., 2010; Sacco et al., 2010). Additionally, hyperserotonaemia is present in approximately 25 per cent of children with ASD and their family members (Cook & Leventhal, 1996; Mulder et al., 2004 ; Schain & Freedman, 1961). Common SLC6A4 variants of platelet antidepressant-sensitive serotonin transporter (SERT; 5-HTT) are only modestly associated with ASD (Devlin et al., 2005), but rare SERT coding variants (conferring increased 5-HT transport in transfected cells as well as in lymphoblasts) derived from SERT variant-expressing probands, have been shown to be over-transmitted to autism probands, and to be associated with both rigid-compulsive behaviour and sensory aversion (Sutcliffe et al., 2005) in humans and to hyperserotonaemia, serotonin receptor hypersensitivity, social impairment, and repetitive behaviour in transgenic mice (Veenstra-VanderWeele et al., 2012).

Studies with the serotonergic tricyclic antidepressant clomipramine have shown contrasting results for anger and ritualized behaviours in ASD: in a 10-week, double-blind placebo-controlled, crossover study, in 24 autistic subjects, clomipramine was superior to both placebo and desipramine on ratings of autistic symptoms (including stereotypies), anger, and compulsive, ritualized behaviours as measured by the Autism Relevant Subscale of the Children's Psychiatric Rating Scale, the Modified Comprehensive Psychopathological Rating Scale–Obsessive-Compulsive Disorder Subscale, with no difference between desipramine and placebo (Gordon et al., 1993). A less significant efficacy for clomipramine was observed in another 7-week RCT on 36 young patients (Remington et al., 2001) and no efficacy was observed (one patient improved, six worsened) in a 5-week open study on 3- to 9-year-old children (Sanchez et al., 1996).

More recently, the SSRI fluvoxamine has been shown to be superior to placebo for repetitive behaviour, aggression, and social relatedness in adults with autism (McDougle et al., 1996); in a similar study in children by the same group, however, only 1 of 18 subjects on fluoxetine showed clinical improvement, whereas significant adverse events were common (Posey et al., 2007). In a 4-month-long open study on 121 children ranging in age from 2 to 8 years fluoxetine induced a good or excellent improvement in almost 70 per cent of patients (De Long et al., 2002), measured by clinical judgment; in an 8-week placebo-controlled double-blind study on 45 children and adolescents liquid fluoxetine (mean final dose: 9.9 ± 4.35 mg/day) was superior to placebo in the treatment of repetitive behaviours by the CY–BOCS compulsion scale, but not on CGI autism score (Hollander et al., 2005) and these results were confirmed by a 12-week double-blind placebo-controlled fluoxetine trial on 36 adult patients (Hollander et al., 2012).

On the other hand, a large double-blind placebo controlled study on 149 ASD patients, aged 5 to 17 years, with high levels of repetitive behaviour, showed that citalopram was not effective in improving results on either the Children's Yale–Brown Obsessive Compulsive Scales for pervasive developmental, or the CGI Improvement Scale (King et al., 2009). Citalopram use was also significantly associated with adverse events, particularly increased energy level, impulsiveness, decreased concentration, hyperactivity, stereotypy, diarrhoea, and insomnia,

A Cochrane review on the efficacy and safety of SSRIs for ASD indicated that there is reasonable support for their use for treating repetitive behaviours and perhaps other core symptoms in adults with ASD, but so far there is a lack of supporting evidence in children and adolescents (Williams et al., 2010).

The lack of evidence of SSRI efficacy in young patients with ASD may be related to heterogeneity in patients and/or assessment tools (Reiersen & Handen, 2011) or wrong symptoms targeting (*i.e.*, repetitive behaviours which the subject enjoys, instead of anxiety, which is distressing). Moreover, outcome measures validated in normally developing patients may not be appropriate to measure anxiety symptoms in ASD youngsters, which may present differently from those in non-ASD children and adolescents. Therefore, an improved definition of target symptoms (specific anxiety symptoms *vs.* repetitive behaviours) and the use of appropriate assessment tools could significantly improve the quality of the trials and lead to more conclusive results. Clinical trials with SSRIs in ASD children and adolescents have used reduction in restricted and repetitive behaviours (RRBs) as a proxy for anxiety. However, not all autistic youngsters with comorbid anxiety disorder, show significant RRBs. It is also important to consider that lower-IQ participants may show lower clinical response to treatments either because of specific difference in brain development or because patients may be unable to correctly report their feeling and may relate behaviour to anxiety when it is actually related to other problems (pain, sadness, etc.). For all these reasons, fluoxetine is also in phase III trials for ASD and benefits from FDA 'Fast Track' and 'Orphan Drug' status.

Research and development trends

Very few drugs with innovative mechanisms of action have been clinically developed in the last 30 years. As an example it could be considered that all the available antipsychotics work by blocking the D2 receptor, such as chlorpromazine, which was discovered in 1954–1956 (second-generation antipsychotic drugs tends to block receptors in the dopaminergic and serotonergic systems). Developing efficacious treatments for the core symptoms of ASDs is considered to be the primary unmet need. Research has changed focus from behavioural observation of ASDs to translating findings from animal models, genomic manipulation studies, and basic science studies to pharmacologic agents with the aim of lessening or reversing the core symptoms of autism.

Although substantial progress has been made in identifying specific aetiologic mechanisms of ASD, most of the genetic risk architecture remains unknown, and the genetic lesions that have been identified are highly heterogeneous. The prevailing view is that the syndrome of autism is a common manifestation of many individually rare gene mutations (Betancur, 2011). Understanding physiologic processes affected by these mutations may establish a molecular logic for development of novel therapeutic interventions, as well as elucidating the pathophysiology of single-gene disorders associated with ASD. Common genetic syndromes associated with ASD include the fragile X syndrome and tuberous sclerosis; the genetic aetiology is known and animal models with similar mutations have been developed to study ASD (Carlson, 2012).

New insight from fragile X syndrome

The fragile X syndrome (FXS) is the most common inherited form of human mental retardation. It is typically caused by a trinucleotide repeat expansion in the X-linked FMR1 gene that prevents expression of the encoded protein, called fragile X mental retardation protein (FMRP; D'Hulst & Kooy, 2009; Hagerman, 2006). The role of the FMRP protein is linked to neurons, astrocytes, dendritic transport, and regulation of synaptic protein synthesis. FMRP inhibits translation by complexing with mRNA associated with polyribosomes in basilar dendrites, leading to unopposed stimulation of protein synthesis, mediated by the mGluR5 subtype of group 1 metabotropic receptors, a receptor Gq-protein linked positively coupled to phospholipase C (Chen, 1992; Darrah *et al.*, 2008; Silverman *et al.*, 2010; Takagi *et al.*, 2010).

It is important to note that the neurotransmitter glutamate is the primary excitatory neurotransmitter in mammalian brain and is responsible for most corticocortical and corticofugal neurotransmission. Glutamate mediates its effects at multiple ionotropic and metabotropic receptors. Ionotropic receptors are characterized by sensitivity to synthetic glutamate derivatives including N-methyl-D-aspartate (NMDA) and 2-amino-3-(5-methyl-3-oxo-1,2-oxazol-4-yl) propanoic acid (AMPA). Both NMDA (NMDAR) and AMPA (AMPAR) receptors are composed by multiple subunits surrounding a central pore, with receptor properties varying, depending upon exact channel composition. Metabotropic glutamate receptors (mGluRs) are divided into groups on the basis of their second-messenger coupling and ligand sensitivity. Group I receptors (mGluR1/5) predominantly potentiate both presynaptic glutamate release and postsynaptic NMDAR currents. In contrast, group II (mGluR2/3) receptors, in general, limit glutamate release, particularly during conditions of glutamate spillover from the synaptic cleft. Group III receptors (mGluR4/6/7/8) show more variable distribution, but also generally inhibit glutamate function. Many of these receptors become rapidly downregulated during stimulation. Thus, positive (PAM) and negative (NAM) allosteric modulators may be more effective in altering receptor activity than more traditional orthosteric agonists, antagonists, and mixed agonists/antagonists (Javitt et al., 2011).

Thus, the absence of the FMRP will result in an upregulating of mGluR5-mediated protein synthesis, leading in turn to abnormal protein synthesis. Much of the mGluR5 hypothesis of fragile X syndrome was established by disrupting FMR1 in mice, zebrafish and *Drosophila* (Bardoni & Mandel, 2002; den Broeder et al., 2009; McBride et al., 2005). FMR1 knock-out (KO) mice showed impaired social interaction and increased seizure susceptibility and anxiety (Westmark et al., 2009). Increased mGluR5 activity in the $FMR1^{-/-}$ mouse led to the prediction that the mGluR5 antagonist may rescue some of these features.

In the brain of an FXS mouse model, total and plasma membrane protein levels of major potassium channel regulating hippocampal neuronal excitability (Kv4.2) are reduced. Antagonizing mGlu5 activity with 2-methyl-6-(phenylethynyl)-pyridine (MPEP) partially rescues reduced surface Kv4.2 levels in Fmr1 KO mice, suggesting that excess mGlu1/5 signal activity contributes to Kv4.2 dysregulation. Absence of FMRP-mediated positive control of Kv4.2 mRNA translation, protein expression, and plasma membrane levels might contribute to excess neuronal excitability in FMR1 KO mice, and thus imply a potential mechanism underlying FXS-associated epilepsy (Meredith et al., 2011).

Burket and colleagues (2011) examined the effects of MPEP (30 mg/kg, intraperitoneally) on sociability and stereotypic behaviours in BTBR T+tfJ mice (a putative mouse model of ASD, derived from Balb/c strain) and Swiss Webster mice in a standard paradigm. MPEP had complex effects on sociability, impairing some measures of sociability in both strains (MPEP-treated mice spent less time engaged in sniffing the enclosed social stimulus mouse), while it reduced the intensity of some spontaneous measures of stereotypic behaviours emerging during free social interaction in Swiss Webster mice. Although stereotypic behaviours may be an important therapeutic target in ASDs, this study showed that medication strategies to attenuate their severity via antagonism of mGluR5 receptors must be pursued cautiously, since their potential to worsen at least some measures of sociability (Burket et al., 2011).

Another recent study (Mehta et al., 2011) analyzed the therapeutic potential of MPEP on repetitive and anxiety-like behaviours in the valproic acid (VPA) mouse model of autism. It was demonstrated that a single prenatal exposure to VPA, which is associated with a 7–10-fold increased relative risk for ASD in humans, induces in mice selective behavioural and electrophysiologic deficits analogous to those seen in the clinical population (Bromley et al., 2008;

Rasalam et al., 2005). In this study mice were exposed prenatally to VPA and assessed for repetitive self-grooming and marble-burying behaviours as adults. VPA-exposed mice displayed increased repetitive and anxiety-like behaviours, consistent with previously published results. MPEP significantly reduced repetitive behaviours in mice, but had no effect on locomotor activity (Mehta et al., 2011). Other biochemical pathways that show promise as pharmacologic targets are receptor-initiated signaling pathways such as the phosphoinositide 3-kinase (PI3K) and mTOR (mammalian target of rapamycin) pathways. Both are linked to mGluR-mediated signaling and also are seen in fragile X and tuberous sclerosis.

Tuberous sclerosis

Tuberous sclerosis complex (TSC) is a single-gene disorder resulting from mutation in the tuberous sclerosis complex-1 or -2 genes (*TSC1* or *TSC2* genes). *TSC* genes encode proteins that are involved in complex signaling pathways that control cell growth and size (Jozwiak, 2006; Kwiatkowski & Manning, 2005). *TSC1* is on chromosome 9q34 and encodes *hamartin*. Hamartin may inhibit tumor formation by regulating cell adhesion through actin-binding proteins of the ezrin–radixin–moiesin (ERM) family. *TSC2* resides on chromosome 16p13 and encodes *tuberin*, a GTPase-activating protein (GAP) that inhibits the RAS-related super-family of small G-proteins such as Rheb (Ras homolog enriched in brain). Hamartin and tuberin form a functional protein complex that constitutively inhibits mTOR. mTOR is a serine-threonine kinase that receives input from multiple signaling pathways to stimulate protein synthesis and hence increase cell proliferation and growth, by phosphorylating key translation regulators.

An important modulator of *TSC1* is AKT, a potent prosurvival and pro-oncogenic protein that is activated by phosphatidylinositol triphosphate. AKT is a protein kinase that directly phosphorylates TSC2 and inhibits its function. mTOR regulates translations of p70S6-kinase and 4EBP1. p70S6-kinase increases ribosome biogenesis by phosphorylating ribosomal protein S6. 4E-BP1 is a eukaryote initiation factor that acts as a translational repressor by binding and inhibiting the eukaryotic translation initiation factor 4E. The loss of TSC1 (hamartin) or TSC2 (tuberin) function leads to selective activation of the mTOR cascade, resulting in a TOR-dependent increase of ribosomal S6, p70S6-kinase, and 4E-BP1 (Inoki et al., 2005).

Loss of function of either gene can lead to the full clinical spectrum of TSC although individuals with TSC2 inactivation tend to have more severe disease manifestations (Ess, 2009; Dabora et al., 2001). TSC has an impact on multiple organs; brain manifestations are especially debilitating on account of a very high prevalence of epilepsy, developmental delay, autism, and mental retardation (Rosser et al., 2006). Individuals with TSC have an approximately 100-fold increase in the probability of being diagnosed with autism compared with the general population (Hunt & Shepherd, 1993).

The use of the mTOR inhibitor rapamycin has been shown to reverse learning and memory impairments in adult mice (Auerbach et al., 2011; Ehninger et al., 2009). Rapamycin (sirolimus) is a macrolide compound obtained from *Streptomyces hygroscopicus* that acts by selectively blocking the transcriptional activation of cytokines, thereby inhibiting cytokine production. Sirolimus is a potent immunosuppressant and possesses both antifungal and antineoplastic properties. Everolimus (RAD-001) is the 40-*O*-(2-hydroxyethyl) derivative of sirolimus and works similarly as an mTOR inhibitor. It is currently used as an immunosuppressant to prevent rejection of organ transplant and the treatment of renal cell cancer. Much research has also been conducted on everolimus and other mTOR inhibitors for use in a number of kinds of cancer.

Recently rapamycin has been shown to reverse impaired social interaction in the Tcs2$^{+/-}$ mouse model of tuberous sclerosis (Sato et al., 2012). Human studies are currently under way to evaluate the potential of rapamycin and similar compounds to produce behavioural improvements in ASD. For example, the trial of RAD001 and neurocognition in the tuberous sclerosis complex (TSC) evaluates the efficacy of RAD001 on neurocognition in patients with TSC compared to placebo as measured by well-validated, standardized, direct and indirect neurocognitive tools (see www.clinicaltrials.gov).

NMDA receptor antagonists

Other targets in this system are also of interest, including memantine hydrochloride (NMDA receptor antagonist that is currently used to treat adults with Alzheimer's disease). Recently, in Fmr1 knockout (KO) mice, a mouse model for the fragile X syndrome (FXS) and syndromic autism, it has been shown that memantine stimulates synapse formation and dendritic spine maturation (Wei et al., 2012). In a large clinical trial involving 151 subjects, Chez and colleagues (2007) observed that open-label use of memantine significantly improved language function, social behaviour, and self-stimulatory behaviours of autistic subjects and similar results have been shown in a small preliminary double-blind placebo-controlled trial (Ghaleiha et al., 2012). Studies are under way with memantine on larger number of autistic subjects (see www.clinicaltrials.gov).

Also D-cycloserine, a partial agonist of NMDA, may be a viable treatment strategy for social deficits of ASD, and studies of this in animal models have led to encouraging results (Deutsch et al., 2012; Modi & Young, 2011). Animal models are powerful tools for investigation of the neurobiological mechanism regulating the cognitive processes leading to the development of social relationships and for potentially extending our understanding of the human condition. Social bonding in the monogamous prairie vole, which is assessed in the laboratory using a partner preference paradigm, is a higher order and multidimensional social cognitive process that involves functional circuits for social recognition, social reward and reinforcement, and associative social learning (Lim & Young, 2006). Modi & Young (2011) showed that a low dose of D-cycloserine administered peripherally enhanced preference formation in prairie voles but not meadow voles under conditions in which it would not otherwise occur. More recently, Deutsch and colleagues (2012) showed that D-cycloserine improved measures of impaired sociability and reduced intensity of stereotypic behaviours in Balb/c mice. Data suggest that targeting the NMDA receptor can have promising therapeutic effects on two prominent domains of psychopathology in ASDs: impaired sociability and spontaneous stereotypic behaviours.

Oxytocin

Oxytocin, a cyclic nonapeptide, has brought new excitement to autism treatment research (Bartz & Hollander, 2008; Hollander et al., 2003) because individuals with ASD have been found to have a reduction in plasma oxytocin concentrations and/or mutations in either the oxytocin receptor or in the peptide itself (Jacob et al., 2007; Modahl et al., 1998). Oxytocin is involved in the development of emotional and social affiliative behaviours including bonding and mating. Therefore, the low levels of oxytocin in persons with ASD were proposed as a plausible cause of some of the social deficits in autism. Thus targeting central oxytocin production or secretion may alter social behaviours in children. A limiting factor is the short half-life of oxytocin when administered either centrally or peripherally. A single intravenous dose of oxytocin has been shown to reduce repetitive behaviours, and improves affective speech comprehension in individuals with ASD (Hollander *et al.*, 2007). Intranasal oxytocin is now being studied as a possible modality for drug administration in children and adolescents with ASD. A recent randomized double-blind crossover trial using intranasal oxytocin showed improvement in emotional recognition in young children with ASD (Guastella *et al.*, 2010). Now an early-stage (Phase I) drug in the pipeline includes a transnasal formulation of the oxytocin receptor agonist carbetocin (Kyalin Biosciences). More information on oxytocin may be found in chapter 20 of this volume.

Conclusions

As shown in this chapter, there are no currently available medications that significantly lessen deficits in social interaction and communication, nor mitigate stereotypies or repetitive behaviours, which are the core symptoms of ASD. Still, fragmentary but accumulating evidence suggests that reducing the interference of repetitive, stereotyped, hyperactive/impulsive, and aggressive behaviours through the judicious administration of psychotropic medications may allow some children with pervasive developmental disorders (PDDs) to more fully access educational and psychosocial interventions.

New molecular targets have been identified in disorders different from "idiopathic" ASDs, but mimicking ASD core features such communicative and social impairment, or repetitive behaviours. Larger controlled comparison trials are urgently needed to both optimize the current pharmacologic armamentarium as well as to confirm the new insights gained from ongoing molecular, genetic, and neuroscientific studies that are crucial for the development of novel and more effective treatments in the future.

Conflicts of interest: Dr Zuddas has received research grants or served as speaker, advisor, or consultant for AstraZeneca, Bristol-Myers Squibb/Otsuka, Lilly, Lundbeck, Schering-Plough, Shire and Vifor.

References

Abikoff, H., McGough, J., Vitiello, B., *et al.*; RUPP ADHD/Anxiety Study Group (2005): Sequential pharmacotherapy for children with comorbid attention-deficit/hyperactivity and anxiety disorders. *J. Am. Acad. Child Adolesc. Psychiatry* **44**, 418–427.

American Psychiatric Association (2000): *Diagnostic and Statistical Manual of Mental Disorders*, 4th ed, Text Revision (DSM-IV-TR). Washington, DC: American Psychiatric Association.

Auerbach, B.D., Osterweil, E.K. & Bear, M.F. (2011): Mutations causing syndromic autism define an axis of synaptic pathophysiology. *Nature* **480**, 63–68.

Bardoni, B. & Mandel, J.L. (2002): Advances in understanding of fragile X pathogenesis and FMRP function, and in identification of X linked mental retardation genes. *Curr. Opin. Genet. Dev.* **12**, 284–293.

Bartz, J.A. & Hollander, E. (2008): Oxytocin and experimental therapeutics in autism spectrum disorders. *Prog. Brain Res.* **170**, 451–462.

Betancur, C. (2011): Etiological heterogeneity in autism spectrum disorders: more than 100 genetic and genomic disorders and still counting. *Brain Res.* **1380**, 42–77.

Brereton, A.V., Tonge, B.J. & Einfeld, S.L. (2006): Psychopathology in children and adolescents with autism compared to young people with intellectual disability. *J. Autism Dev. Disord.* **36**, 863–870.

Bromley, R.L., Mawer, G., Clayton-Smith, J. & Baker, G.A. (2008): Autism spectrum disorders following in utero exposure to antiepileptic drugs. *Neurology* **71**, 1923–1924.

Burket, J.A., Herndon, A.L., Winebarger, E.E., Jacome, L.F. & Deutsch, S.I. (2011): Complex effects of mGluR5 antagonism on sociability and stereotypic behaviors in mice: possible implications for the pharmacotherapy of autism spectrum disorders. *Brain Res. Bull.* **86**, 152–158.

Carlson, G.C. (2012): Glutamate receptor dysfunction and drug targets across models of autism spectrum disorders. *Pharmacol. Biochem. Behav.* **100**, 850–854.

Centers for Disease Control and Prevention. Boyle, C.A., Boulet, S., Schieve, L.A., et al. (2011): Trends in the prevalence of developmental disabilities in US children, 1997–2008. *Pediatrics* **127**, 1034–1042.

Chen, H.S., Pellegrini, J.W., Aggarwal, S.K., et al. (1992): Open-channel block of N-methyl-D-aspartate (NMDA) responses by memantine: therapeutic advantage against receptor-mediated neurotoxicity. *J. Neurosci.* **12**, 4427–4436.

Chez, M.G., Burton, Q., Dowling, T., Chang, M., Khanna, P. & Kramer, C. (2007): Memantine as adjunctive therapy in children diagnosed with autistic spectrum disorders: an observation of initial clinical response and maintenance tolerability. *J. Child Neurol.* **22**, 574–579.

Cook, E.H. & Leventhal, B.L. (1996): The serotonin system in autism. *Curr. Opin. Pediatr.* **8**, 348–354.

Dabora, S.L., Jozwiak, S., Franz, D.N., et al. (2001): Mutational analysis in a cohort of 224 tuberous sclerosis patients indicates increased severity of TSC2, compared with TSC1, disease in multiple organs. *Am. J. Hum. Genet.* **68**, 64–80.

Darrah, J.M., Stefani, M.R. & Moghaddam, B. (2008): Interaction of N-methyl-D-aspartate and group 5 metabotropic glutamate receptors on behavioral flexibility using a novel operant set-shift paradigm. *Behav. Pharmacol.* **19**, 225–234.

de Bruin, E.I., Ferdinand, R.F., Meester, S., de Nijs, P.F. & Verheij, F. (2007): High rates of psychiatric co-morbidity in PDD-NOS. *J. Autism Dev. Disord.* **37**, 877–886.

den Broeder, M.J., van der Linde, H., Brouwer, J.Jr, Oostra, B.A., Willemsen, R. & Ketting, R.F. (2009): Generation and characterization of FMR1 knockout zebrafish. *PLoS One* **4**, e7910.

DeLong, G.R., Ritch, C.R. & Burch, S. (2002): Fluoxetine response in children with autistic spectrum disorders: correlation with familial major affective disorder and intellectual achievement. *Dev. Med. Child Neurol.* **44**, 652–659.

Devlin, B., Cook, E.H., Jr. & Coon, H. (2005): Autism and the serotonin transporter: the long and short of it. *Mol. Psychiatry* **10**, 1110–1116.

Deutsch, S.I., Pepe, G.J., Burket, J.A., Winebarger, E.E., Herndon, A.L. & Benson, A.D. (2012): D-cycloserine improves sociability and spontaneous stereotypic behaviors in 4-week old mice. *Brain Res.* **1439**, 96–107.

D'Hulst, C. & Kooy, R.F. (2009): Fragile X syndrome: from molecular genetics to therapy. *J. Med. Genet.* **46**, 577–584.

Di Martino, A., Melis, G., Cianchetti, C. & Zuddas, A. (2004): Methylphenidate for pervasive developmental disorders: safety and efficacy of acute single dose test and ongoing therapy: an open-pilot study. *J. Child Adolesc. Psychopharmacol.* **14**, 207–218.

Di Martino, A., Dickstein, S.G., Zuddas, A. & Castellanos, F.X. (2007): Psychopharmacology of autism spectrum disorders. In: *Handbook of Contemporary Neuropharmacology*, eds. D. Sibley et al., pp. 319–344. Hoboken, NJ: John Wiley.

Ehninger, D., de Vries, P.J. & Silva, A.J. (2009): From mTOR to cognition: molecular and cellular mechanisms of cognitive impairments in tuberous sclerosis. *J. Intellect. Disabil. Res.* **53**, 838–851.

Ess, K.C. (2009): Tuberous sclerosis complex: everything old is new again. *J. Neurodev. Disord.* **1**, 141–149.

Ghaleiha, A., Asadabadi, M., Mohammadi, M.R., et al. (2012): Memantine as adjunctive treatment to risperidone in children with autistic disorder: a randomized, double-blind, placebo-controlled trial. *Int. J. Neuropsychopharmacol.* **24**, 1–7.

Gordon, C.T., State, R.C., Nelson, J.E., Hamburger, S.D. & Rapoport, J.L. (1993): A double-blind comparison of clomipramine, desipramine, and placebo in the treatment of autistic disorder. *Arch. Gen. Psychiatry* **50**, 441–447.

Guastella, A.J., Einfeld, S.L., Gray, K.M., et al. (2010): Intranasal oxytocin improves emotion recognition for youth with autism spectrum disorders. *Biol. Psychiatry* **67**, 692–694.

Gustavsson, A., Svensson, M., Jacobi, F., et al. (2011): Cost of disorders of the brain in Europe 2010. *Eur. Neuropsychopharmacol.* **21**, 718–779.

Hagerman, R.J. (2006): Lessons from fragile X regarding neurobiology, autism, and neurodegeneration. *J. Dev. Behav. Pediatr.* **27**, 63–74.

Hanley, H.G., Stahl, S.M. & Freedman, D.X. (1977): Hyperserotonemia and amine metabolites in autistic and retarded children. *Arch. Gen. Psychiatry* **34**, 521–531.

Hollander, E., Novotny, S., Hanratty, M., et al. (2003): Oxytocin infusion reduces repetitive behaviors in adults with autistic and Asperger's disorders. *Neuropsychopharmacology* **28**, 193–198.

Hollander, E., Phillips, A., Chaplin, W., et al. (2005): A placebo controlled crossover trial of liquid fluoxetine on repetitive behaviors in childhood and adolescent autism. *Neuropsychopharmacology* **30**, 582–589.

Hollander, E., Bartz, J., Chaplin, W., et al. (2007): Oxytocin increases retention of social cognition in autism. *Biol. Psychiatry* **61**, 498–503.

Hollander, E., Soorya, L., Chaplin, W., et al. (2012): A double-blind placebo-controlled trial of fluoxetine for repetitive behaviors and global severity in adult autism spectrum disorders. *Am. J. Psychiatry* **169**, 292–299.

Hunt, A. & Shepherd, C. (1993): A prevalence study of autism in tuberous sclerosis. *J. Autism Dev. Disord.* **23**, 323–339.

Inoki, K., Corradetti, M.N. & Guan, K.L. (2005): Dysregulation of the TSC-mTOR pathway in human disease. *Nat Genet.* **37**, 19–24.

Jacob, S., Brune, C.W., Carter, C.S., Leventhal, B.L., Lord, C. & Cook, E.H., Jr. (2007): Association of the oxytocin receptor gene (OXTR) in Caucasian children and adolescents with autism. *Neurosci. Lett.* **417**, 6–9.

Jahromi, L.B., Kasari, C.L., McCracken, J.T., et al. (2009): Positive effects of methylphenidate on social communication and self-regulation in children with pervasive developmental disorders and hyperactivity. *J. Autism Dev. Disord.* **39**, 395–404.

Javitt, D.C., Schoepp, D., Kalivas, P.W., et al. (2011): Translating glutamate: from pathophysiology to treatment. *Sci. Transl. Med.* **3** (102),102mr2.

Jozwiak, J. (2006): Hamartin and tuberin: working together for tumour suppression. *Int. J. Cancer* **118**, 1–5.

King, B.H., Hollander, E., Sikich, L., et al., STAART Psychopharmacology Network (2009): Lack of efficacy of citalopram in children with autism spectrum disorders and high levels of repetitive behavior: citalopram ineffective in children with autism. *Arch Gen Psychiatry* **66**, 583–590.

Kwiatkowski, D.J. & Manning, B.D. (2005): Tuberous sclerosis: a GAP at the crossroads of multiple signaling pathways. *Hum. Mol. Genet.* **14**, 251–258.

Levy, S.E., Mandell, D.S. & Schultz, R.T. (2009): Autism. *Lancet* **374**, 1627–1638.

Leyfer, O.T., Folstein, S.E., Bacalman, S., et al. (2006): Comorbid psychiatric disorders in children with autism: interview development and rates of disorders. *J. Autism Dev. Disord.* **36**, 849–861.

Lim, M.M. & Young, L.J. (2004): Vasopresin-dependent neural circuits underlying pair bond formation in the monogamous prairie role. *Neuroscience* **125**, 35–45.

Marcus, R.N., Owen, R., Kamen, L., Manos, G., McQuade, R.D., Carson, W.H. & Aman, M.G. (2009): A placebo-controlled, fixed-dose study of aripiprazole in children and adolescents with irritability associated with autistic disorder. *J. Am. Acad. Child Adolesc. Psychiatry* **48**, 1110–1119.

McBride, S.M., Choi, C.H., Wang, Y., et al. (2005): Pharmacological rescue of synaptic plasticity, courtship behavior, and mushroom body defects in a Drosophila model of fragile X syndrome. *Neuron* **45**, 753–764.

McCracken, J.T., McGough, J., Shah, B., Cronin, P., et al., Research Units on Pediatric Psychopharmacology Autism Network (2002): Risperidone in children with autism and serious behavioral problems. *N. Engl. J. Med.* **34**, 314–321.

McDougle, C.J., Naylor, S.T., Cohen, D.J., et al. (1996): A double-blind, placebo-controlled study of fluvoxamine in adults with autistic disorder. *Arch. Gen. Psychiatry* **53**, 1001–1008.

McDougle, C.J., Erickson, C.A., Stigler, K.A. & Posey, D.J. (2005): Neurochemistry in the pathophysiology of autism. *J. Clin. Psychiatry* **66** (Suppl. 10), 9–1.

McPheeters, M.L., Warren, Z., Sathe, N., et al. (2011): A systematic review of medical treatments for children with autism spectrum disorders. *Pediatrics* **127**, e1312–1321.

Mehta, M.V., Gandal, M.J. & Siegel, S.J. (2011): mGluR5-antagonist mediated reversal of elevated stereotyped, repetitive behaviors in the VPA model of autism. *PLoS One* **6**, e26077.

Meredith, R.M., de Jong, R. & Mansvelder, H.D. (2011): Functional rescue of excitatory synaptic transmission in the developing hippocampus in Fmr1-KO mouse. *Neurobiol. Dis.* **41**, 104–110.

Modahl, C., Green, L., Fein, D., et al. (1998): Plasma oxytocin levels in autistic children. *Biol Psychiatry* **43**, 270–277.

Modi, M.E. & Young, L.J. (2011): D-cycloserine facilitates socially reinforced learning in an animal model relevant to autism spectrum disorders. *Biol. Psychiatry* **70**, 298–304.

Mulder, E.J., Anderson, G.M., Kema, I.P., et al. (2004): Platelet serotonin levels in pervasive developmental disorders and mental retardation: diagnostic group differences, within-group distribution, and behavioral correlates. *J. Am. Acad. Child Adolesc. Psychiatry* **43**, 491–499.

Nakamura, K., Sekine, S. & Ouchi, Y. (2010): Brain serotonin and dopamine transporter bindings in adults with high-functioning autism. *Arch. Gen. Psychiatry* **67**, 59–68.

Nightingale, S. (2012): Autism spectrum disorders. *Nat. Rev. Drug Discov.* **11**, 745–746.

Owen, R., Sikich, L., Marcus, R.N., et al. (2009): Aripiprazole in the treatment of irritability in children and adolescents with autistic disorder. *Pediatrics* **124**, 1533–1540.

Posey, D.J. & McDougle, C.J. (2000): The pharmacotherapy of target symptoms associated with autistic disorder and other pervasive developmental disorders. *Harv. Rev. Psychiatry* **8**, 45–63.

Posey, D.J., Aman, M.G., McCracken, J.T., et al. (2007): Positive effects of methylphenidate on inattention and hyperactivity in pervasive developmental disorders: an analysis of secondary measures. *Biol. Psychiatry* **61**, 538–544.

Rasalam, A.D., Hailey, H., Williams, J.H., *et al.* (2005): Characteristics of fetal anticonvulsant syndrome associated autistic disorder. *Dev. Med. Child Neurol.* **47,** 551–555.

Reiersen, A.M. & Handen, B. (2011): Commentary on 'Selective serotonin reuptake inhibitors (SSRIs) for autism spectrum disorders (ASD)'. *Evid.-Based Child Health* **6,** 1082–1085.

Remington, G., Sloman, L., Konstantareas, M., Parker, K. & Gow, R. (2001): Clomipramine versus haloperidol in the treatment of autistic disorder: a double-blind, placebo-controlled, crossover study. *J. Clin. Psychopharmacol.* **21,** 440–444.

Research Units on Pediatric Psychopharmacology Autism Network [RUPP] (2005): Randomized, controlled, crossover trial of methylphenidate in pervasive developmental disorders with hyperactivity. *Arch. Gen. Psychiatry* **62,** 1266–1274.

Rosser, T., Panigrahy, A. & McClintock, W. (2006): The diverse clinical manifestations of tuberous sclerosis complex: a review. *Semin. Pediatr. Neurol.* **13,** 27–36.

Sacco, R., Curatolo, P., Manzi, B., *et al.* (2010): Principal pathogenetic components and biological endophenotypes in autism spectrum disorders. *Autism Res.* **3,** 237–252.

Sanchez, L.E., Campbell, M., Small, A.M., Cueva, J.E., Armenteros, J.L. & Adams, P.B. (1996): A pilot study of clomipramine in young autistic children. *J. Am. Acad. Child Adolesc. Psychiatry* **35,** 537–544.

Sato, A., Kasai, S., Kobayashi, T., Takamatsu, Y., Hino, O., Ikeda, K. & Mizuguchi, M. (2012): Rapamycin reverses impaired social interaction in mouse models of tuberous sclerosis complex. *Nat. Commun.* **3,** 1292.

Schain, R.J. & Freedman, D.X. (1961): Studies on 5-hydroxyindole metabolism in autistic and other mentally retarded children. *J. Pediatr.* **58,** 315–320.

Silverman, J.L., Tolu, S.S., Barkan, C.L. & Cranley, J.N. (2010): Repetitive self-grooming behaviour in the BTBR mouse model of autism is blocked by the mGluR5 antagonist MPEP. *Neuropsychopharmacology* **35,** 976-989.

Simonoff, E., Taylor, E., Baird, G., *et al.* (2012): Randomized controlled double-blind trial of optimal dose methylphenidate in children and adolescents with severe attention deficit hyperactivity disorder and intellectual disability. *J. Child Psychol. Psychiatry* [E-pub 7 Jun 2012].

Skokauskas, N. & Gallagher, L. (2012): Mental health aspects of autistic spectrum disorders in children. *J. Intellect. Disabil. Res.* **56,** 248–57.

Sutcliffe, J.S., Delahanty, R.J., Prasad, H.C., *et al.* (2005): Allelic heterogeneity at the serotonin transporter locus (SLC6A4) confers susceptibility to autism and rigid-complusive behaviors. *Am J. Hum. Genet.* **77,** 265–279.

Takagi, N., Besshoh, S., Morita, H., Terao, M., Takeo, S. & Tanonaka, K. (2010): Metabotropic glutamate mGlu5 receptor-mediated serine phosphorylation of NMDA receptor subunit NR1 in hippocampal CA1 region after transient global ischemia in rats. *Eur. J. Pharmacol.* **644,** 96–100.

Veenstra-VanderWeele, J. & Blakely, R.D. (2012): Networking in autism: leveraging genetic, biomarker and model system findings in the search for new treatments. *Neuropsychopharmacology* **37,** 196–212.

Veenstra-VanderWeele, J., Muller, C.L., Iwamoto, H., *et al.* (2012): Autism gene variant causes hyperserotonemia, serotonin receptor hypersensitivity, social impairment and repetitive behavior. *Proc. Natl. Acad. Sci. USA* **109,** 5469–5474.

Warren, Z., McPheeters, M.L., Sathe, N., Foss-Feig, J.H., Glasser, A. & Veenstra-Vanderweele, J. (2011): A systematic review of early intensive intervention for autism spectrum disorders. *Pediatrics* **127,** e1303–1311.

Wei, H., Doblein, C., Sheikh, A.M., Malik, M., Brown, W.T. & Li, X. (2012): The therapeutic effect of memantine through the stimulation of synapse formation and dendritic spine maturation in autism and fragile X syndrome. *PLoS One* **7,** e36981.

Westmark, C.J., Westmark, P.R. & Malter, J.S. (2009): MPEP reduces seizure severity in Fmr-1 KO mice over expressing human Abeta. *Int. J. Clin. Exp. Pathol.* **3,** 56–58.

Williams, K., Wheeler, D.M., Silove, N. & Hazell, P. (2010): Selective serotonin reuptake inhibitors (SSRIs) for autism spectrum disorders (ASD). *Cochrane Database Syst Rev.* CD004677.

Wittchen, H.U., Jacobi, F., Rehm, J., *et al.* (2011): The size and burden of mental disorders and other disorders of the brain in Europe 2010. *Eur. Neuropsychopharmacol.* **21,** 655–679.

Zuddas, A., Di Martino, A., Muglia, P. & Cianchetti, C. (2000): Long-term risperidone for pervasive developmental disorder: efficacy, tolerability, and discontinuation. *J. Child Adolesc. Psychopharmacol.* **10,** 79–90.

Zuddas, A., Zanni, R. & Usala, T. (2011): Second generation antipsychotics (SGAs) for non-psychotic disorders in children and adolescents: a review of the randomized controlled studies. *Eur Neuropsychopharmacol.* **21,** 600–620.

Chapter 10

Pharmacologic treatment of autism in clinical practice

Gabriele Masi

*IRCCS Stella Maris, Institute of Child Neurology and Psychiatry,
via dei Giacinti 2, 56018 Calambrone, Pisa, Italy*
gabriele.masi@inpe.unipi.it

Summary

Pervasive developmental disorders (PDDs) always need both pharmacologic and nonpharmacologic interventions. Nonpharmacologic interventions include counseling for the patients and the family, psychological support, behavioural treatments, social and cognitive rehabilitation, assistance in social and scholastic activities, enhancement of social skills, and family support. In selected cases, the appropriate use of pharmacotherapy can alleviate some symptoms and behaviours and increase the efficacy of psychosocial interventions. Available literature on pharmacotherapy in children and adolescents with PDDs is critically reviewed in this chapter. Both first- and second-generation antipsychotics (particularly risperidone and aripiprazole) and selective serotonin reuptake inhibitors, stimulants, and mood stabilizers are principally reviewed and discussed. Randomized, placebo-controlled studies are discussed, as are the most relevant open-label or naturalistic studies. This chapter concludes with a brief discussion of other psychotropic medications, such as opioid antagonists, clonidine, and guanfacine, and glutamatergic agents (amantadine). Finally, practical guidelines for the management of specific clinical situations are provided.

Introduction

Pervasive developmental disorders (PDDs) are severe psychiatric conditions with onset in the first three years of life and are typically marked by impairments in reciprocal social interaction, communication, and cognitive development. Stereotyped behaviour, interest and activities are shared, in different ways and intensity, by the five subtypes of PDDs, that is, autistic disorder (the most severe and prototypical disorder), Asperger's syndrome, Rett syndrome, childhood disintegrative disorder, and PDD not otherwise specified (PDD–NOS). The appropriate use of medications can improve some maladaptive behaviours and increase the person's ability to benefit from nonpharmacologic interventions. Primary behavioural targets of pharmacotherapy in autism include severe behavioural disorders, aggression toward self and others, irritability, hyperactivity, stereotypies, repetitive phenomena and, to a lesser degree, impaired social behaviour (Masi, 2004). Although, to date, no medications have been seen to be effective on the core symptoms of autism, in the United States about 30 to 50 per cent of youth with PDDs take a psychotropic medication for at least 1 year (Aman *et al.*, 2003). The most-frequently prescribed medications are antipsychotics (both atypical and conventional), followed by antidepressants and stimulants. This review will address the available literature on children and adolescents with PDDs.

Atypical antipsychotics

A common feature of the atypical antipsychotics is the ability to produce an antipsychotic effect with lower incidence of acute or subacute extrapyramidal side effects, both in clinical and pre-clinical studies (little or no ability to induce catalepsy is seen in animal models) compared to the side effects that can occur with conventional antipsychotic drugs. It has been suggested that some symptoms of schizophrenia, such as isolation, apathia, and abulia that may respond to atypical antipsychotic drugs, are comparable to some of the core symptoms of PDDs, mainly emotional and social withdrawal, lack of interest in social relationships, stereotyped thinking, blunted affect, and lack of spontaneity and conversation. All these features may be better ameliorated by atypical antipsychotics, compared to conventional antipsychotic agents. To date, reports principally support the use of risperidone and aripiprazole, marketed in the United States for behavioural disorders and irritability in children and adolescents with PDDs.

Risperidone

Risperidone is currently the atypical antipsychotic most frequently used in patients with PDDs. Two controlled studies of risperidone have been published in persons with autism and related PDDs, one in adult patients (McDougle *et al.*, 1998), the other in children and adolescents (Research Units on Pediatric Psychopharmachology [RUPP] Autism Network, 2002). In the latter multi-site, double-blind, placebo-controlled study, 101 children and adolescents (age range 5–17 years, mean age 8.8 years) were randomized to receive risperidone (dose range 0.5 to 3.5 mg/daily) or placebo for eight weeks. On the basis of the CGI–I and the Aberrant Behaviour Checklist–Irritability score (ABC–I), 69 per cent of the patients in the risperidone group and 12 per cent in the placebo group showed a response at the eighth week. At the sixth month, the rate of responders decreased to 47 per cent. Irritability, hyperactivity, and stereotypies were more sensitive to treatment than social withdrawal and inappropriate speech. Increased appetite and weight gain (2.7 ± 2.9 kg), fatigue, and drowsiness were the most commonly reported side effects. In the follow-up, risperidone was effective not only on maladaptive behaviours (aggression, oppositional-defiance, and self-injury), but also on compulsions and repetitive phenomena, while only a trend to significance was found in social relatedness (McDougle *et al.*, 2005). When patients openly and effectively treated for 4 months with risperidone were randomized to risperidone or placebo in a double-blind design, relapse rate was 12.5 per cent in the risperidone group and 62 per cent in the placebo group (McDougle *et al.*, 2005).

In a further development of the RUPP study (Aman *et al.*, 2008), which explored the effect of risperidone on cognitive performance (38 subjects, 8-week study, risperidone dosage up to 3.5 mg/day), eye–hand coordination and spatial memory were not negatively affected by treatment, and there was an increase in sustained attention and verbal learning.

When moderators or mediators of response to risperidone treatment were explored (RUPP Autism Network) (Arnold *et al.*, 2010), a better risk-to-benefit ratio was found in more severely impaired patients and in subjects with lesser weight gain, while comorbidity with anxiety, bipolar disorder, oppositional defiant disorder, and hyperactivity were associated with a poorer response.

Another development of the RUPP study (Aman et al., 2009; Scahill et al., 2012) explored the efficacy of a combined treatment, including both risperidone and parent training, for 24 weeks in 124 children (4–13 years), randomized to medication ($n = 49$) or combined treatment ($n = 75$). The combined treatment was more effective than medication alone on agitation and self-aggressiveness, with a lower dosage of medication. Additional parent training also improved relatedness and communication, according to the Vineland scale, although to a lesser degree.

In summary, empirical evidence supports the efficacy of low-dose risperidone on global measures (CGI). Efficacy is higher in irritability and hyperactivity, while isolation and sterotypies are more refractory to treatment. These positive effects are stable after 6 months, but not when treatment is discontinued (mean suggested duration of treatment 8 to 12 months).

Weight gain is the most frequently reported side effect. All the studies consistently report a significant weight gain, mean 1.7 kg, compared to placebo in the short term, and 8 kg after 8–12 months. The risk of a metabolic syndrome should be actively monitored (obesity, hypertension, hypertriglyceridemia, hypercholesterolemia, hyperglycemia).

Aripiprazole

Two studies ($n = 218$ and $n = 98$, respectively) show short-term (8-week) efficacy of aripiprazole on irritability, hyperactivity, and stereotypies, while lethargy and social isolation are not affected by the treatment. In the first study, Marcus et al. (2009) explored the efficacy of aripiprazole (5–10–15 mg) in a randomized, placebo-controlled study including 218 children and adolescents. All three dose regimens showed better results than did placebo, according to ABC–Irritability and CGI (ES = 0.6–0.9; NNT = 4.7–6.9), with low rates of discontinuation and no significant weight gain (1.3 kg).

Owen et al. (2009) reported a randomized, placebo-controlled 8-week study of 98 children and adolescents given a flexible dose of aripiprazole (5–10–15 mg) or placebo. Aripiprazole was better than placebo according to ABC–I and CGI (ES = 1.23; NNT = 2.6), but with significant residual symptoms. Rate of discontinuation was 8 per cent with placebo, 14.9 per cent with aripiprazole [extrapyramidal side effects (EPS) in 14.9 per cent of the patients]. Weight gain was not relevant (2 kg).

Open studies support the efficacy of aripiprazole (Masi et al., 2009), but report higher rates of agitation, irritability and insomnia in a significant minority of patients.

Olanzapine

Little evidence of efficacy is reported for olanzapine in PDDs. In a small double-blind 8-week study of 11 subjects (Hollander et al., 2006), 50 per cent responded to olanzapine and 20 per cent to placebo, but with a modest global clinical improvement (CGI) and a marked weight gain (3.4 ± 2.2 kg with olanzapine vs. 0.7 ± 0.7 with placebo). Other open-label studies (Kemner et al., 2002) explored efficacy and tolerability of olanzapine, but they reported low rates of responders, and increased appetite and weight gain as the most frequent side effects.

Conventional antipsychotics

The high-potency antipsychotic haloperidol, with a DA (D_2) receptor antagonism, was first extensively studied in controlled trials in children with autism, and remains one of the most studied medications in the treatment of autism. A seminal placebo-controlled, randomized study by Campbell *et al.* (1978) showed efficacy of haloperidol to a maximum of 4 mg/day (mean optimal dose = 1.65 mg/day) in a 12-week study in 40 hospitalized autistic children, aged 2.6 to 7.2 years (mean 4.5 years). Haloperidol treatment was associated with a decrease in stereotypies and withdrawal, but 12 children experienced dose-dependent sedation and two had acute dystonic reactions. In another study from the same research group, Anderson *et al.* (1984) found that haloperidol (maximum dose 4.0 mg/day, optimal dose was 1.1 mg/day) alleviated withdrawal, stereotypies, hyperactivity, abnormal object relationships, negativism, angry affect, and lability of mood, together with discrimination learning in a structured laboratory setting. Acute dystonic reactions occurred in 11 children. A third controlled investigation (Anderson *et al.*, 1989) with lower doses of haloperidol (mean optimal dose 0.8 mg/day) in 45 autistic children showed a significant decrease of hyperactivity, temper tantrums, withdrawal and stereotypies, and an increase in social relatedness, with fewer side effects.

Because long-term medication is often needed in severely affected autistic children, Perry *et al.* (1998) studied the effects of haloperidol (0.5 to 4.0 mg/day, mean optimal dose = 1.23 mg/day) given for 6 months in 60 children with autism. A positive response to treatment was seen in 71.5 per cent of the children, 20 per cent showing no improvement, and 8.5 per cent worsening. Twelve children developed haloperidol-related dyskinesias, 3 during administration and 9 upon discontinuation.

A prospective, longitudinal study specifically addressed the occurrence of drug-related dyskinesias in 118 PDD patients during treatment with haloperidol (mean daily dose = 1.75 mg) (Campbell *et al.*, 1997). The mean duration of treatment was 708.4 days (range 25 to 3,610 days). Forty children (33.9 per cent) developed withdrawal dyskinesias, and 9 developed tardive dyskinesia. However, given the frequency of acute and withdrawal-related dyskinesias, as well as of cognitive toxicity, safer agents, such as the new atypical antipsychotics (risperidone, aripiprazole) have been studied in individuals with autism and other PDDs.

Selective serotonin reuptake inhibitors

Serotonin reuptake inhibitors (SRIs), including the non-selective SRI tricyclic clomipramine and the selective SRIs (SSRIs) are frequently used in children and adolescents with PDDs mostly to alleviate repetitive behaviour and aggression, and possibly to improve aspects of social relatedness. However, definite conclusions cannot be drawn from these studies, because the great majority is uncontrolled, and the similarity of repetitive thoughts and behaviours in PDDs and in obsessive-compulsive disorder is questionable.

Citalopram

King *et al.* (2009) randomized 146 subjects to citalopram ($n = 73$) or placebo ($n = 73$). After a 12-week treatment, no differences in rate of responders according to CGI-I were found between the citalopram group (32.9 per cent) and the placebo group (34.2 per cent) (relative risk, 0.96; $p = 0.99$). The two groups did not differ according to CY–BOCS–PDD improvement [mean (SD) = –2.0 (3.4) in the citalopram group and –1.9 (2.5) in the placebo group, $p = 0.85$]. Finally, according to a combined criterion of response including both CGI–I 1 or 2 and improvement of at least 25 per cent in CY–BOCS–PDD scores, no significant differences were found between citalopram and placebo (20.6 per cent with citalopram, 13.2 per cent with placebo; $p = 0.28$).

Other open studies previously described efficacy and tolerability of citalopram in PDDs. Couturier and Nicolson (2002) retrospectively assessed efficacy of treatment with citalopram (5–40 mg, mean dose 19.7 ± 7 mg) in 17 patients (4–15 years, mean age 9.4 ± 2.9 years). Ten patients (59 per cent) were considered responders according to the CGI-I score in behavioural and anxiety symptoms, even though social relatedness did not improve significantly. Namerow and colleagues (2003) reviewed the medical charts of 15 subjects (aged 6–16 years) with PDDs treated with citalopram (16.9 ± 12.1 mg) for 218 ± 167 days. Eleven subjects showed improvement on CGI at the last visit, with greater improvements in anxiety and mood symptoms, and good tolerability. Finally, Owley *et al.* (2005) treated 28 subjects with low doses of escitalopram, with significant improvement in the ABC irritability score and in CGI–S.

Fluoxetine

Hollander and colleagues (2005) gave fluoxetine or placebo to 45 subjects assessed with CGI Scale–Global Autism Score (CGIS–GAS) and the CY–BOCS in order to lessen repetitive behaviours. The drug was shown to be more effective than placebo ($p = .004$, ES 0.76) in CY–BOCS, but not in the global measures of severity (CGI).

Among the open studies, DeLong and coworkers (2002) treated 37 autistic children (ages 2.25 to 7.75 years) with fluoxetine (0.2–1.4 mg/kg/day), with an excellent response in 11 subjects and good response in the other 11, mainly in behavioural, cognitive, and affective areas, whereas the other 15 children did not respond to treatment. Hyperactivity, aggression, and agitation were the most frequent reasons for discontinuation. These findings have been confirmed by the same research group in an extension of the previous study (DeLong *et al.*, 2002), which considered 129 autistic children (aged 2 to 8 years). Fluoxetine (0.15–0.5 mg/kg) was given for 5–76 months (mean 32 to 36 months), with excellent response in 22 subjects (17 per cent), good response in 67 (52 per cent) and fair-to-poor response in 40 (31 per cent). Response to treatment was highly correlated with familial major affective disorder. Five children (treated for more than 3 years) developed a bipolar disorder during the treatment.

Fluvoxamine

Promising results from a placebo-controlled study (McDougle *et al.*, 1996) in autistic adults treated with fluvoxamine (276.7 mg daily) were not confirmed in a 12-week double-blind, placebo-controlled study in 34 children and adolescents with PDD by the same research group (McDougle *et al.*, 2000); the medication was poorly effective (only one of the 18 treated patients showed significant improvement), and many subjects had significant side effects (insomnia, hyperactivity, agitation, aggression).

Psychostimulants and atomoxetine

Symptoms of attention-deficit/hyperactivity disorder (ADHD) are frequently reported in children with PDDs. Methylphenidate (MPH) (dose 10 or 20 mg b.i.d. for two weeks) was used in a double-blind, placebo-controlled, crossover study of 72 children (aged 5–14 years) with PDDs and ADHD symptoms (ABC Hyperactivity–Impulsivity Subscale) (Research Units of Pediatric Psychopharmacology Autism Network, 2005). After a 7-day test-dose period, patients were randomized with a crossover design (each child received all doses and placebo) in four arms (0.125, 0.25, 0.50 mg/kg/dose or placebo) in random order given three times a day. Raters were teachers and parents. Six of 72 children (8 per cent) were unable to tolerate at least 2 dose levels of MPH (irritability was the most frequent reason for discontinuation), so 66 children entered the crossover study. Using a response criterion of CGI–I 1 or 2 and at least a 25 per cent reduction of hyperactivity scores, 58 subjects completed the crossover phase, and 44 were rated as responders to at least 1 week of treatment (MPH or placebo), 35 to MPH and 9 to placebo. In summary, 35 of 72 subjects (49 per cent) responded to MPH. Thirteen of 72 (18 per cent) exposed to MPH dropped out on account of adverse side effects: irritability ($n = 6$) was the most common reason for discontinuation. Additionally, decreased appetite, delay in falling asleep, and emotional outbursts were more frequent with MPH than placebo. In summary, MPH helps about half of children with PDD + hyperactivity and 18 per cent of children do not tolerate the drug, making the benefit-to-risk ratio less favorable in PDD than in non-PDD ADHD.

These results have been confirmed in other controlled studies. In a study by Posey *et al.* (2007), 66 children and adolescents (mean age 7.5 years) were randomized to MPH (0.125, 0.25, 0.50 mg/kg/dose) or placebo in crossover design, with positive effect on all the ADHD symptoms, and absence of side effects reported in the previous study, such as worsening of repetitive behaviours, stereotypies, and oppositional-defiant behaviours.

In a study by Jahromi *et al.* (2009), 33 children (5–13 years of age) were randomized to MPH (0.125, 0.25, 0.50 mg/kg/dose) or placebo in a crossover design. Social-communication performances, self-regulation, and affective behaviours significantly improved with MPH.

In summary, empirical evidence supports the efficacy of MPH on ADHD symptoms in those with PDDs, although efficacy and tolerability are less favourable then in the general population. Agitation, irritability, aggressiveness, sleep disorders, worsening of repetitive behaviours, and stereotypies are more frequent in severe mental retardation.

Much less evidence is available on the efficacy of atomoxetine in subjects with PDDs with ADHD. In a study by Arnold *et al.* (2006), 16 subjects (age range 5–15 years) took atomoxetine (mean dose 0.8 mg/kg, up to 1.4 mg/kg) for 6 weeks. This drug was more effective than placebo (ABC–Hyperactivity, parent), but improvement was only modest. No differences were apparent with atomoxetine with respect to inattention and cognitive performances.

Mood stabilizers

An emerging literature documents the co-occurrence of mania in children with PDDs, suggesting that up to 21 per cent of children with PDDs may also meet criteria for mania (Wozniak *et al.*, 1997). Identification of this comorbidity may have important therapeutic and theoretical implications, at least for a subgroup of autistic disorders related to bipolar disorder, in terms of occurrence of manic symptoms, extreme hyperactivity nonresponsive to stimulants, the cyclic component of symptomatic behaviours, and/or family history of bipolar disorder. Hollander and colleagues openly assessed the efficacy of divalproex sodium in several small open and controlled studies. In the first study (Hollander *et al.*, 2001), which included 14 patients (age range 5–40 years, mean 17.9 years, mean blood level 75.8 µg/ml), ten patients (71 per cent) were responders according to the CGI–I score. In 2010, in a 12-week study, Hollander and co-workers randomized 55 youth to valproic acid (VPA) or placebo. According to ABC–I, CGI, 63.5 per cent were responders to VPA and 9 per cent to placebo ($p = .008$), with a significant improvement in ABC–I ($p = .048$) and CY–BOCS ($p = .005$, ES = 1.53). In a previous double-blind, 8-week study, including 30 subjects (6–20 years of age), Hellings et al. (2005) failed to show efficacy of valproic acid (20 mg/kg per day) on self- and other-aggression in a double blind placebo-controlled study.

Uvebrant and Bauziene (1994) administered the anticonvulsant lamotrigine to 13 young patients with autism and treatment-refractory epilepsy, and autistic symptoms were significantly decreased in 8 of these patients. This finding has not been confirmed in a more recent double-blind 4-week study of 14 autistic children (age range 3–11 years, mean 5.8 years), without any significant difference from a placebo group, according to the Autism Behaviour Checklist, Aberrant Behavior Checklist, Vineland scales, and CARS (Belsito et al., 2001).

Wasserman et al. (2006) explored the efficacy of levitiracetam (862 ± 279 mg/day) in a double-blind 10–week study including 20 patients (5–17 years of age). According to the CGI and ABC, no differences were found between groups in behaviour and aggression; furthermore CY–BOCS and Conners' scales scores did not differ.

Evidence supporting the use of mood stabilizers is still scarce. The prevailing indication for valproic acid is the co-occurrence of mood dysregulation and irritability/impulsivity, possibly with familial loading for bipolar disorders.

Other medications

Opioid antagonists

Early findings from animal models suggested that exogen opioids may induce socio-emotional blindness and absence of separation distress in animal models, and these phenomena can be reversed by opioid receptor blockage (Panksepp, 1979). These features have suggested that an excess of opioid system activity in the brain may contribute to the genesis of autistic symptoms. On the basis of these findings, the opioid antagonist naltrexone has been investigated as a potential treatment for self-injurious behaviour, social deficits, and aggressiveness. Controlled studies failed to confirm efficacy (Willemsen-Swinkels et al., 1996). Open studies have reported transient and moderate results on hyperactivity, but in some subjects there was a worsening of behavioural symptoms and stereotypies (Campbell et al., 1993; Kolmen et al., 1995).

Clonidine and guanfacine

The alpha-adrenergic agent (transdermal) clonidine, usually used in subjects with hyperactivity and impulsivity, was explored in two small double-blind, placebo-controlled studies, with mixed results regarding hyperactivity, anxiety, and global functioning (Fankhauser et al. 1992; Jaselskis et al., 1992). Hypotension, fatigue, and sedation are frequent side effects. Furthermore, many patients tend to develop tolerance to the positive effects of clonidine during the first months of treatment.

The efficacy of guanfacine in 80 children and adolescents (age range 3–18 years, mean 7.7 years) with PDDs has been retrospectively assessed by Posey and coworkers (2004). At a mean dose of 2.6 mg/day (range 0.25–9 mg), only 19 subjects (23.8 per cent) were responders according to the CGI score, with some improvement with respect to hyperactivity, inattention, insomnia, and tics. Subjects with Asperger's syndrome or PDD Not Otherwise Specified (PDD–NOS) demonstrated greater improvement.

Glutamatergic compounds

The hypothesis of a glutamatergic component in the pathophysiolgy of autism (Carlsson, 1998) stimulated interest in the efficacy of glutamatergic compounds like lamotrigine and amantadine in the treatment of autism and has led to specific studies of these agents. Data on lamotrigine were discussed in the section on mood stabilizers (see above). The efficacy of amantadine has been assessed in a double-blind placebo-controlled study in 39 autistic children and adolescents (age range 5–19 years, mean 7 years) (King et al., 2001). After a 1–week trial of placebo, patients were randomized to placebo or amantadine (2.5 mg/kg/day) in one daily dose for one week, and then placebo or amantadine (5 mg/kg per day) in two daily doses for 3 weeks. A significant decrease in hyperactivity and inappropriate speech was found, according to the clinician-rated Aberrant Behavior Checklist–Community Version, even though the corresponding parent-rated measure failed to show any clinical effect. Amantadine was well tolerated.

Discussion

Pharmacologic treatment can be considered a symptomatic intervention in children and adolescents with behavioural disorders associated with core autistic symptomatology. Hyperactivity, aggression, lability of mood, and repetitive phenomena are the most sensitive target symptoms, while social impairment is more resistant to pharmacologic intervention.

Atypical antipsychotics are drugs that act on a broad range of symptoms, and they are particularly indicated when more serious behavioural symptoms, such as aggression, self-injurious behaviour, hyperactivity, and tantrums are prominent. In addition, atypical antipsychotics may be beneficial in repetitive behaviours. On the basis of empirical evidence, risperidone should be considered as the first-choice medication, while aripiprazole can be considered next, when risperidone is not effective or is poorly tolerated (on account of weight gain, increased prolactin levels, etc.). The main indication for aripiprazole is in children who are not severely aggressive and in those in whom repetitive behaviours and isolation are prevalent. Increased irritability and agitation should be monitored. When risperidone is associated with intolerable side effects, and aripiprazole is not effective in controlling behavioural disorders, conventional antipsychotics (haloperidol, chlorpromazine) may be considered as they are associated with a lesser weight gain and risk of metabolic syndrome.

On the basis of an analysis of controlled and non-controlled studies, including those of citalopram, fluoxetine, and fluvoxamine, there is not sufficient evidence that SSRIs are effective as a treatment for children with autism. Furthermore, their use is associated with an increased risk of side effects, mostly irritability. Behavioural activation (irritability, agitation, hyperactivity, aggressiveness) is frequently reported during SSRI treatment, and at least in some cases this may represent a pharmacologic hypomania. Decisions about the use of SSRIs for established clinical indications that may co-occur with autism, such as obsessive–compulsive disorder and depression and anxiety, should be made on a case-by-case basis.

When hyperactivity and inattention are prominent features, stimulants such as methylphenidate are recommended, and their efficacy is supported by empirical evidence, although their efficacy and tolerability profile is less favorable in children with PDDs than in other children. Evidence for the efficacy of mood stabilizers, particularly valproic acid, is limited, and VPA should be used when irritability, mood lability, and anxiety are associated, as when there is an associated familial history of mood disorders.

Further research is warranted, mainly to determine the efficacy and safety of medications for specific subtypes of patients, according to age and clinical profile. Long-term data are needed, given the paucity of information about the pharmacodynamic effect on the developing brain of drugs administered for extended periods of time during the first years of life, when dramatic developmental changes in neurotransmitters and receptors occur. These considerations are not limited to psychotropic medications, but indeed apply to the entire field of pediatric pharmacology.

Long-term, well-designed controlled studies on large samples of affected young children should expand current knowledge on psychopharmacology in the treatment of PPDs. Although the randomized, placebo-controlled clinical trial is the gold standard, when data about safety and efficacy are lacking and/or when there is uncertainty regarding whether a medication is a valid alternative, an interesting question is how far the results of controlled studies on very selected populations, intensively studied for short periods, can apply to everyday care. Systematic naturalistic observations of long-term outcome in routine care can yield their own specific kind of essential information needed to practice evidence-based health care.

Conflicts of interest: The author declares no conflicts of interest.

References

Aman, M.G., Mam, K.S. & Collier-Crespia, A. (2003): Prevalence and patterns of psychoactive medicines among individuals with autism in the Autism Society of Ohio. *J. Autism Dev. Disord.* **33**, 527–534.

Aman, M.G., Hollway, J.A. & McDougle, C.J., *et al.* (2008): Cognitive effects of risperidone in children with autism and irritable behaviour. *J. Child Adolesc. Psychopharmacol.* **18**, 227–236.

Aman, M.G., McDougle, C.J., Scahill, L., *et al.* (2009): Medication and parent training in children with pervasive developmental disorders and serious behaviour problems: results from a randomized clinical trial. *J. Am. Acad. Child Adolesc. Psychiatry* **48**, 1143–1154.

Anderson, L., Campbell, M., Grega, D., *et al.* (1984): Haloperidol in the treatment of infantile autism: effects on learning and behavioral symptoms. *Am. J. Psychiatry* **141**, 1195–1202.

Anderson, L., Campbell, M., Adams, P., *et al.* (1989): The effects of haloperidol on discrimination learning and behavioral symptoms in autistic children. *J. Autism Dev. Disord.* **19**, 227–239.

Arnold, L.E., Aman, M.G., Cook, A.M., *et al.* (2006): Atomoxetine for hyperactivity in autism spectrum disorder: placebo-controlled, cross-over pilot trial. *J. Am. Acad. Child Adolesc. Psychiatry* **45**, 1196–1205.

Arnold, L.E., Farmer, C., Kraemer, H.C., *et al.* (2010): Moderators, mediators and other predictors of risperidone response in children with autistic disorder and irritability. *J. Child Adolesc. Psychopharmacol.* **20**, 83–93.

Belsito, K.M., Law, P.A., Kirk, K.S., *et al.* (2001): Lamotrigine therapy for autistic disorder: a randomized, double-blind, placebo-controlled trial. *J. Autism Dev. Disord.* **31**, 175–181.

Campbell, M., Anderson, L., Meier, M., *et al.* (1978): A comparison of haloperidol and behavior therapy and their interaction in autistic children. *J. Am. Acad. Child Psychiatry* **17**, 640–655.

Campbell, M., Anderson, L.T., Small, A.M., *et al.* (1993): Naltrexone in autistic children: behavioral symptoms and attentional learning. *J. Am. Acad. Child Adolesc. Psychiatry* **32**, 1283–1291.

Campbell, M., Armenteros, J.L., Malone, R.P., *et al.* (1997): Neuroleptic-related dyskinesias in autistic children: a prospective, longitudinal study. *J. Am. Acad. Child Adolesc. Psychiatry* **36**, 835–843.

Carlsson, M.L. (1998): Hypothesis: is infantile autism a hypoglutamatergic disorder? Relevance of glutamate-serotonin interactions for pharmacotherapy. *J. Neural Transm.* **105**, 525–535.

Couturier, J.L. & Nicolson, R. (2002): A retrospective assessment of citalopram in children and adolescents with pervasive developmental disorders. *J. Child Adolesc. Psychopharmacol.* **12**, 243–248.

DeLong, G.R., Teague, L.A. & Kamran, M.M. (1998): Effects of fluoxetine treatment in young children with idiopathic autism. *Dev. Med. Child Neurol.* **40**, 551–562.

DeLong, G.R., Ritch, C.R. & Burch, S. (2002): Fluoxetine response in children with autistic spectrum disorder: correlation with familial major affective disorder and intellectual achievement. *Dev. Med. Child Neurol.* **44**, 652–659.

Fankhauser, M.P., Karumanchi, V.C., German, M.L., et al. (1992): A double-blind, placebo-controlled study of the efficacy of transdermal clonidine in autism. *J. Clin. Psychiatry* **53**, 77–82.

Hellings, J.A., Weckbaugh, M., Nickel, E.J., et al. (2005): A double-blind, placebo-controlled study of valproate for aggression in youth with pervasive developmental disorders. *J. Child Adolesc. Psychopharmacol.* **15**, 682–692.

Hollander, E., Dolgoff-Kaspar, R., Cartwright, C., et al. (2001): An open-trial of divalproex sodium in autism spectrum disorders. *J. Clin. Psychiatry* **62**, 530–534.

Hollander, E., Phillips, A., Chaplin, W., et al. (2005): A placebo-controlled crossover trial of liquid fluoxetine on repetitive behaviors in childhood and adolescent autism. *Neuropsychopharmacology* **30**, 582–589.

Hollander, E., Wasserman, S., Swanson, E., et al. (2006): A double blind, placebo controlled pilot study of olanzapine in childhood/adolescent pervasive developmental disorder. *J. Child Adolesc. Psychopharmacol.* **16**, 541–548.

Hollander, E., Chaplin, W., Soorya, L., et al. (2010): Divalproex sodium versus placebo for the treatment of irritability in children and adolescents with autism spectrum disorders. *Neuropsychopharmacology* **35**, 990–998.

Jahromi, L.B., Kasari, C.L., McCracken, J.T., et al. (2009): Positive effects of methylphenidate on social communication and self-regulation in children with pervasive developmental disorders and hyperactivity. *J. Autism Dev. Disord.* **39**, 395–404.

Jaselskis, C.A., Cook, E.H., Jr., Fletcher, K.E., et al. (1992): Clonidine treatment of hyperactive and impulsive children with autistic disorder. *J. Clin. Psychopharmacol.* **12**, 322–327.

Kemner, C., Willemsen-Swinkels, S., DeJonge, M., et al. (2002): Open-label study of olanzapine in children with pervasive developmental disorders. *J. Clin. Psychopharmacol.* **22**, 455–460.

King, B.H., Wright, D.M., Habden, J., et al. (2001): Double-blind, placebo-controlled study of amantadine hydrochloride in the treatment of children with autistic disorder. *J. Am. Acad. Child Adolesc. Psychiatry* **40**, 658–665.

King, B.H., Hollander, E., Sikich, L., et al. (2009): STAART Psychopharmacology Network. Lack of efficacy of citalopram in children with autism spectrum disorder and high levels of repetitive behavior: citalopram ineffective in children with autism. *Arch. Gen. Psychiatry* **66**, 583–590.

Kolmen, B.K., Feldman, H.M., Handen, B.L., et al. (1995): Naltrexone in young autistic children: a double blind, placebo-controlled, cross-over study. *J. Am. Acad. Child Adolesc. Psychiatry* **34**, 223–231.

Marcus, R.N., Owen, R., Kamen, L., et al. (2009): A placebo-controlled, fixed study of aripiprazole in children and adolescents with irritability associated with autistic disorder. *J. Am. Acad. Child Adolesc. Psychiatry* **48**, 1110–1119.

Masi, G. (2004): Pharmacotherapy of pervasive developmental disorders in children and adolescents. *CNS Drugs* **18**, 1031–1052.

Masi, G., Cosenza, A., Millepiedi, S., et al. (2009): Aripiprazole monotherapy in children and young adolescents with pervasive developmental disorders: a retrospective study. *CNS Drugs* **23**, 511–521.

McDougle, C.J., Naylor, S.T., Cohen, D.J., et al. (1996): A double-blind, placebo-controlled study of fluvoxamine in adults with autistic disorder. *Arch. Gen. Psychiatry* **53**, 1001–1008.

McDougle, C.J., Holmes, J.P., Carlson, D.C., et al. (1998): A double-blind, placebo-controlled study of risperidone in adults with autistic disorder and other pervasive developmental disorders. *Arch. Gen. Psychiatry* **55**, 633–641.

McDougle, C.J., Scahill, L., McCracken, J.T., et al. (2000): Research Units on Pediatric Psychopharmacology–Autism Network: background and rationale for an initial controlled study of risperidone. *Child Adolesc. Psychiatr. Clin. N. Am.* **9**, 201–224.

McDougle, C.J., Scahill, L., Aman, M.G., et al. (2005): Risperidone for the core symptom domains of autism: results from the study by the autism network or the research units on pediatric psychopharmacology. *Am. J. Psychiatry* **152**, 1142–1148.

Namerow, L.B., Thomas, P., Bostic, J.Q., et al. (2003): Use of citalopram in pervasive developmental disorders. *J. Dev. Behav. Pediatr.* **24**, 104–108.

Owen, R., Sikich, L., Marcus, R.N., et al. (2009): Aripiprazole in the treatment of irritability in children and adolescents with autistic disorder. *Pediatrics* **124**, 1533–1540.

Owley, T., Walton, L., Salt, J., et al. (2005): An open trial of escitalopram in pervasive developmental disorders. *J. Am. Acad. Child Adolesc. Psychiatry* **44**, 343–348.

Panksepp, J. (1979): A neurochemical theory of autism. *Trends Neurosci.* **2**, 174–177.

Perry, R, Campbell, M, Adams, P., et al. (1998): Long-term efficacy of haloperidol in autistic children: continuous versus discontinuous drug administration. *J. Am. Acad. Child Adolesc. Psychiatry* **28**, 87–92.

Posey, D.J., Puntney, J.I., Sasher, T.M., et al. (2004): Guanfacine treatment for hyperactivity and inattention pervasive developmental disorders: a retrospective analysis of 80 cases. *J. Child Adolesc. Psychopharmacology* **14**, 233–241.

Posey, D.J., Aman, M.G., McCracken, J.T., et al. (2007): Positive effects of methylphenidate on inattention and hyperactivity in pervasive developmental disorders: an analysis of secondary measures. *Biol. Psychiatry* **61**, 538–544.

Research Units on Pediatric Psychopharmacology (RUPP) Autism Network (2002): Risperidone in childen with autism and serious behavioral problems. *N. Engl. J. Med.* **347,** 314–321.

Research Units on Pediatric Psychopharmacology (RUPP) Autism Network (2005): Randomized, controlled, crossover trial of methylphenidate in pervasive developmental disorders with hyperactivity. *Arch. Gen. Psychiatry* **62,** 1266–1274.

Scahill, L., McDougle, C.J., Aman, M.G., *et al.* (2012): Effects of risperidone and parent training on adaptive functioning in children with pervasive developmental disorders and serious behavioral problems. *J. Am. Acad. Child Adolesc. Psychiatry* **51,** 136–146.

Uvebrant, P. & Bauziene, R. (1994): Intractable epilepsy in children: the efficacy of lamotrigine treatment, included non-seizure-related benefits. *Neuropediatrics* **25,** 284–289.

Wasserman, S., Iyengar, R., Chaplin, W.F., *et al.* (2006): Levitiracetam versus placebo in childhood and adolescents autism: a double-blind placebo-controlled study. *Int. Clin. Psychopharmacol.* **21,** 263–267.

Willemsen-Swinkels, S.H.N., Buitelaar, J.K. & van Engeland, H. (1996): The effects of chronic naltrexone treatment in young autistic children: a double-blind placebo-controlled crossover study. *Biol. Psychiatry* **39,** 1023–1031.

Wozniak, J., Biederman, J., Faraone, S.V., *et al.* (1997): Mania in children with pervasive developmental disorders revisited. *J. Am. Acad. Child Adolesc. Psychiatry* **36,** 1552–1559.

Rehabilitation

Chapter 11

The TEACCH approach to working with individuals on the autism spectrum: understanding, educating, empowering

Steven E. Kroupa*

*Department of Psychiatry, University of North Carolina at Chapel Hill,
Chapel Hill, North Carolina 27599, USA*
Steve_Kroupa@med.unc.edu

Summary

The TEACCH approach to working with individuals with autism spectrum disorder (ASD) is based on a best practices model that integrates empirical research and expert-validated principles of clinical and educational practice. A central feature of the model is the development of strategies and techniques that allow for a multifaceted and detailed understanding of shared diagnostic symptoms, of individualized strengths and challenges, and of respect for the uniqueness of each individual. The overall goal of the TEACCH approach is to develop competencies in all aspects of the person's life and to provide environmental supports so that the individual is able to function at the highest levels of independence, social connectedness, and self-determination. This article provides a brief review of the historical and conceptual foundation of the TEACCH model along with a description of current services and practices. The main components of the psychoeducational intervention known as Structured Teaching will be defined. Some recent findings from neurobiological and neuropsychological research will be integrated into the discussion as they relate to the biopsychosocial understanding of autism and effective treatments. Finally, a critical analysis of the current state of treatment outcome research will be presented and the existing empirical support for the TEACCH approach will be referenced.

Introduction

If, as many have suggested, Leo Kanner's robust descriptions (Kanner, 1943) of eleven children in the 1930s and '40s initiated the modern era of autism spectrum disorder (ASD) diagnostics, then it might also be said that the early challenges of a small group of empirically minded professionals to the prevailing psychogenic theories of autism led to the current state of more effective psychosocial (including applied behavioural) interventions for individuals with ASD. Eric Schopler, a graduate of the University of Chicago (where the psychoanalytic conceptions of the nature of autism became personified in faculty member Bruno

---

*Emeritus Professor; correspondence concerning this article should be addressed to Steve Kroupa, 153 Lumina Place, Holly Springs, North Carolina 27540, USA.

Bettelheim) and later co-founder of Division TEACCH, was one of the more vocal and persistent critics of the 'refrigerator mother' metaphor (Mesibov, 2006; Mesibov et al., 2005). Schopler died in 2006, after having made numerous significant contributions to the established view that autism is fundamentally a neurodevelopmental disorder that has a profound impact on families, educational systems, communities, and public policy makers. It is within this broad and rich historical context of nearly seven decades of advances in autism research and practice that a representative from the TEACCH program is honored to be among the invited participants at the 2012 Mariani Foundation conference who are discussing the current state of autism research and practice.

Both Kanner's description of autism and the reaction to misguided theories and practices represent significant paradigm shifts in how autism has come to be viewed and treated. Since that time, a number of less dramatic but still significant shifts in thinking and practice have occurred. The importance of early identification of children at risk for developing ASD and the association of early intervention programs with improved developmental outcomes seems especially notable, as do the periodic changes to the Diagnostic and Statistical Manual (DSM) system of categorizing behavioural and developmental disorders in children. For example, the fourth revision to the DSM (American Psychiatric Association, 2000) expanded the clinical definition of 'pervasive developmental disorder' by including a subtype (Asperger's disorder) for individuals who do not also have a significant intellectual disability or history of language impairment. Indeed, the recognition of intelligent, articulate, and high-functioning individuals with autism as published authors, public speakers, and recognized authorities (*e.g.*, Temple Grandin) led to what, for many, was a *second wave* of insights into the behaviour and information-processing characteristics of individuals with ASD. And finally, recent technological and conceptual advances in a number of biomedical specialties have, for the first time, positioned genetic and neurobiological assessment techniques and interventions to be of greater clinical utility in the coming years. Although there does not appear to be a medical 'cure' for ASD anywhere on the near horizon, there is increased optimism that newly developed biomedical interventions will augment the behavioural and psychoeducational interventions that comprise the most effective treatments available today.

The proposed biopsychosocial model of autism assessment and intervention (explicitly identified here by me, but which is implicit in the TEACCH approach) begins with an attempt to understand how ASD affects the individual's biological, psychological, and social systems, and then integrates that understanding into highly individualized interventions that are sensitive to the specific contexts in which the individual lives. The TEACCH approach is, in my estimation, inherently *trans*-theoretical, multimodal, and multisystemic (*cf.* Mesibov et al., 2005).

Although this article retains the basic outline of the presentation made in Rapallo, Italy, its present written form allows increased latitude for crafting ideas and additional space for listing a small number of selected references. However, this format does not lend itself to displaying visual examples of specific techniques and strategies (which is a bit out of character for an approach that espouses the power of the image to convey meaning). For that, there are a number of other TEACCH publications that can be consulted (*e.g.*, Boswell, 2009), as well as numerous other sources, such as the *Tasks Galore* series of books (*e.g.*, Eckenrode et al., 2003). The TEACCH approach is a dynamic one which is, in part, interpreted anew by each person who finds that this approach 'fits like a comfortable pair of jeans.' It should, then, not be surprising that some of the descriptions of the TEACCH approach in this paper are somewhat novel but, it is hoped, still resonate with its essential principles and values.

Following this introduction, I will briefly define TEACCH as a physical organization and as an organized framework of concepts and clinical priorities that shape its methods. As the current understanding of ASD expands to accommodate the remarkable advances being made in the areas of genetics, neurology, and immunology, TEACCH strategies are re-framed as tools for enhancing the efficiency with which the person with autism understands and values the world of people and its social 'artifacts' – language, mores, customs, and relationships. Some of the core components of Structured Teaching are described, with a final, brief discussion of the issues involved in empirical studies evaluating the effectiveness of the TEACCH approach in particular, and of autism services in general.

An inclusive and integrative TEACCH approach

TEACCH is both a community-based program for residents of North Carolina that is administered by faculty at the University of North Carolina at Chapel Hill, and a clearly defined theoretical framework for understanding and treating individuals on the autism spectrum. TEACCH services are philosophically and practically collaborative – empowering clients, families, community professionals, and public policy makers to participate as full partners and tasked with meeting the various challenges that individuals with autism face on a daily basis. TEACCH clinical services include diagnostic and psychological evaluations, individual and group treatment, parent education, professional training, school and agency consultation, and research collaboration. Recently expanded programs target very young children (early intervention), adults in work (supported employment) and residential settings, and a broad range of university students, interns, and other professionals in training. Historically, most regional clinic services were funded through yearly legislative grants, although recent reductions in funding have necessitated fee-for-service payments for some services. As a university program, TEACCH has been in the forefront of disseminating the latest research and accurate information about ASD, and in advancing the field with innovations in assessment techniques (*e.g.*, Childhood Autism Rating Scales, Psychoeducational Profile) and educational strategies (*e.g.*, Structured Teaching) (Mesibov *et al.*, 2005). TEACCH workshops for parents and professionals have been well received in all 50 U.S. states and in more than 30 countries worldwide.

In contrast to some other theoretical perspectives, the TEACCH framework is essentially inclusive and integrative, with the primary determinant of intervention strategies being what is in the best interest of the individual with ASD, especially when viewed ecologically. This *client-centered* approach is based on a thorough understanding of how autism affects the individual (*assessment-driven*); on the individual's internal resources for coping (*strength-based*); and on sensitivity to the various family, community, and cultural values, needs, and priorities operating at all levels of caregiving (*systems-sensitive*).

The TEACCH approach is also inclusive and integrative in its commitment to the *whole* person – seeking to enhance all aspects of each person's functioning and quality of life – by incorporating the most salient features and effective strategies (*treatment effects*) from the various existing psychological theories (paradigms) of learning and behaviour. TEACCH practitioners strive to understand an individual's behaviour from a variety of theoretical perspectives (*e.g.*, cognitive-behavioural, developmental, social-psychological, systems, humanistic, and behavioural) and develop intervention plans with the knowledge of the individual gained from an integration of these perspectives. (I prefer the term 'integrative' to 'eclectic' and refer the reader to the literature on integrative psychotherapy for a more detailed discussion.) Integration also occurs at a level that maximizes the beneficial *nonspecific treatment effects* by emphasizing the qualities of an effective practitioner (*e.g.*, excellent listening and communication skills, empathy, honesty, congruence, resourcefulness) and the development of a supportive and *therapeutic* relationship with all clients (individuals, families, other professionals) (*relationship-based*).

The emerging neurobiological basis of ASD

One of the core principles of the TEACCH approach is an affirmation of the importance of empirical research in *informing* both conceptual models of ASD, and clinical and educational best practices. In recent years remarkable advances have been made in understanding genetic and neurobiological factors in the development of autistic traits and tendencies. For the most part, these advances in our understanding of the neurobiology of ASD seem to have produced findings that are remarkably consistent with the information-processing paradigms derived from cognitive and neuropsychological research, first-person accounts, and clinical inferences made based on behavioural observations. In general, the brains of individuals affected by ASD seem to have developed in ways that some information-processing functions are notably less efficient (*e.g.*, social and pragmatic language skills, complex learning, applied skills), some may be notably more efficient (*e.g.*, rote memory, visual/spatial abilities, routinized learning), and some may be similarly efficient as compared to other individuals of the same developmental age. The range of affected functions (*pervasiveness*) and the degree to which specific functions are more or less efficient (*atypicality*) seems to characterize the ASD condition in contrast to general intellectual disability (more pervasive, less atypical) or specific learning disabilities (less pervasive, specific inefficiency).

At the biological level it seems self-evident, given the social context of conception and the human infant's dependence on caretaking for an extended period of time (relative to other mammals), that humans have innate social needs. Indeed, the identification of humans as inherently social creatures has been well established by various branches of the biological and social sciences, and through compelling models of human development, such as the attachment theory of human social behaviour (*e.g.*, Bowlby, 1969). More recently, advances in neurobiological research have begun to associate social behaviours with specific brain structures and functions, and to lay the foundation for a neurobiological understanding of ASD.

The evolving neurobiological picture suggests that the human brain is organized to select, prioritize, and integrate social information (specific, detailed, and intricate information about people as a special category of 'objects'), and it is this organization and functioning that is most affected by ASD. For example, diminished eye contact with primary caregivers and diminished social smile response in infants, selective inattention to people in both familiar and unfamiliar contexts (*e.g.*, Osterling *et al.*, 2002), and atypical activation of the regions of the brain associated with the recognition of objects when presented with pictures of people (*e.g.*, Schultz *et al.*, 2000) all indicate an early pattern of marked differences in the *social interest* in individuals with ASD. Presumably, these differences eventually contribute to higher-level social information-processing and skill deficits, such as the reduced ability to identify emotions in facial expressions (*e.g.*, Harms *et al.*, 2010), to imitate the actions of others, to initiate interactions, and to regulate one's thinking and behaviour according to social feedback and expectations (reciprocity).

Further, by definition, communication is a social behaviour. One of the most established research findings is that general verbal and nonverbal communication challenges are a core component of the ASD diagnostic criteria. More specifically, the ability to form abstract language concepts (*e.g.*, Minshew *et al.*, 2002), or to use language as a basis for imagining perspectives other than one's own (theory of mind) (*e.g.*, Colle *et al.*, 2007) and developing empathy appear to be underdeveloped in many individuals with ASD. Furthermore, inefficiencies in social and pragmatic communication (*e.g.*, Lord & Paul, 1997) and in imaginative play skills (*e.g.*, Wolfberg, 1999) have been well documented in individuals with ASD, including those with age-level or advanced verbal vocabularies.

Whatever differences in neural circuitry (*e.g.*, mirror neurons, 'white matter', neurotransmitter regulation) or other aspects of neurobiology that may eventually explain ASD, advances in the understanding of the neurobiology of ASD may not only lead to promising new biomedical technologies and interventions, but also encourage a re-examination of existing assessment and treatment protocols in order to *justify* current practices and to refine strategies and implementation. To some degree, the fundamental problem to be solved appears to be – to borrow an analogy from computer science – that there are *compatibility* issues between the brains of individuals with ASD and the conventional ways the (social) world and social expectations are structured. Given this perspective, the most direct paths of resolution would appear to be: (1) restructure the 'ASD brain' (primarily through treatment and education); (2) restructure the world (primarily through environmental modifications and social change); or (3) restructure both. The TEACCH approach advocates the third option.

TEACCH strategies: enhancing compatibility

During the introduction to training workshops, I sometimes suggest that the initial goal for someone using the TEACCH approach is to make the world seem more *Windows-based* (computer operating system using visual supports or icons that can be accessed easily) than *DOS-based* (an operating system requiring the precise use of language), especially the world involving people and implied social expectations. Historically, TEACCH has organized its interventions around an assumption, supported in part by research findings (briefly summarized in Mesibov *et al.*, 2005) and based on clinical experience that many people on the autism spectrum process certain kinds of visual information more efficiently than they do auditory information. Further compelling anecdotal evidence supporting these visual information-processing efficiencies has emerged from credible, first-person accounts of the autistic experience, such as Temple's Grandin's book, *Thinking in Pictures* (Grandin, 1995). Some studies have suggested that basic visual information-processing, especially regarding objects, appears to be largely intact in many individuals with ASD (*e.g.*, Schultz *et al.*, 2000), although other aspects of visual information processing (*e.g.*, visual scanning and central coherence, visual/spatial memory) may be negatively affected (*e.g.*, Behrmann *et al.*, 2005).

Although TEACCH strategies emphasize the use of visual supports for people with ASD, I suggest that the TEACCH approach should still be tailored to the needs of the individual, which may mean adapting environmental supports to the most intact sensory/processing modality as a way of compensating for a less-efficient modality. Indeed, TEACCH practitioners have reported success using auditory supports for individuals with ASD who are visually impaired, or tactile supports for individuals with ASD who are both visually and aurally impaired. Although the main emphasis is always in helping the person with ASD more meaningfully engage in the world, the strategic core of the TEACCH model, called Structured Teaching, emphasizes an increased use of visual supports, not unlike what would be helpful for 'neurotypical' travelers to unfamiliar cultures (*e.g.*, picture restaurant menus, international traffic symbols, pictures and diagrams for accessing public services).

Structured Teaching might be thought of as a way of organizing and presenting information to individuals with ASD in order to *increase their degree of cooperation with others*, to *increase their ability to function more independently*, and to *increase their overall quality of life*. Historically, four components of Structured Teaching are typically described: physical structure, individualized daily schedules, work/activity systems, and visual structure (of specific tasks and activities). All four of these components together enhance the social information-processing capabilities of the person with ASD by making implicit social 'rules' much more salient and potentially more pertinent. Together these four components restructure the implicit *social contract* that characterizes interactions and situations involving people (the 'who', 'what', 'when', 'where', 'how', and 'why' of social expectations):

1. *What* activity you need to be doing;
2. *When* you need to be doing the activity;
3. *Where* you need to be doing the activity; and
4. *How* you need to be doing the activity.

Individualizing the message clarifies the 'who' of social expectations. Informing the individual about 'why' he needs to be doing the activity may be partly addressed in the structuring of activities (*e.g.*, intrinsic meaning and rewards, extrinsic incentives), or through more direct strategies (*e.g.*, social narratives). Of course, part of this largely implicit social contract is that the needs and desires of the individual, his ability to delay gratification of those needs/desires, and her ability to act on those needs/desires in a socially acceptable manner are also intentionally integrated into the structure of the day and setting.

Physical structure

In the TEACCH model, *physical structure* refers to the way in which the physical setting is optimized for specific individuals with ASD. It is the nature of autism that special precautions need to be taken to ensure the *safety* of the individuals with ASD and those who work with them; to arrange the *placement* of furniture and materials to address individual educational goals; to 'engineer' the learning environment to focus *attention* and minimize distractions; to help the student regulate his emotions through *'calming'* centers and activities; and to maximize the *efficient* use of movement, materials, and resources (*e.g.*, individual instruction time). (I use the key words Safety, Placement, Attention, Calming, and Efficient or *SPACE* as the mnemonic acronym for these special considerations.)

Once again, the specific challenges and strengths of the individuals involved determine the exact 'prescription' of how the physical setting is arranged and organized to ensure safety. For example, some beginning learners may need a less 'open' classroom to prevent easy access to exits or to the activities of other students. At home, heavy objects (*e.g.*, flat panel TVs, tall shelves) might need to be secured so that they cannot be easily pulled down on a child who has yet to learn not to climb on furniture. In the community, an adult with pica may need to have unsupervised access to an environment, but certain kinds of inedible materials must be nevertheless limited by removal of the materials or placing them in secure containers.

In school, at home, or in the community, many individuals with autism have specific goals for what they are to be working on while in those settings. In schools in the United States the student's specific goals are based in her individualized education plan (IEP), and these goals may be addressed in a variety of learning formats (*e.g.*, one-on-one teaching, small group instruction, play-based learning, the teaching of special subjects or special therapies, independent work), each of which may require a designated place in the classroom, as well as specific furniture and materials. Placement of furniture and materials to accomplish specific goals then becomes an important consideration when working with individuals with ASD, especially given that different degrees of supervision are associated with some of these learning formats and that individual learners are likely to have different monitoring requirements. For example, a high-functioning student with ASD might need a special study carrel provided in a quiet corner of the room for his independent work. A beginning learner might be more inclined to stay in a gross-motor play area if his favorite play materials are in the area and some small, stabilized bookshelves form a perimeter around the area. And a mother might find that her young son with autism is much more willing to join the family for dinner if he sits at a small table and chair similar to what he uses at school.

Individuals with ASD are frequently described as inattentive, in spite of the fact that they may have the ability to spend long periods of time engaged in high-interest activities, oblivious to everyone and everything around them. The key, of course, is what captivates their interest, and to what degree some of their interests have been 'socialized' or shaped by the expectations and interests of others. The lack of 'common interests', of interest in others, and in pleasing others contributes to the frequently observed inattention and distractibility in many individuals with ASD. 'Engineering' an individual's environment to attract the student to places and activities that are appropriate and to minimize distractions that lead to inappropriate behaviours are primary considerations in a well-structured setting. Focusing an individual's attention may involve creating a clearly defined and distinctive appearance to the different areas (and expectations) in the classroom, and incorporating the individual's interests (if not obsessive) in the area's décor. Minimizing distractions within a setting may involve identifying any challenges to sensory integration and filtering that the individual may have and eliminating overwhelming sensory stimulation, and blocking competing interests with *sensory barriers* (*e.g.*, tall shelves, facing away from the distraction, noise-reducing head phones, sensory neutral clothing).

Finally, arranging the physical setting so that the available resources (*e.g.*, space, materials, and the teacher's time) are used in the most efficient and stress-minimizing fashion may need to be informed by the particular challenges and strengths of the individuals in that setting, especially in individuals with ASD. Making transitions in the setting easy and predictable (*e.g.*, having a relatively short distance for highly distractible learners to travel between activities), regulating access to materials and 'activity stations' (*e.g.*, computers and video games), and organizing play and break areas so that they can be student-maintained (*e.g.*, photos of objects on storage shelves to indicate return placement) may all help to contribute to efficient, easy-to-maintain settings for persons with ASD.

Individualized daily schedules

Inefficiencies in executive functioning likely contribute to many of the observed challenges individuals with ASD have in organizing time internally, sequencing activities and events, and anticipating the social demands that are inherent in specific situations and times of the day. The TEACCH strategy of providing an individualized daily schedule supports an individual's ability to remain focused and relaxed as he proceeds through the various demands of the day, in the same way that external written and electronic schedules help individuals without autism stay organized and efficient in meeting their daily responsibilities. External schedules are used when the demands for staying organized and recalling important appointments exceed a person's cognitive capabilities or when limited cognitive resources can be freed up for essential and creative activities, with the management of daily details routinized into the habit of keeping an external schedule. Because persons with ASD sometimes have more limited cognitive resources, the individualized daily schedule tends to be more of a necessity, to be used more pervasively throughout the individual's day, and for a longer period in the individual's development. Some individuals with autism may never develop the cognitive capacities to function effectively without an external schedule and, of course, special circumstances with heightened demands for personal organization and information processing (*e.g.*, a new job, work overload, impaired health) may require temporary use of an external schedule.

In addition, a schedule also functions as an effective tool to teach individuals with ASD about the expectations that others have for them (social agenda) throughout their day and to better manage their level of stress around meeting the expectations of others. In other words, use of an external schedule can promote social development, improve behaviour, and enhance self-control in individuals with ASD. Paradoxically, routinized use of a daily schedule can also be employed to increase efficiency in independent functioning and to teach flexibility in overly rigid individuals. As before, the key to an effective schedule is that it uses an individual's information-processing strengths to help compensate for his area of challenge in the same way that properly prescribed eyeglasses improve an individual's vision. For someone with ASD a generic schedule may not be any more helpful than a pair of magnifying lenses purchased in a drug store would be for someone with an atypical visual impairment.

In the traditional TEACCH model, schedules are 'prescribed' according to information gained from a detailed assessment of an individual's strengths and weaknesses in independently following another person's agenda. Specifically, how will the expectations for the person with ASD be communicated (type of schedule)? How many specific activities of the day should be presented to the individual at any given time (length of schedule)? How should the responsibility of keeping track of one's own schedule be ingrained in the individual (tracking of schedule)? And, how can the teacher or parent efficiently and effectively cue the individual to use her schedule for activities that she should not initiate herself (cueing the schedule)?

A final point: autism, by itself, often dictates that a schedule is necessary; however, the level of intellectual deficit usually determines how the schedule is presented. For an individual at the sensorimotor stage of development, handing him a functional object (what to do), at the specified time (when to do it), with a similar object clearly visible in the designated area (where to do it) may provide him with information about what is expected of him in a way that can be efficiently processed by his brain. More-capable individuals may readily understand more abstract, visual communications (*e.g.*, pictures or written words), and expanded 'listings' (multiple events) of what is expected of them throughout the day.

Task/activity visual structure

Practitioners of the TEACCH approach have learned this important lesson from working with students with ASD: by better organizing task materials, modifying instructions, and highlighting key information, a task can be more easily understood, made more interesting, and completed more independently, thereby enhancing the intrinsic motivation for being meaningfully and appropriately engaged in one's own learning. An intended benefit of this approach is that time off-task or otherwise inappropriate behaviour is greatly reduced.

Most consumer product manufacturers recognize that even among the general population there are distinct preferences in how instructions are to be presented in order to complete new and complex tasks (*e.g.*, putting together a bicycle, setting up a new computer). Typically, both written and picture instruction options are included and, more recently, video demonstrations can be accessed on YouTube or on company websites. Adapting a set of task instructions to make completing a task particularly *user-friendly* is one of the Structured Teaching strategies for working with individuals with ASD. However, when working with these individuals, modifying a task or activity may need to be specific to each individual, and generic modifications (like adding line-drawing picture instructions) may not be useful for all of the individuals who might be asked to work that task.

Traditionally, the types of modifications that can be made to tasks or activities for individuals with ASD are sorted into three categories: *task instructions, material organization*, and *highlighting key information*. Decisions about the amount and type of task 're-structuring' that needs to take place is usually based upon an intimate knowledge of how the individual best processes information (*e.g.*, the ability to imitate actions, to understand pictures, or to read words) and through careful observation and an *informal assessment*. A range of restructuring options is available, including allowing the materials to define the task, providing object or picture 'product samples' of completed work, constructing inset or picture jigs for assembly tasks; or using pictures, written words, or a combination of pictures/words to guide multiple-step activities.

Many individuals with ASD, especially beginning learners, have difficulty with visual/spatial scanning and organization. They may also be more attracted to the sensory features of items loosely organized than they are to a higher-cognitive-level purpose (*e.g.*, matching colors or shapes) for the materials. Providing additional organizational structure of the task can help the individual *F*ind the materials needed to complete a task more easily, *U*se the materials in an appropriate manner, and k*N*ow when a task has been completed successfully (mnemonic acronym *FUN*). When tasks are properly organized, the individual is much more likely to enjoy the 'work' and the endogenous reward system of the brain may be activated, thus making learning fun. Techniques for helping an individual find materials easily include isolating and securing (*e.g.*, with Velcro) small pieces, limiting the amount of materials used, sorting and 'containerizing' materials, and labeling containers with pictures or words. Techniques for reducing the inappropriate use of some materials include separating and stabilizing loose items so that a pincer grasp is necessary to manipulate the objects, limiting learning trials to reduce frustration (and the throwing of materials), and securing lids to task receptacles (*e.g.*, put-in container) to minimize perseveration with materials. Techniques for helping the individual know when the task is completed might be separate start and finish containers for materials, arranging all of the possible 'answers' in a display panel which empties as the answers are used up, or breaking a complex task into clearly defined and sequentially worked sections until the entire task is completed.

Finally, given what we are learning about the neurobiology of the brain it seems likely that social factors have shaped the development of brain structures and functions at all levels, including the level of *perceptual selection bias* – the innate tendencies of the brain to attend to sensory information that has social significance, such as quickly scanning a room full of objects and people to determine social intent (*e.g.*, attending to a lecturer at the front of the room). Inefficiencies in these tendencies may contribute to the ways in which individuals with ASD appear to see the world differently. The TEACCH strategy of highlighting important aspects of tasks so that they are more likely to be completed in the (socially prescribed) manner intended has proven useful in working with many individuals with ASD. Highlighting typically includes sharpening the contrast in boundaries around an important feature of a task (*e.g.*, outlining a receptacle opening in black ink) or drawing attention to an important feature by modifying a pertinent attribute (color, shape, size) (*e.g.*, placing a colored background into containers used for color-matching specific objects).

Work/activity systems

To parents and practitioners alike, one of the most perplexing (and sometimes frustrating) characteristics of individuals affected by ASD is their inconsistent performance of skills that are well within their abilities. From a behavioural perspective, this is the equivalent of the failure-to-generalize phenomenon. This tendency also accounts for the typically counterproductive 'can't-*versus*-won't' debate that repeatedly plays out in households and school conference rooms across the country. In normal development consistency of performance is the direct result of the socialization process in which society's expectation that we always 'do our best' becomes mostly internalized and eventually self-reinforced. Parents come to expect a particular level of consistency from their children, teachers from their students, supervisors from their supervisees, and, yes, wives from their husbands (and *vice versa*). Autism seems to short-circuit this process, leaving the person much less interested in pleasing others and preferring to 'do what I want to do all of the time'.

The TEACCH strategy of using work/activity systems seems to address this functional incompatibility between the brains of individuals with ASD and the social expectation to work consistently across settings by making work expectations more visual, developmentally appropriate, and inherently rewarding. The work/activity system is essentially a 'to do' list, not unlike what is found in calendar organizers, typed into meeting agendas, or handwritten on a note pad before the beginning of a busy day. Work tasks for a beginning learner may be organized on the actual workspace ('task on table' [ToT]), or next to the workspace and moved onto the workspace ('left to right'). For an intermediate learner, work may be just outside the immediate workspace necessitating a 'move and match' maneuver to find the work and bring it back to the workspace. Work systems for advanced learners tend to be written lists with materials situated in a variety of places in and even out of the room.

Once again, the individual's cognitive abilities determine what level of abstraction (concrete object to abstract written symbol) can be used to represent the work that needs to be done and how the system is set up. In addition, the system incorporates the brain's tendency to repeat efficient routines, gain *confidence through competence* (self-efficacy) by seeing work completed, respond to the natural incentives of one's own special interests, and boost performance by designating an extrinsic 'reward' when all of the work is done. In a very practical and efficient manner a properly prescribed work/activity system compensates for many of the performance deficits due to lower levels of social motivation. (Of course, praise and other social reinforcers are paired with an individual's *efforts* to use the work/activity system in order to build the individual's capacity to internalize and respond to positive social expectations.)

Because work/activity systems are intended to address some of the deficits in social development and to prepare the individual for the highest levels of independent functioning, they are integrated into a treatment/educational program at the earliest of ages and designed at the child's emerging level of frustration tolerance that results from not getting one's way – 'first do what I want you to do, then you get to do what you want to do'. This is the first rule of learning to cooperate with others. As the person's ability to delay gratification and consistently perform independent work develops, the structure of the work/activity systems may be modified and, perhaps, eventually 'faded' out in some settings. But like with 'neurotypical' individuals, once a work/activity system has become a useful tool, it can be reintroduced when the demands of a given situation either exceed the functional capabilities of the person's brain or when an external system is preferred in order to offer greater reliability, to enhance the satisfaction that comes with seeing work 'checked off', or to preserve cognitive energies for other tasks.

Empirical evidence for the TEACCH approach and future research considerations

The TEACCH autism program is somewhat unique given its longevity, broad spectrum of services and products, integrative theoretical framework, and diversity of clientele (*cf.* Odom *et al.*, 2010). With this uniqueness come particular challenges in program evaluation, in general, and in separating out and evaluating individual components or strategies. Further, it is probably the case that data that might have, at one time, provided reasonable 'evidence' in support of an intervention may no longer conform to contemporary standards of evidence. This is likely true for some of the early studies 'demonstrating' the effectiveness of the TEACCH program (Mesibov & Shea, 2010), as it is for research supporting the effectiveness of early programs based in, for example, discrete trial training (*i.e.*, the Lovaas model) (*cf.* Rutter, 2011). An updated accounting of both the concept of 'evidence based' and a summary of the studies of the effectiveness of strategies based in the TEACCH approach can be found in two related articles by Mesibov and Shea (2010, 2011).

Given the current state of evaluation of comprehensive interventions for ASD (*e.g.*, Odom *et al.*, 2010; Rogers & Vismara, 2008), it can be argued that nearly every empirical study done to date has employed a *quasi-experimental design* (Campbell & Stanley, 1963) with potentially confounding variables insufficiently controlled. Although randomly assigning subjects to treatment and comparison groups (randomized controlled trials or RCTs) should, *theoretically*, equally distribute (and, therefore, neutralize) the effects of variables that cannot be otherwise controlled, rarely is there sufficient information available that would allow for this assumption to be tested. Moreover, experimental methodology is designed not to determine *directly* whether a treatment is effective (experimental hypothesis), but to evaluate the hypothesis that the treatment is not effective (null hypothesis) for a large group of individuals who share a similar 'condition' (*cf.* Campbell & Stanley, 1963). Therefore, interpretations of experimental data tend to be more useful in telling us what we *should not do* for a large group of people (*e.g.*, prescribing secretin for individuals with autism or discontinuing vaccines for all children), than they are at telling us precisely what we *should do* for an individual person. Perhaps, the most optimistic statement that can be made about a particular intervention (from an empirical perspective) is that it is 'promising' and needs further study. Claims based upon an interpretation of experimental data that a particular approach leads to 'recovery' or is the 'only scientifically proven' treatment for autism are unfounded.

Moving forward, a number of researchers have offered several suggestions that have the potential to enhance the empirical basis for prescribing autism treatments. First, priority for funding 'end-stage' treatment-outcome studies (Smith *et al.*, 2007) should be given to independent evaluators. The common practice of developers conducting research on their own treatment protocols is akin to pharmaceutical companies evaluating their own 'new drug in the pipeline' – the potential for even unintended bias is high and it may not be identified in peer review. Second, with independent evaluations, in particular, comes the need for the development of quality fidelity measures and monitoring (*e.g.*, Hume *et al.*, 2011).

Third, most experienced clinicians-as-researchers recognize the potential significance of the interpersonal context of treatment delivery (*nonspecific treatment effects*), even though few of them identify these confounding variables in the discussion of study limitations, and fewer still attempt to measure these variables and control for them in some fashion (*e.g.*, by entering them as covariates in the statistical analysis). For example, it seems very likely that the treatment providers differ on a range of characteristics such as enthusiasm, belief in the method, interpersonal skills, and job satisfaction, especially when they have been hand-picked and trained by a charismatic leader with the promise of an innovative approach; in contrast to a comparison group of providers made up of a particular group of dedicated community service workers who may be poorly supported by their overwhelmed administration, may not receive adequate continuing education (*cf.* Odom *et al.*, 2012), and may be at risk for professional 'burnout'. The failure to account for interpersonal and other contextual variables may be one of the reasons why significant results are often not fully replicated (*cf.* Ozonoff, 2011).

And finally, treatment programs that afford greater ecological validity, such as those implemented by TEACCH, are much more difficult to evaluate than, for example, a single-subject experiment employing behavioural methods conducted in a specialized learning lab. Until new methods of assessing multifaceted treatments in community settings are developed and validated, a reasonable 'facsimile' of current best practice may reside in clinical expertise (informed by clinical experience, empirical research and expert consensus opinion), a clear statement of treatment principles and rationale, and an ethical commitment to ongoing client monitoring using both quantitative and qualitative measures.

The temptation to suggest that using the term 'evidence-based' in the description of an intervention somehow equates with a higher level of 'objectivity' or validity *without a critical analysis of the limitations of experimental methods* should be resisted, even by well-meaning providers who every day join clients and families in the desperate search for 'answers'. In the end, it is partly the work of science *to quantify uncertainty, not to deny it.* Scientists engaged in public policy discussions regarding funding for ASD services should be cautious about overstating what is currently known, and what can be known through empirical methods.

Acknowledgments: I would like to thank Greg Rich for assistance in preparing this manuscript.

Conflicts of interest: The author declares no conflicts of interest.

References

American Psychiatric Association (2000): *Diagnostic and Statistical Manual of Mental Disorders (4th Edition, Text Revision).* Washington, DC: APA.

Behrmann, M., Thomas, C., Kimchi, R. & Minshew, N. (2005): Visual perceptual organization in adults with autism. *J. Vis.* **5,** 283.

Boswell, S. (2009): *Let's Get Started! Visually Structured Tasks from the TEACCH Early Childhood Demonstration Program.* Chapel Hill, NC: Susan Boswell.

Bowlby, J. (1969): *Attachment and Loss.* New York: Basic Books.

Campbell, D.T. & Stanley, J.C. (1963): *Experimental and Quasi-Experimental Designs for Research.* Boston: Houghton, Mifflin.

Colle, L., Baron-Cohen, S. & Hill, J. (2007): Do children with autism have a theory of mind? A non-verbal test of autism *vs.* specific language impairment. *J. Autism Dev. Disord.* **37,** 716–723.

Eckenrode, L., Fennell, P. & Hearsey, K. (2003): *Tasks Galore.* Raleigh, NC: Tasks Galore Publishing Inc.

Grandin, T. (1995): *Thinking in Pictures and Other Reports from my Life with Autism.* New York: Doubleday.

Harms, M., Martin, A. & Wallace, G. (2010): Facial emotion recognition in autism spectrum disorders: a review of behavioral and neuroimaging studies. *Neuropsychol. Rev.* **20,** 290–322.

Hume, K., Boyd, B., McBee, M., *et al.* (2011): Assessing implementation of comprehensive treatment models for young children with ASD: reliability and validity of two measures. *Res. Autism Spect. Disord.* **5,** 1430–1440.

Kanner, L. (1943): Affective disturbances of affective contact. *Nerv. Child* **2,** 217–253.

Lord, C. & Paul, R. (1997): Language and communication in autism. In: *Handbood of Autism and Pervasive Developmental Disorders*, 2nd ed., eds. D.J. Cohen & F.R. Volkmar. New York: Wiley.

Mesibov, G.B. (2006): A tribute to Eric Schopler. *J Autism Dev. Disord.* **36,** 967–970.

Mesibov, G.B. & Shea, V. (2010): The TEACCH program in the era of evidence-based practice. *J. Autism Dev. Disord.* **40,** 570–579.

Mesibov, G.B. & Shea, V. (2011): Evidence-based practices and autism. *Autism* **15,** 114–133.

Mesibov, G., Shea, V. & Schopler, E. (2005): *The TEACCH Approach to Autism Spectrum Disorders.* New York: Kluwer Academic/Plenum.

Minshew, N.J., Meyer, J. & Goldstein, G. (2002): Abstract reasoning in autism: a disassociation between concept formation and concept identification. *Neuropsychology* **16,** 327–334.

Odom, S.L., Boyd, B.A., Hall, L.J. & Hume, K. (2010): Evaluation of comprehensive treatment models for individuals with autism spectrum disorders. *J. Autism Dev. Disord.* **40,** 425–436.

Odom, S., Hume, K., Boyd, B. & Stabel, A. (2012): Moving beyond the intensive behavior treatment versus eclectic dichotomy. *Behav. Mod.* **36,** 270–297.

Osterling, J., Dawson, G. & Munson, J. (2002): Early recognition of 1-year-old infants with autism spectrum disorder versus mental retardation. *Dev. Psychopathol.* **14,** 239–251.

Ozonoff, S. (2011): Editorial: the first cut is the deepest: why do the reported effects of treatments decline over trials? *J. Child Psychol. Psychiatry* **52,** 729–730.

Rogers, S.J. & Vismara, L.A. (2008): Evidence-based comprehensive treatments for early autism. *J. Clin. Child Adolesc. Psychol.* **37,** 8–38.

Rutter, M. (2011): Progress in understanding autism: 2007–2010. *J. Autism Dev. Disord.* **41,** 395–404.

Schultz, R., Gauthier, I., Klin, A., *et al.* (2000): Abnormal ventral temporal cortical activity during face discrimination among individuals with autism and Asperger syndrome. *Arch. Gen. Psychiatry* **57,** 331–340.

Smith, T., Scahill, L., Dawson, G., *et al.* (2007): Designing research studies on psychosocial interventions in autism. *J. Autism Dev. Disord.* **37,** 354–366.

Wolfberg, P.J. (1999): *Play and Imagination in Children with Autism.* New York: Columbia University Teacher's College Press.

Chapter 12

Experience using the TEACCH program at the Autism Centre of AO San Paolo in Milan: applications and critical aspects

Monica Saccani

*Center for Autism and Developmental Disability, Azienda Ospedaliera San Paolo,
via Di Rudinì 8, 20142 Milan, Italy*
monica.saccani@ao-sanpaolo.it

Summary

This paper outlines developments in provision for people with autism spectrum disorders (ASDs) that have occurred over the last ten years within the Autism Centre of San Paolo Hospital (CTR). The intervention approach of the Centre refers to the TEACCH program, which was introduced in Italy in the 1980s. TEACCH (Treatment and Education of Autistic and Related Communication-Handicapped Children) is an evidence-based service, training, and research program for individuals of all ages and skill levels with autism spectrum disorders (Mesibov & Shea, 2010). This program is based at the University of North Carolina at Chapel Hill, and was established in the early 1970s by Eric Schopler and colleagues. The TEACCH program has been used in thousands of individuals with autism spectrum disorders. Our Centre has been inspired by TEACCH with regard to its neuropsychological framework and treatment. Significant improvements, both in levels of diagnosis and of service provision, have been achieved since its initiation both generally and at AO San Paolo. Recent literature on autism spectrum disorders suggests different developmental trajectories when an early diagnosis of an ASD is made and treatment is quickly provided (Wallace & Rogers, 2010; Warren *et al.*, 2011). The Autism Centre has moved to early intervention based on shared attention development, imitation, and intersubjective relations, which are carried out, when possible, within an environment familiar to the child. The paper goes on to discuss the challenges that have been faced and overcome as well as remaining areas of need.

Introduction

Autism is a developmental disability characterized by difficulties and abnormalities in several areas: communication skills, social relationships, cognitive functioning, sensory processing, and behaviour. Approximately 10–15 per cent of individuals with autism have average or above-average intelligence: 25 to 35 per cent function in the range of borderline to mild mental retardation, while the remainder are moderately to profoundly mentally retarded. The TEACCH approach is called Structured Teaching, which is based on evidence and observation that individuals with autism share a pattern of neuropsychological deficits and strengths called the 'culture of Autism' (Mesibov et al., 2005). The following items list these characteristics of autism that are at the heart of CTR's intervention approach, based on the principles of Structured Teaching:

1. Relative strength in and preference for processing visual information (compared to difficulties with auditory processing, particularly of language).
2. Heightened attention to details, but difficulty with sequencing, integrating, connecting, or deriving meaning from them.
3. Enormous variability in attention.
4. Communication problems, which vary by developmental level, but always include impairments in the initiation and social use of language (pragmatics).
5. Difficulty with concepts of time and having problems recognizing the beginning or end of an activity, how long the activity will last, and when it will be finished.
6. Tendency to become attached to routines and the settings where they are established, so that activities may be difficult to transfer or generalize from the original learning situation, and disruptions in routines can be uncomfortable or upsetting.
7. Very intense interests and impulses to engage in favored activities and difficulties disengaging once engaged.
8. Marked sensory preferences and aversions (see Dawson, 1996; Ozonoff et al., 2005; Tsatsanis, 2005).

The principles of Structured Teaching allow us to structure the environment and activities in ways that are understandable to the individual; for example, we use individual relative strengths in visual skills and interests in visual details to supplement relatively weaker skills, as well as individual special interests to engage autistic patients in learning and supporting self-initiated use of meaningful communication.

Because autistic organically-based disabilities are non-reversible, the TEACCH Program does not take 'being normal' as the goal of its educational and therapeutic efforts. Rather, the long-term goal of the TEACCH program is for youths with autism to fit as well as possible into our society as they grow into adulthood. Recently considerable progress in early detection of ASD has been made thanks to the productiveness of infant sibling studies and early screening studies (Yirmiya et al., 2006; Zwaigenbaum et al., 2005, 2010). As a consequence, early interventions with children need to be oriented to develop joint attention and communication skills as well as social interests (and thus not just independence and functional behaviour).

Review of the topic

Over the last ten years, diversity in behavioural phenotypes of ASDs has become a central issue to setting a comprehensive assessment and a tailored intervention. As mentioned, considerable progress has been achieved in the early detection of ASD by means of infant sibling studies and early screening studies. The primary purpose of such early detection is to prevent or mitigate symptoms and severity of disability associated with ASDs through early and intensive intervention (Wallace & Rogers, 2010).

For this reason, CTR turned to a more specific set of interventions dealing exclusively with ASDs (since the beginning of the 2000s CTR carried on its activity in children with ASDs, integrating TEACCH multi-professional programs with early intervention, while the outpatient department screened children with all kinds of developmental delays.

At the same time we set a screening program for early identification of signs of ASD in infants from 6 months to 2 years old, which was composed of two steps:
(1) training for the pediatric professionals who alert our district by 'red flagging' cases where they suspect communicative and social interaction disorders; and
(2) and an outpatient department for monitoring infants and toddlers with developmental disorders and supporting their parents' competencies (Olivari et al., 2012). A subset of children with ASDs is found on screening and then selected for the structured teaching program at CTR.

Systematic literature research and effect size analysis of interventions for infants and toddlers with developmental disorders revealed that the most efficacious interventions routinely used a combination of four specific intervention procedures including (1) parental involvement in intervention, ongoing coaching of the parent focused both on parental responsivity and sensitivity to the child's cues, and on teaching families to provide the infant interventions; (2) individualization of the singular infant's developmental profile; (3) focus on a broad rather than a narrow range of learning targets; and (4) characteristics that are noticed as early as the risk is detected, allowing greater intensity and duration of the intervention (Wallace & Rogers, 2010).

When diagnosis of an ASD is confirmed, according to scientific evaluation, we schedule individual sessions for parents in order to: (*a*) improve their understanding of their child's behaviour and characteristics; (*b*) teach them how to set the environment to improve the child's attention and comprehension, turning a normal situation into a motivational one; (*c*) help parents to recognize the communication skills of their child within a natural setting; and (*d*) develop parental skills to handle the child's behaviour within the domestic milieu.

CTR patients' ages range from 3 to 15 years, and different ages are associated with different interventions. We have two main goals: (1) assessment of the individual child's strengths and needs in order to develop effective teaching strategies (especially for preschoolers); and (2) engaging the parents in the work, as suggested by the TEACCH philosophy, as if they are co-therapists.

The TEACCH staff shares knowledge about autism and effective intervention strategies. Parents are encouraged in turn to share their detailed knowledge of their child and family and to observe, give feedback, and gradually apply principles of Structured Teaching in activities with their child. Intervention with preschoolers consists of an ongoing assessment of social and communicative competences and behaviour. We use PEP-3 for assessing expressive and receptive communication, play, social interaction and learning abilities (attention, self-organizational and generalizing competence according to the principles of Structured Teaching), and then we create a curriculum with a singular evaluation of each kind of competence (Schopler et al., 2006).

Spontaneous communication is a vital goal for all people with ASDs. We suggest that activities for learning language and/or social communication have a visual or physically concrete component because visual processing is relatively easier to comprehend and makes a stronger impression than auditory processing does in children with ASDs.

Furthermore, Structured Teaching can be an excellent foundation for facilitating social activities that would otherwise be too unpredictable and confusing for children with ASDs. And, while Structured TEACCHing values independence highly and has established it as an important educational priority, developing enjoyable social interaction and meaningful social relationships are also important priorities.

With 5- to 8-year-old children, education becomes the primary form of treatment: Each student is unique, and multiple developmental needs call for a variety of educational options, so educators must be familiar with theory and research concerning best practices and be able to implement them accurately.

Individual treatment is associated with small group treatment (therapist-to-child ratio between 2:4 and 2:5), and groups are composed of patients with similar functional levels meeting from two to five times per week. A session usually lasts between 1.5 and 2.5 hours. Individual goals, sharing communication with peers, and imitation play are all fundamental aspects in generalizing learned abilities.

Small groups and individual interventions use strategies and methods based on Structured Teaching, including physical organization and environmental supports, a picture exchange communication systems, and an independent work system. *Physical organization and environmental supports* refers to visual supports and schedules that assist children in organizing daily events, knowing what will happen next, and facilitating transition from one activity to the next. Visual support forms include iconic pictures of scheduled activities, sequential pictures of scheduled activities, and transportable schedules that children carry from one setting to another. The *pictures exchange communication system* is a systematic method of teaching students a socially interactive and functional communication system. The *independent work system* is designed to assist children in understanding the questions (*1*) What do I have to do? (*2*) How much do I do? (*3*) How will I know I'm finished? and (*4*) What happens when I'm finished?

All these strategies and visual supports increase understanding, facilitate learning and independence, and decrease behavioural problems.

An effective ASD program also includes 'home base programs', 'safe-harbor programs', competent buddy pairing, and protection from teasing and bullying. Parent and teacher training and support are fundamental parts of this effective ASD program, because they allow patients to apply their learned abilities into protective and natural environments. Teachers and parents, because of their deep knowledge of the child, are able to suggest the best strategies for different social contexts.

Teachers in Italy are not specifically trained to deal with autism so this training has to be completely supplied by the Centre. This program involves teachers who work with children in treatment and informs them about the characteristics of ASDs along with the principles of Structured Teaching. We noticed that visual strategies that support communicative issues are more often used than ones that support the whole working system, and are so-called 'Augmentative Alternative Communication/PECS/PCS').

Recent literature shows that from childhood to adulthood, there is a general tendency toward modest improvement and alleviation of symptoms across studies despite a wide variation in design, measurement, and diagnostic criteria. Shattuck *et al.* (2007) found, in adolescent and adult patients, a greater prevalence of impairment in nonverbal communication and social reciprocity than in verbal communication or repetitive behaviours and stereotyped interests. This pattern of findings lends support to the idea that impaired social reciprocity is both more central and more persistent than the other core symptoms of the autism behavioural phenotype (Mesibov *et al.*, 1989; Volkmar & Klin, 2005). The most robust predictor of change in both autism symptoms and maladaptive behaviours seems to be whether or not there is a comorbid diagnosis of mental retardation, which is similar to what has been found in autism in children at earlier stages of life.

Transition planning from adolescence to adulthood for individuals with autism spectrum disorders should comprise a coordinated set of activities for a student, designed within a result-oriented process which facilitates movement from school to post-school activities. Transition from rehabilitation structures and schools to adult services is a major life cycle change: families must be prepared, gather information and be informed, and develop a network of 'natural support' systems. Families must be involved in developing a clear picture of their son or daughter with regard to postsecondary education, work, and housing; they should be helped to be clear about expectations and have a life plan.

Transition planning is a big challenge facing services for children with ASDs in implementing effective practices. Because the skills needed for learners with ASDs are not optimal, how do we decide what to teach? It depends on the desired post-school outcomes and on the degree to which the typical curriculum can be adapted to meet the needs of a particular student. We should consider and promote those basic living (functional) skills, the social and self-determination skills that a specific student can achieve. CTR therapists usually evaluate a wide range of competences regarding occupational and social domains through TTAP (TEACCH-Transition Assessment Profile; Mesibov et al., 2007). We focus on self-protection abilities and a degree of autonomy in order to decide whether to enter the student into neurotypical groups (for high functioning individuals) or another program (for severely intellectually impaired ones).

Effective transition practices should begin early to conduct person-centered planning that addresses the personal interests and unique characteristics, skills, and talents of the student. Transition planning has to be built on the patient's personal experiences and create opportunities that increase strengths and minimize weaknesses: It requires effective collaboration among agencies, schools, and community members.

In Italy transition is carried out within scholastic contexts which are not oriented to the development of the Individualized Education Plan (IEP) beyond their specific learning domain. Moreover, there are few community services that are set up to guarantee intervention and continuity of care for adolescents and adults with ASDs.

Conclusions

The two main aspects for effective ASD treatment are (1) early intervention and (2) transition planning from school age to adolescence and adulthood.

Early intensive treatment, delivered within an affectively rich relationship-focused context, can be effective for improving outcomes of young children with autism. Parents' use of these strategies at home during their daily activities is an important ingredient for successful outcomes. As reported by other authors who work with persons with ASDs during transitional ages, effective transition planning has a positive impact on students, their families, and their communities. It is important to include students and their families as active participants in planning and to offer them real choices coming from real experiences, including work and supported-work experiences or inclusion in day-care services. We think that we can reach the long-term goal of the TEACCH program for youths with autism 'to fit as well as possible into our society as an adult' only by combining these two main aspects.

Acknowledgments: The work with families and their children was partially supported by a grant (A11-59 – 2011) from the Mariani Foundation (Milan), Progetto Assistenza.

Conflicts of interest: The author declares no conflicts of interest.

References

Dawson, G. (1996)· Brief report: neuropsychology of autism: a report on the state of the science. *J. Autism Dev. Disord.* **26**, 179–184.

Mesibov, G.B. & Shea, V. (2010): The TEACCH Program in the era of evidence-based practice. *J. Autism Dev. Disord.* **40**, 570–579.

Mesibov, G.B., Schopler, E., Schaffer, B. & Michal, N. (1989): Use of the Childhood Autism Rating Scale with autistic adolescents and adults. *J. Am. Acad. Child Adolesc. Psychiatry* **28**, 538–541.

Mesibov, G.B., Shea, V. & Schopler, E. (2005): *The TEACCH Approach to Autism Spectrum Disorders.* New York: Springer.

Mesibov, G.B., Thomas, J.B., Chapman, S.M. & Schopler, E. (2007): *TTAP: TEACCH Transition Assessment Profile* (2nd ed.). Austin, TX: Pro-Ed.

Olivari, B., Olgiati, P., Grossi, M.L., Saccani, M. & Lenti, C. (2012): Indicatori e rischio di disturbo dello spettro autistico: studio longitudinale dei primi due anni di vita. *Autismo e Disturbi dello Sviluppo* **10**, 53–69.

Ozonoff, S., South, M. & Provençal, S. (2005): Executive functions. In: *Handbook of Autism and Pervasive Developmental Disorders (3rd ed.) – Vol. 1: Diagnosis, Development, Neurobiology, and Behaviour*, eds. F.R. Volkmar, R. Paul, A. Klin & D. Cohen, pp. 606–627. Hoboken, NJ: Wiley.

Shattuck, P.T., Seltzer, M.M., Greenberg, J.S., et al. (2007): Change in autism symptoms and maladaptive behaviours in adolescents and adults with an autism spectrum disorder. *J. Autism Dev. Disord.* **37**, 1735–1747.

Schopler, E.,Villa, S. & Micheli, E. (2006): *PEP 3 Profilo Psicoeducativo*, 3rd ed. Brescia, Italy: Vannini Ed.

Tsatsanis, K.D. (2005): Neuropsychological characteristics in autism and related conditions. In: *Handbook of Autism and Pervasive Developmental Disorders (3rd ed.) - Vol. 1: Diagnosis, Development, Neurobiology and Behaviour*, eds. F.R. Volkmar, R. Paul, A. Klin & D. Cohen, pp. 365–381. Hoboken, NJ: Wiley.

Volkmar, F.R. & Klein, A. (2005): Issues in the classification of autism related conditions. In: *Handbook of Autism and Pervasive Developmental Disorders*, eds. F.R. Volkmar, R. Paul, A. Klin & D.J. Cohen, pp. 5–41. Hoboken, NJ: Wiley.

Wallace, K.S. & Rogers, S.J. (2010): Intervening in infancy: implications for autism spectrum disorders. *J. Child Psychol. Psychiatry* **51**, 1300–1320.

Warren, Z., McPheeters, M.L., Sathe, N., et al. (2011): A systematic review of early intensive intervention for autism spectrum disorders. *Pediatrics* **127**, 1303–1311.

Yirmiya, N., Gamliel, I., Pilowsky, T., Feldman, R., Baron-Cohen, S. & Sigman, M. (2006): The development of siblings of children with autism at 4 and 14 months: social engagement, communication, and cognition. *J. Child Psychol. Psychiatry* **47**, 511–523.

Zwaigenbaum, L. (2010): Advances in the early detection of autism. *Curr. Opin. Neurol.* **23**, 97–102.

Zwaigenbaum, L., Bryson, S., Rogers, T., Roberts, W., Brian, J. & Szatmari, P. (2005): Behavioural manifestations of autism in the first year of life. *Int. J. Dev. Neurosci.* **23**, 143–152.

Chapter 13

Applied Behaviour Analysis and the analysis of verbal behaviour in treating autism

Judah B. Axe

*Department of Education, Simmons College, 300 The Fenway, W304A,
Boston, Massachusetts 02115, USA*
judah.axe@simmons.edu

Summary

Applied Behaviour Analysis (ABA) is an assessment and treatment approach to alleviating problems of human behaviour, most commonly in individuals with autism. It is derived from the basic experimental work of B.F. Skinner and the 45-year history of publications on the subject in the *Journal of Applied Behavior Analysis*. Three applications of ABA are described in this chapter: First, discrete trial training is an intensive, one-on-one approach to teaching language and academic skills. Second, ABA is used to conduct functional behaviour assessments and function-based interventions to understand the causes of challenging behaviours, and to treat them using preventive methods. Third, the analysis of verbal behaviour is a conceptual analysis used to understand the environmental variables evoking and maintaining instances of communication, and to alter those variables to produce desired communicative repertoires. All ABA approaches analyze behaviour using the basic principles of behaviour (*e.g.*, positive reinforcement, extinction, stimulus control, motivating operations), make programmatic changes using carefully collected data, and evaluate treatments using rigorous research methods. Practice based on ABA has been validated in numerous research studies using single-subject design, randomized clinical trials, and meta-analysis. Autism practitioners should adopt ABA methods not only because they are effective, but also because practitioners can derive the benefits of joining the profession of practicing behaviour analysts.

Introduction

Treatments based on Applied Behaviour Analysis (ABA) have the most research evidence amongst other treatments for children diagnosed with autism (National Research Council, 2001; Surgeon General, 1999). Applied behaviour analysis is derived from the work of B.F. Skinner (1938, 1953), who outlined the science of operant conditioning, the concepts of positive reinforcement, and the philosophy of behaviourism. His basic science approach, *the experimental analysis of behaviour*, allowed discoveries to be made about the fundamental laws of behaviour, including positive reinforcement, extinction, and stimulus control. In 1968, Baer, Wolf, and Risley took Skinner's experimental approach and founded the *Journal of Applied Behavior Analysis*, which published studies applying that science to solving problems of human behaviour. Early examples of such challenges were reducing disruptive behaviours in classrooms, increasing cooperative play of preschool children, and improving mathematics skills. The current chapter describes three major ABA approaches derived from this early work: discrete trial training, function-based reductions of challenging behaviour, and the analysis of verbal behaviour.

Building on the ABA foundation, Lovaas's (1987) seminal study documented improvements in communication, play, challenging behaviours, and IQ (*e.g.*, the Wechsler Intelligence Scale for Children–Revised; Wechsler, 1974) in children diagnosed with autism who received intensive training based on the principles of ABA. The intensiveness of this *discrete trial training* (DTT) approach was in the form of 40 hours per week of one-on-one, direct teaching of individual skills, such as matching pictures, receptively identifying objects, and imitating motor movements. The major goals of the treatment were to increase expressive and receptive communication, verbal and motor imitation, play skills, academic skills, and other conceptual skills. Lovaas's study, along with Catherine Maurice's (1993) personal account of her experience witnessing the vast benefits achieved by DTT in her child with autism, spawned a movement of parents and teachers seeking this intensive approach for their children. Discrete trial training continues to be popular and has gained further research support (Eikeseth *et al.*, 2002; Howard *et al.*, 2005; Sallows & Graupner, 2005) summarized in meta-analyses (Kuppens & Onghena, 2012; Peters-Scheffer *et al.*, 2011; Virués-Ortega, 2010).

A second development in applying behaviour analysis to treating children with autism was the work of Iwata *et al.* (1982/1994), who developed a methodology for analyzing the environmental events that evoked and maintained challenging behaviour. Common forms of such behaviour in children with autism are loud vocalizations, destruction of property, aggression, and self-injury. The methodology of Iwata *et al.* and Vollmer *et al.* (2001), *functional behaviour assessment*, involves observing a child's challenging behaviour and noting the environmental events that immediately precede and follow those behaviours. Such observations allow a therapist to determine the function, or cause, of the problem behaviour, such as to gain attention or escape from demands. Understanding the function of a challenging behaviour, a therapist can design a *function-based intervention* to alter the environmental variables affecting this behaviour, thereby reducing its instances. Studies on analyzing and treating difficult behaviour have dominated the *Journal of Applied Behavior Analysis* and related journals (see Hanley *et al.*, 2003 and Mueller *et al.*, 2011 for reviews).

A third application of behaviour analysis is Sundberg and Michael's (2001) description of applying Skinner's (1957) analysis of verbal behaviour to treating communication skills in children with autism. The basic approach is similar to the analysis of problem behaviour in that the therapist directly analyzes the environmental variables evoking and maintaining instances of ineffective communication, and alters those environmental variables to produce desired communicative repertoires. A hallmark of this approach is determining whether a word is controlled by the variables that control a request, a label, a response to someone else's communication, text, and so on. This *analysis of verbal behaviour* borrows methodology from DTT and also emphasizes teaching in the natural environment. Like the other two applications of ABA, the analysis of verbal behaviour has a rich research base (see Sautter & LeBlanc, 2006 for a review).

Review of the topic

This chapter reviews the defining features of, and research evidence for, three primary applications of ABA: discrete trial training, behaviour management, and the analysis of verbal behaviour.

Discrete trial training

A discrete trial is defined as a single instance of an antecedent, a behaviour, and a consequence (Cooper *et al.*, 2007). This *ABC paradigm* is inherent in all analyses of ABA and will be discussed throughout this chapter. The behaviour (B) is the behaviour of the child or of the person whose behaviour is being analyzed or treated; and the antecedent (A) and consequence (C) occur in the child's environment, and usually as another person's behaviour. In discrete trial training (DTT), an antecedent is usually a question or an instruction, such as 'What's your name?', 'Match these colours', or 'Where is the shoe?'. The behaviour is responding to this question or instruction, such as telling one's name, matching the colors, or pointing to the shoe. Finally, the consequence is the delivery of a preferred item or event given a correct response, or an error correction for an incorrect response. This delivery of a preferred item is perhaps the most important part of DTT because it is what makes a child respond correctly more often, and it establishes connections between antecedent events and behaviours.

Understanding the effects of that preferred item requires understanding the definition of *positive reinforcement*: the process of delivering an item or event immediately following a behaviour and observing a future increase in that behaviour (Skinner, 1953). Most simply, this can be applied to a casual occurrence of a behaviour, such as a child approaching a teacher. If a preferred event, such as the teacher's blowing bubbles, is delivered when a child approaches the teacher, there is positive reinforcement if the child approaches the teacher more often in the future. The teacher can blow bubbles simply when a child gets a little closer to a teacher and withhold bubbles when the child walks away from the teacher. The process is termed *differential reinforcement* because one behaviour is reinforced and another behaviour is not. If the teacher differentially reinforces successive approximations of this approach behaviour until the child completely approaches a teacher, the process is termed *shaping*. Positive reinforcement is applied in a DTT format when there is first an instruction, such as 'come here'. When a reinforcer (*e.g.*, bubbles) is delivered for a behaviour (*e.g.*, approaching a teacher) only in the presence of an antecedent (*e.g.*, 'come here'), the A–B connection is reinforced, and the child will approach the teacher when she says, 'come here' more often in the future.

Applying this most important concept of positive reinforcement requires identifying effective, potent reinforcers for students. For most typically-developing children, praise and attention from adults function as reinforcers. However, these consequences often do not function as reinforcers for children diagnosed with autism, and teachers and therapists must identify consequences that will function as reinforcers by increasing the future likelihood of behaviour they follow. Therapists should consider the full range of senses when identifying reinforcers: sight (*e.g.*, bubbles, spinning objects), taste (*e.g.*, pretzels, juice), sound (*e.g.*, music), smells (*e.g.*, perfumes), and touch (*e.g.*, tickles, shoulder rubs, engagement with toys). Therapists can identify reinforcers by displaying items and observing how long a child spends with each item (Sautter *et al.*, 2008). Therapists can also use trial-based procedures by systematically presenting 2–10 items and collecting data on particular selections (DeLeon & Iwata, 1996; Fisher *et al.*, 1992). This systematic method of identifying reinforcers is known as *preference assessment*.

In addition to positive reinforcement, a basic concept required for DTT is *stimulus control*. That is, a therapist aims to establish the reliable control of an antecedent over a particular response. This is accomplished most generally through *discrimination training*, in which a response is reinforced in the presence of the correct antecedent, but not in the presence of other antecedents. For example, a therapist will reinforce a child saying 'car' in the presence of a car, but not in the presence of a hat. This history of reinforcement establishes the car–'car' (A–B) connection. However, reinforcement alone is often insufficient to promote these connections, and prompts are often needed. A *prompt* is a supplementary stimulus used to gain stimulus control (*i.e.*, of an antecedent over a response). Prompts can be physical (*i.e.*, hand-over-hand guidance of a response), gestural (*i.e.*, pointing to the correct response), and verbal (*i.e.*, giving more verbal information that helps a child arrive at a response). Once inserted, prompts must eventually be faded.

There are three common *prompt-fading* techniques in ABA and DTT. First is *least-to-most prompting*, in which an instruction is given and progressively more-helpful prompts are given with incorrect or no responses (Murzynski & Bourret, 2007). For example, a child is asked to 'Find car' from an array of other objects. If he is incorrect or makes no response, the therapist says, 'Find car' and points to the car. If the child is still incorrect, the therapist says, 'Find car' and guides the child's hand to the car. A second technique is *most-to-least prompting* in which the therapist gradually moves from more-helpful prompts to less-helpful prompts (Libby *et al.*, 2008). In the example above, the therapist would first say, 'Find car', and immediately physically guide the child's hand to the car. After repeated experiences at this prompt level, the therapist would say, 'Find car', and use a gestural prompt. Finally, the therapist would only say, 'Find car', and reinforce correct responses. A third prompt-fading method is *time delay*, in which the therapist gradually increases the delay between the instruction and the prompt (Heckaman *et al.*, 1998). For example, the therapist would say, 'Find car', and use a 0-second delay by immediately prompting the child, perhaps with a gestural prompt. Given repeated success, the therapist then increases the delay to 2 s between the instruction and the prompt, and so on. Most-to-least prompting and time delay are used as *errorless teaching* approaches which help students gain success with learning new skills (Mueller & Palkovic, 2007).

A final hallmark of DTT, and all methods using ABA, is data collection. Applied behaviour analysts carefully define all targeted behaviours, set goals for how much to increase or decrease those behaviours, and carefully specify the methods used to measure behaviours. Therapists using DTT typically collect data on every trial presented to a child. When conducting a session on teaching animal sounds, for example, a therapist might present 10 trials with the sounds of a cow, dog, and pig. For every antecedent (*e.g.*, 'What sound does a dog make?'), the therapist records a + if the child makes the correct response and a − if the response is incorrect. Therapists usually convert these records from a session into a percentage correct (*e.g.*, 80 per cent correct). Therapists can graph those records to make data-based decisions. That is, if a child is progressing steadily and reaching high percentages of correct responses in sessions, the therapist would introduce new skills. However, if graphs indicate slow or minimal progress, the therapist would make changes to the teaching strategy to increase the likelihood of progress. Trial-by-trial data also allow therapists to closely examine response patterns to make specific adjustments to children's training. Some programs use probe data, in which only a sample of responses are measured, which then frees up more time for teaching (Lerman *et al.*, 2011). There are many variations of data collection methods, but ABA therapists must collect data to ensure children make progress.

Managing challenging behaviour

Even though most forms of challenging behaviour are not diagnostic criteria for autism, many children with autism exhibit destructiveness (of property), aggression, and/or self-injurious behaviour. These problems are obvious priorities for treatment, as they disrupt education and community involvement, and they cause harm to the child and others. The major ABA approach to reducing challenging behaviours is to first determine *why* they occur (*i.e.*, identifying the environmental variables evoking and maintaining the behaviours), and second to prevent future instances of these problem behaviours by altering the environmental variables evoking and maintaining them (Iwata *et al.*, 1982/1994). This approach is contrasted with more common reactive approaches, which are limited to reacting to the behaviours, usually by reprimands. Instead, the ABA approach puts the emphasis on the *antecedent* side of the ABC paradigm and designs interventions to prevent the challenging behaviours from arising. This is accomplished in two phases: functional behaviour assessment and function-based intervention.

The purpose of a *functional behaviour assessment* is to gain information about a child's challenging behaviour: what it looks like, how often it occurs, with whom and where it occurs, and why it occurs (Vollmer *et al.*, 2001). Like all ABA methods, this begins with carefully defining what the challenging behaviour looks like (*e.g.*, 'the child picks up a toy and throws it in the direction of another person; it must travel at least 1 m'). A second step is measuring the challenging behaviour by counting instances of it (and often converting the count to a rate), or using time-sampling methods (*e.g.*, counting how many 1-min intervals contained challenging behaviour in a 30-min observation session). As in DTT, challenging behaviour is graphed to make data-based decisions on interventions. A third step is interviewing people who commonly interact with the child (*e.g.*, parents, teachers), and having them complete questionnaires (*e.g.*, the functional analysis interview form; O'Neill *et al.*, 1997) to gain information about where, when, and why the challenging behaviours most often occur. A fourth, and perhaps most important, step is directly observing the child and recording instances of his challenging behaviour, as well as what occurred right before and right after those instances. This is called *ABC observations*.

ABC observations are extremely useful for determining why challenging behaviours occur, and they require understanding the basic concepts of positive reinforcement and stimulus control described earlier. When conducting ABC observations, a therapist is aiming to determine whether a child's challenging behaviours serve one of four functions: (1) to gain attention from others; (2) to gain a tangible item, such as a toy or food; (3) to escape from an unpleasant situation, such as work demands; or (4) to gain sensory stimulation, such as the stimulation produced by body rocking and hand flapping. These are four common consequences that maintain the challenging behaviour of children with autism. The antecedent variables (called *motivating operations*) are also influential in evoking challenging behaviour (*e.g.*, child has not had attention in a while; child has not had a preferred tangible item in a while; child is given difficult work demands). Attention is common because adults often approach or reprimand children when they engage in challenging behaviour, and that attention might reinforce the aberrant behaviour. If a child has not had access to a preferred toy in some time, he may engage in challenging behaviour to gain access to the toy or he may tear up a worksheet to escape from work demands.

Once the function of the problem behaviour is determined (and this can often be difficult to discern, thus requiring careful analysis), a *function-based intervention* can be designed and implemented. There are many types of function-based interventions, and three are described here. First, *differential reinforcement* involves reinforcing one behaviour, but not reinforcing another (Vollmer et al., 1999). Not reinforcing a behaviour and observing its decrease is referred to as *extinction*. For example, if a child screams to gain the teacher's attention, the teacher could use differential reinforcement by withholding attention for screaming and reinforcing an alternative behaviour, such as completing schoolwork. Given proper analysis and implementation, this procedure will result in more completed schoolwork and less screaming. A second preventive strategy is *functional communication training*, in which a challenging behaviour is not reinforced and a communicative behaviour *is* reinforced (Carr & Durand, 1985). For example, if a functional behaviour assessment indicates a child's self-injurious behaviour is maintained by access to food items, functional communication training is withholding food for self-injurious behaviour and reinforcing the request, 'Food, please'. A third strategy is *self-management* in which the child records instances of his behaviour and this leads to reinforcement (Koegel et al., 1992). For example, a child whose problem behaviour functions to escape difficult work could be given a short list of academic assignments that he can check off as they are completed. When he checks off the last assignment, he gets access to a preferred activity, such as a computer game. There are more variations of function-based interventions, but the principles are similar: identify the function and arrange the environment to prevent further occurrences of challenging behaviours while reinforcing desired behaviours.

The analysis of verbal behaviour

A third application of behaviour analysis is using the analysis of verbal behaviour to assess and treat communication skills with children with autism. As in DTT and function-based interventions, the crux of the *analysis of verbal behaviour* is identifying the environmental variables evoking and maintaining poor communicative behaviour and altering those variables to produce desired repertoires (Skinner, 1957; Sundberg & Michael, 2001). Traditional treatments of language categorize communication into receptive language and expressive language. The analysis of verbal behaviour builds on this by sub-classifying expressive language, while always defining types of language by their antecedent and consequence controlling variables. One critical type of expressive language is the *mand*, defined as a verbal response whose antecedent is a motivating operation (*i.e.*, deprivation, aversive stimulation), and whose consequence is a reinforcer specific to the motivating operation and the verbal response. For example, 'cookie' is a mand if it is controlled by deprivation of a cookie (*i.e.*, hunger) and receipt of a cookie. A second type of expressive language is the *tact*: a verbal response whose antecedent is a nonverbal stimulus (*i.e.*, an object) and whose consequence is general, social reinforcement (*e.g.*, 'that's right', 'thank you'). Saying 'cookie' as a tact might be to inform someone else that a cookie is present, not because one wants a cookie. A third classification of language is the *intraverbal*, defined as a verbal response whose antecedent is someone else's verbal behaviour and whose consequence is general, social reinforcement. An example is saying 'cookie' when someone says, 'What is your favorite dessert?' or 'What do you think goes well with milk?'. The reinforcer might be 'Interesting', or 'Good idea'. A fourth type of expressive language is different from the others because it is controlled by an antecedent that matches the response, and is called the *echoic* (*i.e.*, saying 'cookie' when someone else says 'cookie'). Learning the other types of language is often dependent on a strong echoic repertoire. A final type of verbal response is controlled by textual stimuli (*i.e.*, reading). This is referred to as *textual* behaviour.

The heart of the analysis of verbal behaviour is analyzing the variables controlling a child's communicative behaviour. When a child says, 'truck,' is he saying it because he wants a truck (a mand), because he sees a truck (a tact), because someone said truck (an echoic), because someone asked a question about a truck (an intraverbal), or because he see the printed word, 'truck' (textual)? For example, a mother comes to a clinic with her child and says, 'He can request preferred items – watch this.' The mom holds up a toy truck and says, 'Do you want truck?' the child says, 'Truck' and the mom hands him the truck. This is good in the sense that the child talked to receive a preferred item, but what were the sources of control over the utterance? Presumably the child wanted the truck (motivating operation; mand); the child saw the truck (nonverbal stimulus; tact); and the mom said, 'truck' (verbal stimulus matching the response; echoic). Therefore, the child's utterance, 'truck', was part mand, part tact, and part echoic. In other words, it was *multiply-controlled*, and verbal behaviour under natural circumstances is almost always multiply-controlled. However, when the mother said her child can request preferred items, a therapist would want to see a clean, or pure, mand controlled only (or primarily) by the motivating operation (*i.e.*, the child wants the truck; hasn't had it in a while). The role of the applied behaviour analyst would be to fade out those supplementary sources of control (*i.e.*, the presence of the truck and the adult saying 'truck'), using fading procedures described earlier.

Before developing treatment based on the analysis of verbal behaviour, it is important to assess a child's verbal behaviour repertoire. The goal of such an assessment is to determine which of those verbal skills (*e.g.*, mands, tacts, intraverbals) are strong in a child's repertoire and which are more delayed. The best tool we currently have for conducting such an assessment is the Verbal Behaviour Milestones Assessment and Placement Program (VB-MAPP; Sundberg, 2008), which has four parts. First, the Milestones Assessment contains 170 learning and language milestones taken from normative child data across three age ranges: 0–18 months, 18–30 months, and 30–48 months. In addition to the verbal skills discussed earlier, the Milestones Assessment assesses play, social, imitation, receptive, group, reading, math, writing, and linguistic skills. Conducting tests in this section allows a therapist to identify the age range and skill levels within each of those skill domains. Second, the Barriers Assessment examines repertoires that are barriers to a child's rapid progress, such as challenging behaviours, dependency on prompts, dependency on atypical reinforcers, limited eye contact, and difficulties generalizing skills across people and places. Third, the Transition Assessment documents a child's functioning level in repertoires needed to transition from intensive teaching environments to more natural teaching environments (*e.g.*, general education classrooms): completing independent work, learning skills quickly, retaining skills, spontaneously using desired behaviours, and demonstrating independence with self-help skills. Finally, the Task Analysis provides long lists of skills that can be targeted in a child's education plan. The results of all four parts of the VB-MAPP allow the design of an individualized education plan based on ABA and the analysis of verbal behaviour.

The actual teaching in a model based on the analysis of verbal behaviour is similar to teaching based on DTT, though there are important exceptions. First, in the approach based on the analysis of verbal behaviour, mands are taught first (Carbone *et al.*, 2010). This is because the mand directly benefits the child by allowing him access to preferred items. Mands are relatively easy to teach when motivation for a particular item is strong, and it is best to teach a specific word as a mand (*e.g.*, 'cracker' to mand for a cracker). For children who cannot produce speech sounds, mands can also take the form of signs (*e.g.*, the American Sign Language sign for 'cracker'; Valentino & Shillingsburg, 2011), picture exchange (*i.e.*, handing someone a picture of a cracker; Bondy & Frost, 2001; Ziomek & Rehfeldt, 2008), or using a voice-output device (Schepis *et al.*, 1998). Because mands are associated with motivation, they are often taught in a child's natural environment, rather than while sitting at a table. Second, the careful analysis of verbal behaviour has permitted the development of other prompt-fading techniques than those used in DTT. One example is the *quick transfer of stimulus control procedure* (Axe et al., 2012; Barbera & Kubina, 2005; Bloh, 2008), in which an instruction with a prompt is given, a child responds, the instruction is quickly repeated without the prompt, the child responds, and the therapist delivers a reinforcer. A final distinction is programs using the analysis of verbal behaviour have found that mixing different types of skills in one teaching session is superior to teaching only one type of skill in a teaching session (Volkert *et al.*, 2008).

Conclusions

Using discrete trial training to impart linguistic and academic skills, functional behaviour assessment and function-based interventions to manage challenging behaviour, and the analysis of verbal behaviour to analyze and teach communication skills are three ways of employing applied behaviour analysis to treat the core symptoms of autism. They all rest on Skinner's basic principles of behaviour – positive reinforcement, extinction, stimulus control, and motivating operations – derived from basic research. The strategies are all also based on applied, single-subject design research published in the *Journal of Applied Behavior Analysis* and similar journals, as well as on randomized clinical trials published in more mainstream autism journals (*e.g.*, *Clinical Psychology Review, Journal of Autism and Development Disorders, Journal of Consulting and Clinical Psychology, Research in Autism Spectrum Disorders*). Although procedures come in different forms, all treatments based on ABA require analyzing the antecedents and consequences evoking and maintaining a child's behaviour, dividing skills into small parts and teaching individual behaviours, and altering environmental contingencies (the antecedents and consequences) to promote desired behaviours.

Does ABA need to be one-on-one? The primary treatment that has substantial research evidence – DTT – prescribes one-on-one intervention. However, what makes ABA effective is the analysis of the basic concepts operating on a child, and not the form of the intervention. In fact, ABA has been effective during group instruction and as a way to improve a child's inclusion in mainstream education (Carnahan *et al.*, 2009; Chan & O'Reilly, 2008; Charania *et al.*, 2010; Kamps *et al.*, 1999). Social skills instruction is also incorporated into ABA programs and is critical for children with autism. Researchers have taught the following social skills to children with autism using ABA techniques: reciprocal pretend play (MacDonald *et al.*, 2009), sharing (Marzullo-Kerth *et al.*; Reeve *et al.*, 2011), giving and accepting compliments (Kamps *et al.*, 1992), showing empathy (Schrandt *et al.*, 2009), responding to facial expressions (Axe & Evans, 2012), and perspective-taking (LeBlanc *et al.*, 2003). One final point here: ABA is not only for autism. It has been used to treat problems related to smoking (Romanowich & Lamb, 2010), obesity (VanWormer, 2004), staff training (Haberlin *et al.*, 2012), and more.

Autism practitioners should adopt practices based on ABA not only because they are highly effective, but also because practitioners can join the profession of ABA. The Behaviour Analyst Certification Board (BACB) has conferred certification to nearly 10,000 individuals internationally. Becoming a Board Certified Behaviour Analyst (BCBA) requires coursework, clinical supervision, and passing a written examination. Coursework is offered in numerous online graduate training programs, including ones offered by the University of North Texas, the Florida Institute of Technology, and Pennsylvania State University. Continuing education occurs at the annual conferences of the Association for Behaviour Analysis International (ABAI), and at annual conferences of 81 affiliated chapters worldwide. The Association for Professional Behaviour Analysts (APBA) is a new organization that provides continuing education and advocacy specifically targeting the practice of behaviour analysis. Dissemination of theory, research, and practice also happens through Division 25 of the American Psychological Association (APA), the Cambridge Center for Behavioural Studies (CCBS), and the Autism Special Interest Group of ABAI. Given the strong research foundation and support of professionals, treatments based on the science and practice of ABA should be used to improve the lives of individuals with autism.

Conflicts of interest: The author declares no conflicts of interest.

References

Axe, J.B. & Evans, C.J. (2012): Using video modeling to teach children with PDD-NOS to respond to facial expressions. *Res. Autism Spect. Dis.* **6,** 1176–1185.

Axe, J.B., Markovits, R.A. & Koenig, S. (2012): Comparative analysis of the quick transfer of stimulus control procedure with students with severe disabilities. Paper presented at the Symposium *Analysis of transfer-of-stimulus control procedures: Effective teaching practices for children with autism spectrum disorders*, A. Kisamore (Chair), at the annual conference of the Association for Behavior Analysis International, Seattle, WA.

Baer, D.M., Wolf, M.M. & Risley, T.R. (1968): Some current dimensions of applied behaviour analysis. *J. Appl. Behav. Anal.* **1,** 91–97.

Barbera, M.L. & Kubina, R.M. (2005): Using transfer procedures to teach tacts to a child with autism. *Anal. Verbal Behav.* **21,** 155–161.

Bloh, C. (2008): Assessing transfer of stimulus control procedures across learners with autism. *Anal. Verbal Behav.* **24,** 87–101.

Bondy, A. & Frost, L. (2001): The picture exchange communication system. *Behav. Modif.* **25,** 725–744.

Carbone, V.J., Sweeney-Kerwin, E.J., Attanasio, V. & Kasper, T. (2010): Increasing the vocal responses of children with autism and developmental disabilities using manual sign mand training and prompt delay. *J. Appl. Behav. Anal.* **43,** 705–709.

Carnahan, C., Musti-Rao, S. & Bailey, J. (2009): Promoting active engagement in small group learning experiences for students with autism and significant learning needs. *Educ. Treat. Child.* **32,** 37–61.

Carr, E.G. & Durand, V. (1985): Reducing behaviour problems through functional communication training. *J. Appl. Behav. Anal.* **18,** 111–126.

Chan, J.M. & O'Reilly, M.F. (2008): A Social Stories' intervention package for students with autism in inclusive classroom settings. *J. Appl. Behav. Anal.* **41,** 405–409.

Charania, S.M., LeBlanc, L.A., Sabanathan, N., Ktaech, I.A., Carr, J.E. & Gunby, K. (2010): Teaching effective hand raising to children with autism during group instruction. *J. Appl. Behav. Anal.* **43,** 493–497.

Cooper, J.O., Heron, T.E. & Heward, W.L. (2007): *Applied Behaviour Analysis* (2nd ed.), p. 800. Upper Saddle River, NJ: Merrill/Prentice Hall.

DeLeon, I.G. & Iwata, B.A. (1996): Evaluation of a multiple-stimulus presentation format for assessing reinforcer preferences. *J. Appl. Behav. Anal.* **29,** 519–533.

Eikeseth, S., Smith, T., Jahr, E. & Eldevik, S. (2002): Intensive behavioural treatment at school for 4- to 7-year-old children with autism: a 1-year comparison controlled study. *Behav. Modif.* **26,** 49–68.

Fisher, W., Piazza, C.C., Bowman, L.G. & Hagopian, L.P. (1992): A comparison of two approaches for identifying reinforcers for persons with severe and profound disabilities. *J. Appl. Behav. Anal.* **25,** 491–498.

Haberlin, A.T., Beauchamp, K., Agnew, J. & O'Brien, F. (2012): A comparison of pyramidal staff training and direct staff training in community-based day programs. *J. Organ. Behav. Manage.* **32,** 65–74.

Hanley, G.P., Iwata, B.A. & McCord, B.E. (2003): Functional analysis of problem behaviour: a review. *J. Appl. Behav. Anal.* **36,** 147–185.

Heckaman, K.A., Alber, S., Hooper, S. & Heward, W.L. (1998): A comparison of least-to-most prompts and progressive time delay on the disruptive behaviour of students with autism. *J. Behav. Educ.* **8,** 171–201.

Howard, J.S., Sparkman, C.R., Cohen, H.G., Green, G. & Stanislaw, H. (2005): A comparison of intensive behaviour analytic and eclectic treatments for young children with autism. *Res. Dev. Disabil.* **26,** 359–383.

Iwata, B.A., Dorsey, M.F., Slifer, K.J., Bauman, K.E. & Richman, G.S. (1994): Toward a functional analysis of self-injury. *J. Appl. Behav. Anal.* **27**, 197–209 (reprinted from *Anal. Intervent. Dev. Disabil.* **2**, 3–20, 1982).

Kamps, D.M., Leonard, B.R., Vernon, S. & Dugan, E.P. (1992): Teaching social skills to students with autism to increase peer interactions in an integrated first-grade classroom. *J. Appl. Behav. Anal.* **25**, 281–288.

Kamps, D.M., Dugan, E., Potucek, J. & Collins, A. (1999): Effects of cross-age peer tutoring networks among students with autism and general education students. *J. Behav Educ.* **9**, 97–115.

Koegel, L.K., Koegel, R.L., Hurley, C. & Frea, W.D. (1992): Improving social skills and disruptive behaviour in children with autism through self-management. *J. Appl. Behav. Anal.* **25**, 341–353.

Kuppens, S.S. & Onghena, P.P. (2012): Sequential meta-analysis to determine the sufficiency of cumulative knowledge: the case of early intensive behavioural intervention for children with autism spectrum disorders. *Res. Autism Spect. Dis.* **6**, 168–176.

LeBlanc, L.A., Coates, A.M., Daneshvar, S., Charlop-Christy, M.H., Morris, C. & Lancaster, B.M. (2003): Using video modeling and reinforcement to teach perspective-taking skills to children with autism. *J. Appl. Behav. Anal.* **36**, 253–257.

Lerman, D.C., Dittlinger, L., Fentress, G. & Lanagan, T. (2011): A comparison of methods for collecting data on performance during discrete trial teaching. *Behav. Anal. Pract.* **4**, 53–62.

Libby, M.E., Weiss, J.S., Bancroft, S. & Ahearn, W.H. (2008): A comparison of most-to-least and least-to-most prompting on the acquisition of solitary play skills. *Behav. Anal. Pract.* **1**, 37–43.

Lovaas, I.O. (1987): Behavioural treatment and normal educational and intellectual functioning in young autistic children, *J. Consult. Clin. Psych.* **55**, 3–9.

MacDonald, R., Sacramone, S., Mansfield, R., Wiltz, K. & Ahearn, W.H. (2009): Using video modeling to teach reciprocal pretend play to children with autism. *J. Appl. Behav. Anal.* **42**, 43–55.

Marzullo-Kerth, D., Reeve, S.A., Reeve, K.F. & Townsend, D.B. (2011): Using multiple-exemplar training to teach a generalized repertoire or sharing to children with autism. *J. Appl. Behav. Anal.* **44**, 279-294.

Maurice, C. (1993): *Let Me Hear Your Voice: A Family's Triumph over Autism*, p. 400. New York: Ballentine.

Mueller, M.M. & Palkovic, C.M. (2007): Errorless learning: review and practical application for teaching children with pervasive developmental disorders. *Psychol. Schools.* **44**, 691–700.

Mueller, M.M., Nkosi, A. & Hine, J.F. (2011): Functional analysis in public schools: a summary of 90 functional analyses. *J. Appl. Behav. Anal.* **44**, 807–818.

Murzynski, N.T. & Bourret, J.C. (2007): Combining video modeling and least-to-most prompting for establishing response chains. *Behav. Intervent.* **22**, 147–152.

National Research Council (2001): *Educating Children with Autism*, p. 324. Washington, DC: National Academy Press.

O'Neill, R.E., Horner, R.H., Albin, R.W., Sprague, J., Storey, K. & Newton, J.S. (1997): *Functional Assessment and Program Development for Problem Behaviour: A Practical Handbook* (2nd ed.), p. 144. Pacific Grove, CA: Brooks/Cole Publishing.

Peters-Scheffer, N., Didden, R., Korzilius, H. & Sturmey, P. (2011): A meta-analytic study on the effectiveness of comprehensive ABA-based early intervention programs for children with autism spectrum disorders. *Res. Autism Spect. Dis.* **5**, 60–69.

Romanowich, P. & Lamb, R.J. (2010): Effects of escalating and descending schedules of incentives on cigarette smoking in smokers without plans to quit. *J. Appl. Behav. Anal.* **43**, 357–367.

Sallows, G.O. & Graupner, T.D. (2005): Intensive behavioural treatment for children with autism: four-year outcome and predictors. *Am. J. Ment. Retard.* **110**, 417-438.

Sautter, R.A. & LeBlanc, L.A. (2006): Empirical applications of Skinner's analysis of verbal behaviour with humans. *Anal. Verbal Behav.* **22**, 35–48.

Sautter, R.A., LeBlanc, L.A. & Gillett, J.N. (2008): Using free operant preference assessments to select toys for free play between children with autism and siblings. *Res. Autism Spect. Dis.* **2**, 17–27.

Schepis, M.M., Reid, D.H., Behrmann, M.M. & Sutton, K.A. (1998): Increasing communicative interactions of young children with autism using a voice output communication aid and naturalistic teaching. *J. Appl. Behav. Anal.* **31**, 561–578.

Schrandt, J.A., Townsend, D.F. & Poulson, C.L. (2009): Teaching empathy skills to children with autism. *J. Appl. Behav. Anal.* **42**, 17–32.

Skinner, B.F. (1938): *Behaviour of Organisms*, p. 472. New York: Appleton-Century-Crofts.

Skinner, B.F. (1953): *Science and Human Behaviour*, p. 461. New York: The Free Press.

Skinner, B.F. (1957): *Verbal Behaviour*, p. 514. New York: Appleton-Century-Crofts.

Sundberg, M.L. (2008): *The Verbal Behaviour Milestones Assessment and Placement Program: The VB-MAPP*. Concord, CA: AVB Press.

Sundberg, M.L. & Michael, J. (2001): The value of Skinner's analysis of verbal behaviour for teaching children with autism. *Behav. Modif.* **25,** 698–724.

Surgeon General (1999): *Mental Health: A Report of the Surgeon General.* Washington, DC: Department of Health and Human Services.

Valentino, A.L. & Shillingsburg, M. (2011): Acquisition of mands, tacts, and intraverbals through sign exposure in an individual with autism. *Anal. Verbal Behav.* **27,** 95–101.

VanWormer, J.J. (2004): Pedometers and brief e-counseling: increasing physical activity for overweight adults. *J. Appl. Behav. Anal.* **37,** 421–425.

Virués-Ortega, J. (2010): Applied behaviour analytic intervention for autism in early childhood: meta-analysis, meta-regression and dose–response meta-analysis of multiple outcomes. *Clin. Psychol. Rev.* **30,** 387–399.

Volkert, V.M., Lerman, D.C., Trosclair, N., Addison, L. & Kodak, T. (2008): An exploratory analysis of task-interspersal procedures while teaching object labels to children with autism. *J. Appl. Behav. Anal.* **41,** 335–350.

Vollmer, T.R., Roane, H.S., Ringdahl, J.E. & Marcus, B.A. (1999): Evaluating treatment challenges with differential reinforcement of alternative behaviour. *J. Appl. Behav. Anal.* **32,** 9–23.

Vollmer, T.R., Borrero, J.C., Wright, C.S., Van Camp, C. & Lalli, J.S. (2001): Identifying possible contingencies during descriptive analyses of severe behaviour disorders. *J. Appl. Behav. Anal.* **34,** 269–287.

Wechsler, D. (1974): *Manual for the Wechsler Intelligence Scale for Children–Revised.* New York: Psychological Corporation.

Ziomek, M.M. & Rehfeldt, R. (2008): Investigating the acquisition, generalization, and emergence of untrained verbal operants for mands acquired using the Picture Exchange Communication System in adults with severe developmental disabilities. *Anal. Verbal Behav.* **24,** 15–30.

Chapter 14

Applied Behaviour Analysis: the Italian experience of the Scuolaba Model for children with autism spectrum disorders

Lucia D'Amato

Associazione Scuolaba ONLUS, via del Carso 4, 25124 Brescia, Italy;
Fondazione Stefano e Angela Danelli, largo Stefano e Angela Danelli 1, 26900 Lodi, Italy

Summary

Applied Behaviour Analysis (ABA) is the applied science derived from behaviourism. It studies the behaviour of the organism and its interactions with the environment. In Italy, the linking between ABA and autism is both common and strong. Since the 1980s, the scientific literature on behaviourism has increased, applying its principles to such socially significant behaviour of human beings as communication, self-help skills, stimulatory behaviours, and academic and cognitive skills (Cooper *et al.*, 2007).
In Europe and all around the world, there are centres that specialize in the rehabilitation of children with autism and the support of their families using the methodology of ABA. In Italy, the first experience in this direction was started with the Scuolaba Project in Lodi in 2008, followed by two similar programs in Brescia and Milan. The only model before the Scuolaba one was the Home-Based Model of rehabilitation through ABA.
In the following article, the results with 30 children are discussed. Fifteen of these children were assessed after undergoing two years of treatment (Lodi), and the other 15 were assessed after one year of treatment (Brescia). The Scuolaba Model is compared to the Home-Based one, evaluating positive and negative aspects of the two.

ABA: an introduction

Applied Behaviour Analysis is a science of human behaviour. It began with the work of Dr. B.F. Skinner 70 years ago. In 1938, Skinner published *The Behavior of Organisms*, which described operant conditioning, the process by which learning occurs as the result of consequences of selecting certain behaviours. Skinner also discussed how antecedent stimuli, when correlated with the function altering effects of consequences, also alter future occurrences of that behaviour.

Later applications of this science to education and to other matters of socially significant behaviour, by behavioural analysts led to what is now known as Applied Behaviour Analysis (ABA).

In 1957, Skinner published *Verbal Behavior*, which elaborated the functional analysis of behaviour. In his text he extended operant conditioning to verbal behaviour in order to fully describe the series of human behaviours. He described several components of language as 'verbal operants' or functional units of language. This abstract model of language classification was seldom found in educational intervention programs until recently.

Now, however, many applied behaviour analysts, including Mark Sundberg, Jim Partington, Vincent Carbone, and Jack Michael (Carbone *et al.*, 2006; Michael, 1984; Partington, 2006; Sundberg, 1998; Sundberg & Partington, 1998; Sundberg & Michael, 2001) have conducted and published research on verbal behaviour. Applied Verbal Behaviour (AVB) is the application of the science of behavioural analysis to teaching 'verbal behaviour', binding it to motivational variables (Carbone *et al.*, 2006; Carr *et al.*, 1994).

ABA/VB addresses difficulties in the area of communication observed in individuals with developmental disorders like autism spectrum disorders (ASDs). Behavioural analysts have developed teaching strategies that demand a very high degree of creativity and flexibility in order to proceed with the student's motivational variables. ABA/VB has brought about dramatic results for many people with these disorders.

ABA is a mixture of psychological and educational techniques that are modified to the needs of each individual child to change his or her behaviours. The basics of ABA involve the use of behavioural methods to measure behaviour, teach functional skills, and evaluate progress through data analysis.

ABA in Italy

ABA techniques have been proven in many studies to be the methodology of choice in treating deficits in the behaviour of children with autism spectrum disorder (ASD) at any level. The ultimate goal is to find a way of motivating the child and using a number of different strategies and positive reinforcement techniques to ensure that the sessions are enjoyable and productive and then to test for efficacy of the results obtained in changing behaviour.

In Italy, services for individuals with autism and their families are very scant and, most of the time, not agreeing in principle with the Autism Guidelines set out by the Istituto Superiore della Sanità (SIS) in 2011. According to these guidelines, ABA is recommended as the first choice treatment for individual with ASD and is to be prefered to eclectic models of treatment.

ABA services started late in Italy compared to those in other parts of the world, because there was not much Italian expertise until the first years after 2000; the consultants [or Board-Certified Behaviour Analysts (BCBAs) or Board-Certified Assistant Behaviour Analysts (BCaBAs)] (Behavioural Analyst Certification Board, 2004) came mainly from the United States and Northern Europe, beginning as private services for families of children with ASD. I'll refer to this model as the Home-Based program of intervention.

The main characteristics of the Home-Based Model are the following:
- therapy setting is within the house (a bedroom converted into a therapeutic setting or a studio used mainly used for this purpose);
- therapists are recruited by the family and can be also (most of the time) family members;
- the consultant visits the family and assesses the child once every 2 to 3 months;
- staff training is infrequent and there are no parameters of basic knowledge of therapists;
- materials and teaching tools are provided by the family.

In Europe and the United States, the Centre-Based Model of service for individuals with ASD is used together with the Home-Based one since services started to be more accessible for individuals with ASD and their families.

The main characteristics of the Centre-Based Model are the following:
- therapy setting is a space within a centre;
- therapists are recruited by the centre;
- consultant works in the centre together with the therapists;
- staff training is provided on a regular basis;
- material and teaching tools are provided by the centre.

In Italy, the Centre-Based Model of services for children with ASD did not exist until 2008, when the first Scuolaba Project was put in place.

The Scuolaba Model

Considering the different circumstances of the Italian services and the culture around ASD, a new model of service for these children and their families needed to consider very important aspects, such as school integration, family support, staff training and, last but not least, evidence-based methodology and data-collecting procedures, which are not a fundamental part of any rehabilitation service for children with ASD within the public sphere (Stokes & Osnes, 1988).

The Scuolaba Model is a Centre-Based service for children with ASD aged 2 to 12 years old and their families.

Fig. 1 depicts a schematic model of the Scuolaba Centre-Based service.

The main characteristics of the Scuolaba Model are the following:
- the therapy space is a big room (min. 100 m^2), where all the children have all the space they need for working and playing. The space is shared by children and therapists; it's a colourful room filled with stimuli, with lots of distracters, in order to emulate school settings, for generalization purposes (Fig. 2, here in black and white version);
- teaching is conducted on a 1:1 ratio;
- staff training is provided on a regular basis;
- a BCBA consultant is in the centre at least twice a week;
- therapists receive 150 hours of training (theory and practice) at the beginning of their work experience;
- parent training and follow-up meetings are held monthly with each family, by the Consultant or the therapists;
- school consultant attends official meetings for the drawing up of the PEI and its revision.

The Scuolaba Projects: Lodi and Brescia

In 2008, the Cooperativa Sociale Il Paguro ONLUS fostered the first Scuolaba Project and in 2009 the same project came under the direction of the Stefano and Danelli Foundation, which guaranteed its continuity and still does.

The Scuolaba Lodi Project started with 20 children, all diagnosed with disorders on the autistic spectrum; these children were aged between 3 and 12 years old. Children arrived at the centre with a diagnosis given at a qualified public service.

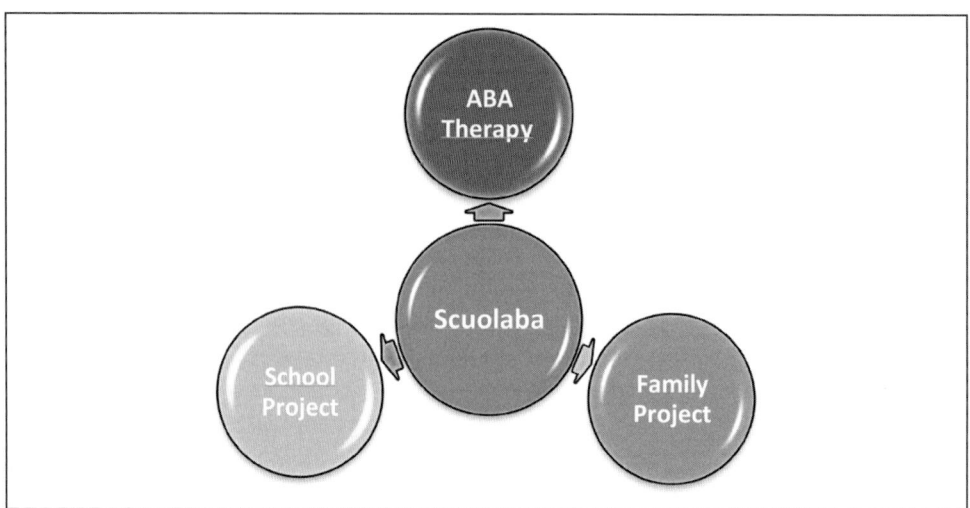

Fig. 1. Outline of the Scuolaba Model.

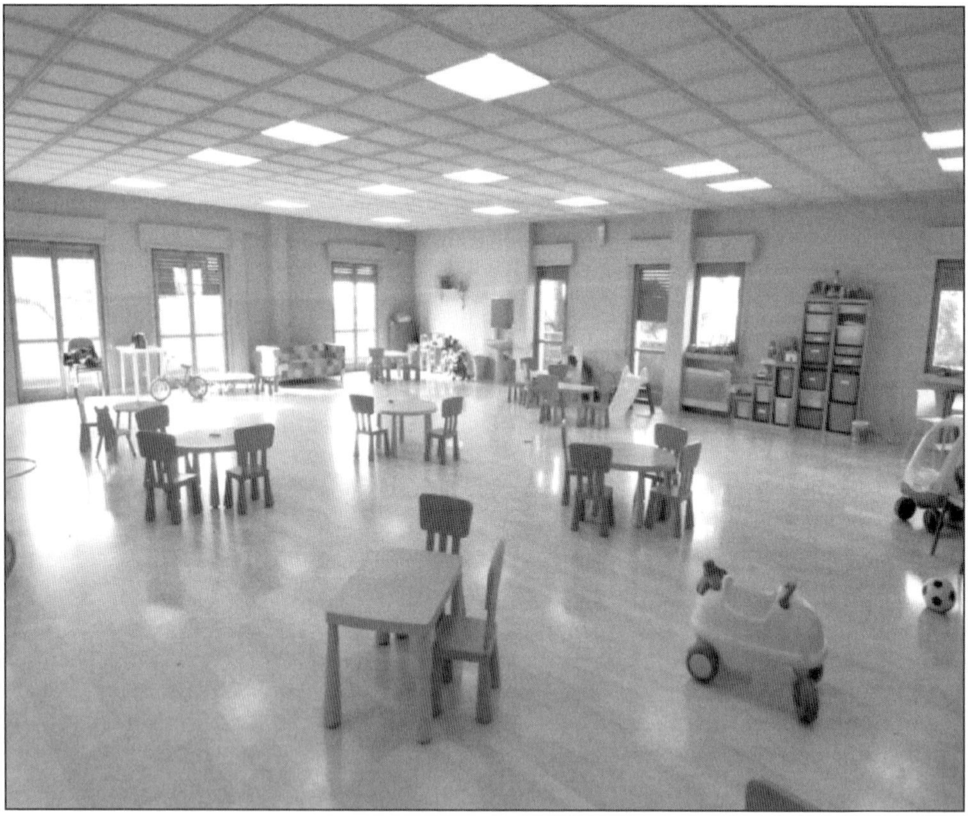

Fig. 2. Therapy room.

The children were divided into four groups (two in the morning and two in the afternoon), each composed of 5 children. The schedule was worked on a 1:1 basis 5 days a week, with 1 h 45 min per child per day.

Staff training at the beginning of the project was provided by a Board-Certified Behavior Analyst to the five therapists for four months.

The children's skills were assessed at the beginning of the project, using the Assessment of Basic Language and Learning Skill (ABLLS–R; Partington, 2006) and the Verbal Behavior Milestones Assessment and Placement Program (VB–MAPP; Sundberg, 2008).

An assessment was then made again for each child at the end of each year of attendance in the program in order to evaluate each child's progress.

In 2010, the second Scuolaba Project was established: the Scuolaba Brescia Project. This project was fostered by the Associazione Scuolaba ONLUS, which was founded in 2009 in order to promote similar projects in Italy.

The main characteristics of the Brescia Project were the same as for the Lodi one, except that the length of therapy was increased to 2 hours and the number of participating children was 18 (currently 28), coming to therapy Monday to Friday.

For all the children in both projects, programs were individualized and based on the results of the evaluation mentioned above; they included the following areas, as suggested by Sundberg & Michael (2001):
- verbal operants (mand, tact, echoic, intraverbal) (Sundberg, 1998);
- listener behaviour;
- social and group skills;
- play skills;
- imitation skills;
- attentive skills;
- visual performance and matching-to-sample skills;
- managing challenging behaviour through functional assessment and behaviour intervention plans.

Teaching is based on the principles of Applied Behaviour Analysis, such as *reinforcement, prompting, extinction, fading, shaping, generalization,* and *maintenance of skills acquired*, and on strategies like errorless teaching, teaching to fluency, DTT (discrete trial training), NET (natural environmental teaching) (Smith *et al.*, 2002) and the Learn Unit (Greer & McDonough, 1999).

For both projects, a great deal of attention is given to the Families and School projects, in order to create a real NET of people around the child that talk to each other and share the same objective, working to the same aim.

Study and results

Data collected at the beginning of each course, for each child, allowed the comparison of data after two years of treatment for children in the Lodi Project and after one year for children in the Brescia project.

Subjects and treatment

Table 1 shows the main information about subjects and treatment in the two projects.

Data were collected referring to the VB–MAPP grid in which each filled-in square was counted as a single unit (one filled-in square = 1). The count of the squares filled in at the beginning of treatment is the comparison data for the following evaluations.

Data are presented for 15 children of the Scuolaba Lodi Project and 15 children of the Scuolaba Brescia Project. The first graph (Fig. 3) shows results at the beginning of treatment for each child and data after one year and two years of treatment. Data are derived by counting the number of filled-in squares at the beginning, after one and after two years of treatment by the VB–MAPP grid.

Fig. 4 represents results in 15 subjects in the Scuolaba Brescia Project after one year of treatment; all were obtained in the same way as the one described for Fig. 3.

Table 1. Data for the two studies

Scuolaba Lodi Project	Scuolaba Brescia Project
15 children (diagnosed with ASD)	15 children (diagnosed with ASD)
Age: 4 to 12 years old	Age: 3 to 12 years old
Daily therapy time: 1 h 45 min (Mon. to Fri.)	Daily therapy time: 2 h (Mon. to Fri.)
1:1 ratio of child to therapist	1:1 ratio of child to therapist

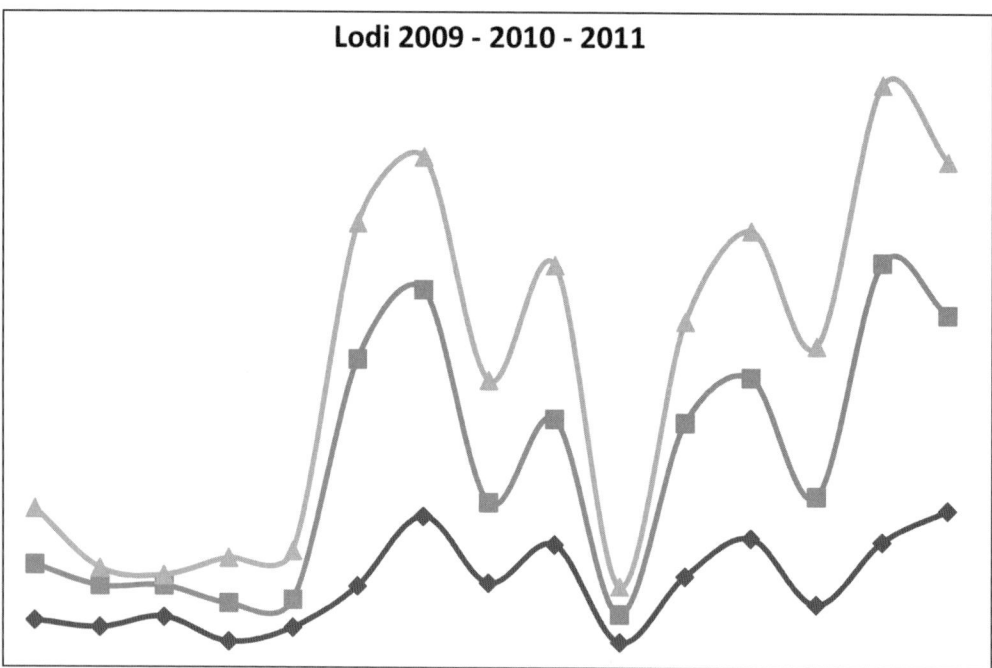

Fig. 3. Data of 15 children at beginning of treatment (diamonds), *and after one* (squares) *and two years of treatment* (triangles).

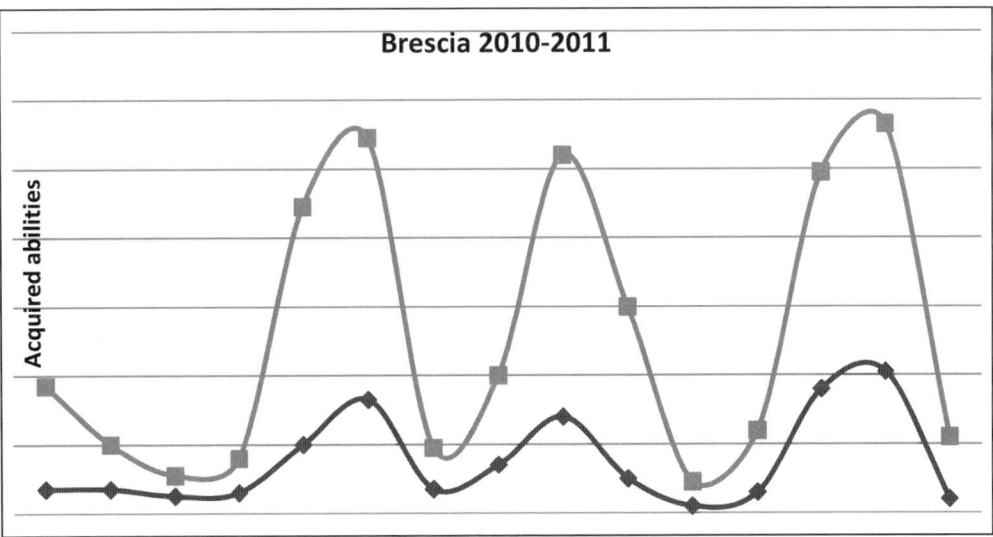

Fig. 4. Data at beginning of treatment (diamonds) *and after one year of treatment* (squares).

Conclusions

Applied Behaviour Analysis is recognized as the first treatment of choice for individuals with ASD. Public rehabilitative and educational services in Italy have not yet embraced it as a possible option, although private institutions and organizations are providing these sorts of services in a home-based setting. The Scuolaba Project is trying to offer a different perspective, believing that home is not the right place for initial rehabilitation because of likely stress and management problems that are difficult for the family alone to overcome. At the same time the home is the perfect place for generalizing and maintaining skills acquired in a structured setting, is a place where to work on self-help skills, managing challenging behaviour following a plan that has been given by the consultant and yet is in effect in every place the child lives. A Centre-Based Model allows constant training for the staff and provides stability for the staff because the therapist is seen as a professional, and not just as a babysitter who sits at a table with a child, ask him to match banana with banana.

Stability allows consistency in treatment and improvement in staff abilities and skills. These advantages are very important when dealing with children with ASD and it takes time to build relationships and trust with the adult and peers. Data have shown that important results have been made in the acquisition of crucial developmental skills for all children in the study.

Future research could compare acquisition of skills for children attending Home-Based *versus* Centre-Based intervention programs. It could also investigate correlations between age at start of treatment and skills acquired.

A Centre-Based program allows for better control of all the variables involved in rehabilitating a child with ASD, together with good and intense work with families in order to support them and allow for generalization of all the skills acquired by the child.

Conflicts of interest: The author declares no conflicts of interest.

References

Behavior Analyst Certification Board (2004): *Guidelines for Responsible Conduct for Behavior Analysts*. Tallahassee, FL: BACB (www.bacb.com).

Carbone, V.J., Lewis, L., Sweeney-Kerwin, E.J., Dixon, J., Louden, R. & Quinn, S. (2006): A comparison of two approaches for teaching VB functions: total communication vs. vocal-alone. *J. Speech Lang. Pathol. Appl. Behav. Anal.* **1**, 181–192.

Carr, E.G., Levin, L., McConnachie, G., Carlson, J., Kemp, D.C. & Smith, C. (1994): *Communication-Based Intervention for Problem Behavior: A User's Guide for Producing Positive Change*. Baltimore, MD: Paul H. Brookes.

Cooper, J.O., Heron, T.E. & Heward, W.L. (2007): *Applied Behavior Analysis*, 2nd ed. Upper Saddle River, NJ: Pearson/Merrill-Prentice Hall.

Greer, R.D. & McDonough, S.H. (1999): Is the learn unit a fundamental measure of pedagogy? *Behav. Analyst* **22**, 5–16.

Istituto Superiore della Sanità (2011): Il trattamento dei disturbi dello spettro autistico nei bambini e negli adolescenti. http://www.snlg-iss.it/lgn_disturbi_spettro_autistico

Michael, J. (1984): Verbal behavior. *J. Exp. Anal. Behav.* **42** (3), 363–76.

Partington, J. (2006): *Assessment of Basic Language and Learning Skills-Revised (ABLLS®-R)*. [Italian translation and adaptation by L. D'Amato (2011): ORMA Editing].

Skinner, B.F. (1938): *The Behavior of Organisms: An Experimental Analysis*. Oxford, England: Appleton-Century.

Skinner, B.F. (1957): *Verbal Behavior*. Englewood Cliffs, NJ: Prentice-Hall.

Smith, L.D., Best, L.A., Stubbs, D.A., Archibald, A.B. & Robertson-Nay, R. (2002): The role of graphs and tables in hard and soft psychology. *American Psychologist* **57**, 749–751.

Stokes, T.F. & Osnes, P.G. (1988): The developing applied technology of generalization and maintenance. In: *Generalization and Maintenance: Life-style Changes in Applied Settings*, eds. R.H. Horner, G. Dunlap & R.L. Koegel. Baltimore, MD: Paul H. Brookes.

Sundberg, M.L. (1998): Realizing the potential of Skinner's analysis of verbal behavior. *Anal. Verb. Behav.* **15**, 9143–9147.

Sundberg, M.L. (2008): *VB-MAPP: Verbal Behavior Milestones Assessment and Placement Program*. Concord, CA: AVB Press. [Italian adaptation by P. Moderato & L. Copelli (2011): Vannini Editoria Scientifica].

Sundberg, M. & Partington, J. (1998): *Teaching Language to Children with Autism or Other Developmental Disabilities*. Pleasant Hill, CA: Behavior Analyst, Inc.

Sundberg, M.L. & Michael, J. (2001): The value of Skinner's analysis of verbal behavior for teaching children with autism. *Behav. Modificat.* **25**, 698–724.

Chapter 15

DIR–Developmental, Individual Difference, Relationship-Based Model: the sensory-motor affect connection to progress

Serena Wieder

Profectum Foundation, 140 Riverside Drive, New York, NY 10024, USA
Serena.Wieder@Profectum.org

Summary

Establishing the foundations for emotional and cognitive development for children identified with autism spectrum disorders is more compelling than ever. Given the complexity and individual variations of autism, the guidance of a dynamic model that embraces the critical elements of development and functional competence that can be applied in educational, family, clinical and research settings is imperative. DIR*, the $\underline{D}$evelopmental, $\underline{I}$ndividual Difference, $\underline{R}$elationship-Based Model, provides a dynamic comprehensive framework for understanding the child and his or her family and culture, including diagnostic developmental profiles and comprehensive interventions. It enables educators, clinicians, and parents to design a program tailored to the child's unique challenges and strengths. The $\underline{D}$ refers to fundamental capacities for joint attention and regulation, engagement across a wide range of emotions, two-way communication, and complex social problem-solving, all of which underlie the development of symbol formation, language, and intelligence. Intervention starts with pleasurable interactions between children and parents, which are at the heart of building the relationships that support developmental progress. The $\underline{I}$ refers to individual differences related to sensory reactivity and regulation, visual-spatial and auditory/language processing, and purposeful movement. Challenges in these neurobiological factors make it difficult for the child to participate in the emotional interactions that enable mastery of the developmental capacities (the $\underline{D}$). The $\underline{R}$ refers to relationships with caregivers that provide affect-based developmentally appropriate interactions and learning experiences. Parents and families are central to this model because of their ongoing opportunities to support their child's everyday functioning to carry out emotionally meaningful goals based on developmental levels. Cultural and environmental influences are also considered. By taking all three areas of DIR into account, the foundation for functioning, learning, and relating to others in meaningful ways is established and will support progress. Research has not yet been able to compare different approaches or explain the different responses of individuals to the same approach, but no one approach has been demonstrated to be better than others. It is therefore important to have a model that embraces the complexity of ASD and provides comprehensive interventions to address the unique learning challenges of each individual.

---

*DIR® is the registered trademark of ICDL, founded by Stanley Greenspan and Serena Wieder.

Introduction

DIR introduced major paradigm shifts from behavioural to dynamic developmental systems for the treatment of autism. These revolutionized the concept of development by recognizing:
- that affect was central to relating, learning, and understanding–emotions drive early cognitive development;
- that we were now treating *relationships* and not just the child–relationships are the vehicle for learning;
- that every child has an inner world of feelings and sense of self and so does each parent in relation to their child that influences development;
- that emotional experiences and emotional development is best expressed through symbolic development;
- that everyone has individual differences that need tailored and integrated interventions to address poor neurologic connectivity in processing areas;
- that integrated interdisciplinary models are needed in assessment, treatment, and education;
- that competencies come from meaningful experience – not training or rote learning;
- that development builds on what has already developed and is not 'taught';
- that developmentally-appropriate approaches are needed to address developmental challenges in meaningful ways;
- and that development is a life-long process and developmental goals should be pursued at all ages.

The components of the DIR Model have long theoretical, clinical, and research traditions. Psychodynamic developmental frameworks go as far back as Freud, were expanded by Erikson, Piaget, Anna Freud, Mahler, Pine and Bergman and others who looked at early experience. Later clinical reports of Spitz, Bowlby, Winnicott, Fraiberg, Lourie, and Provence showed the critical impact disrupted and impoverished environments had on early relationships and development. Meanwhile, Escalona, Murphy, Brazelton, Ayres, Tomaso, and others were identifying neurobiological factors and opening the door to understanding individual differences.

DIR's initial formulation was based on both theory and experience during a preventive-intervention NIMH research study on multi-risk families, where the objective was to establish foundations for a better future for their infants. This study led to the developmental structuralist theory describing the emotional capacities that organize experience at successively higher levels and provide the structure for development (Greenspan & Wieder, 2011). Three dynamically related influences on development were identified: biological and genetic influences which affect what the child brings into his interactive patterns through individual differences in regulation and sensory motor processing; cultural, environmental, and family factors which influence what the parent or caregiver brings into the interactions; and child-caregiver interactions that determine the relative mastery of six core developmental capacity/processes. These were called the Functional Emotional Developmental Levels: regulation and shared attention, engaging and relating; simple two-way gesturing, complex social problem-solving, creative use of ideas and symbols, and analytic/logical thinking.

A comprehensive approach evolved with a range of unstructured and semi-structured interventions that utilized affect-based interactions to strengthen each child's developmental capacities. Affect was the critical component and is described below. DIR is also commonly known as

Floortime, which is the central component of its model. Floortime™ is both a philosophy and a specific technique where parents and other members of the intervention team both follow the child's natural emotional interests and at the same time challenge the child towards greater mastery of social, emotional, and intellectual capacities by tailoring interactions to the child's unique motor and sensory-processing profile. Emphasis is placed on developmental process, including child initiation, intentionality, reciprocity, continuous flow of purposeful interactions, reasoning and symbolic thinking, engagement and empathy, and self-reflection. These developmental capacities constitute the foundation for functioning, learning, and relating to others in meaningful ways (Greenspan & Wieder, 1998, 2006; Wieder, 2011, 2012).

DIR theory and practice: the role of affect transformations to advance development

DIR theory proposes that in autism children have biological/neurological difficulties in connecting affect/intent to their emerging ability to plan and sequence their actions and subsequent difficulty in relating, communicating, and thinking. Affect involves the emotional signals conveyed through looks, tone of voice, movement, timing, and synchrony that activate development and organize the sequence necessary from the start (initiation) to the finish (*i.e.*, the execution of intent necessary for engagement, communication, and problem-solving interactions). From the beginning an infant usually connects the sensory system to the motor system through affect, *e.g.*, seeing the caregiver's smiling face or hearing her wooing voice entices the infant to turn and look and listen and smile back.

Through many of these interactions the infant begins to recognize patterns as they share attention, take pleasure in interactions, read each others' cues and respond to each other over and over again through gaze, vocalizations, and gestures. Even at a few days infants react to sensations emotionally–suck harder to focus the picture of the mother's image and prefer the mother's touch and smell. Later they learn hot and cold from the many affect-based signals they receive during baths and bottles/food, and learn a little or a lot based on how much they like what they get! Intelligence is forming as the baby discriminates these differences based on the emotional or affective cues, be it between mother's and father's voice and touch, sensations that are pleasurable or not, and later the meaning of ideas. It is this dual coding of experience that is key to understanding how emotions organize intellectual abilities.

By the end of the first year the infant recognizes variations in his caregiver's affect as well as his own feelings related to love, anger, feeling proud, disapproved of, *etc.* By the second year of life, these patterns lead to a sense of self as purposeful and a differentiated sense of others. By the third year of life these affect-based meaningful interactions enable a child to form and give meaning to symbols leading to higher levels of thinking. For example, 'safe or not safe' will depend on how you show that the tiger is not a kitty cat or that the pirate is deceiving as he attempts to take your treasure. All of the child's senses work with his motor system as he interacts with others to solve problems. Difficulties arise when he becomes aware that things are not as they should be based on his memory of prior experiences, and he encounters new difficulties to solve as his experience expands.

DIR theory identifies six fundamental capacities or levels that emerge in infancy and expand in duration, range, and stability as the child grows and reaches across the life span:

I. Regulation and joint attention (between infant and caretaker)

From birth to 3 months, an infant's capacity grows for calm, focused interest in the sights and sounds of the outer world while she begins to share her interests with the caregiver.

II. Forming attachments and engaging in relationships

During the first 4 months, infant and parents become more intimate as they interact with warmth, trust and intimacy. They each use their senses to enjoy each other through looks, hugs, songs, and dancing together. Over time the infant will need to remain related and engaged across the full range of emotions, even when disappointed, scared, angry, or feeling other stresses.

III. Intentional two-way affective communication

Between 4 and 10 months, purposeful, continuous flow of interactions with gestures and reciprocating emotions gets under way. The infant begins to act purposefully, now that she has matured and is more aware of her body and the functions it can perform. As the infant gains motor control over her body and intent, she is better able to communicate her desires. With emerging abilities to reach; sit and turn; crawl and creep; and give and take or drop objects, the infant's awareness of the interpersonal world is growing, as is her awareness of her body in space and in relation to others who may also be moving.

IV. Complex social problem solving

Between 9 and 18 months, an infant has learned the back-and-forth rhythm of interactive emotional signaling and begins to use this ability to think about and solve problems that are emotionally meaningful to get what he wants, such as pulling mommy to the door to go outside and play. All of the child's senses work with his motor system as he interacts with others to solve problems. Difficulties arise when he becomes aware that things are not as they should be, based on his memory of prior experiences, and he encounters new difficulties to solve as his experience expands. Level IV provides the key to competence and reasoning in that it is at this stage that capacities are launched for longer sequences, independent movement in space, purposeful behaviour and reasoning, integration of feelings and communication of thoughts and feelings. Complex gestures are the bridge to expanded language and ideas where symbols begin to take priority and experiences lead to competence.

V. Creating emotional ideas

Between 18 and 36 months, the toddler begins to represent or symbolize intentions, feelings and ideas in imaginative play and/or language, using gestures, words, and symbols. The toddler now calls on a toy phone, sets up a picnic or tea party, takes the sick baby to the doctor or repairs his car before driving somewhere, and enters fantasy. These first ideas come from experiences in real life that can now be enacted in pretend dramas as the child experiments with different roles and feelings.

The child develops a continuous flow in his or her interactions. Longer chains of co-regulated affective gesturing will enable the child to recognize the variations in the caregiver's gestures, facial expressions, and tone of voice and to become aware of his anxiety and repetitive behaviour. The relationship becomes the vehicle for affect transformations that allow the child to negotiate each of the above functional emotional developmental levels. It is affect that transforms labels into meanings leading to symbolic thinking and more complex and abstract reasoning (Greenspan & Wieder, 1998; Wieder & Greenspan, 2003).

VI. Emotional thinking, logic, and sense of reality

At about 3 years of age, the child begins to combine ideas to tell a story as he develops more logic and understanding of himself and others, and of what is real or not real. His stories use imaginative characters and animal figures who talk and may have magic as he discovers he needs more power to encounter the fears and conflicts in life, but reasoning skills click in to elaborate sequences, and stories become increasingly logical and realistic. Over the next few years, the child's emotional and mental abilities move toward abstract thinking and he develops the ability to distinguish reality from fantasy, self from non-self, and one feeling from another; and to make distinctions concerning time and space.

Three additional levels build on Level VI, starting at age 6 when the child goes to school. These include:

VII. Multi-causal and comparative thinking

At this level the child 'deepens the plot' as she can explore multiple motives, get opinions, and compare and contrast ideas. The child can express how she would feel 'in [another person's] shoes' and can predicts what the other will do based on the other's 'affect cues' such as deception, fairness, and justice.

VIII. Relativistic or gray-area thinking

Here, the child differentiates more of his thoughts, rather than thinking only in 'black and white' terms. The lion may pay a price for killing the zebra, or the bear devouring all the honey will disappoint his friend. The child now considers different possibilities and contingencies, and is aware of different outcomes and of how he would feel under different circumstances.

IX. Self-reflection or thinking using an internal standard

Now the child has a sense of herself; she can look at and reflect on her performance and feelings. She can question why she is feeling a certain way and contrast this with how she usually feels, or she can compare her current efforts with earlier ones. This kind of thinking allows her to make inferences about herself and others, and creates new choices and ideas.

The DIR Profile

Unlike some other diagnostic criteria, DIR functional profiles capture the complexity and heterogeneity of the child's developmental capacities, underlying biological processes, functioning and adaptation, and relationships. DIR can guide each family to identify the most appropriate program for the child and family based on their individual profiles and can help to set priorities. This would include exploring the following items:

– *Functional emotional developmental levels* identifying child's interests and loves.
– *Individual differences* in regulation, sensory integration, movement (praxis), language and visual spatial abilities.
– *Family relationships*, including caregiver and social profile, parenting challenges, and typical days and adaptations.
– *Educational, executive functions*, including cognitive and learning profiles and use assessments.
– *Biomedical/neurologic profile*, including allergies, gastrointestinal problems, and seizures.

The child's evolving DIR Profile determines the individualized intervention as he progresses. The DIR Model can also be brought in at older ages (children, adolescents, and adults) when gaps in development are identified, rate of progress is less than expected, plateaus are reached and the client 'gets stuck' or other barriers to development are identified. It is important to go back to core developmental capacities that need strengthening and also to identify various other interventions that are in order, such as those for specific learning disabilities, visual spatial challenges, social challenges, *etc.*

DIR Comprehensive Intervention

A comprehensive approach is necessary to meet individual needs and Floortime™ principles inform all education and therapies. Interventions are perforce of a moving target, but most critical is establishing the first four Functional Emotional Developmental Levels that focus on relating and communicating, opening the doors to higher levels. Interventions include:
- floortime: (6–8 twenty-minute daily sessions at the start, when spontaneous engagement and communication is a priority) and Talktime™, ongoing reality-based problem-solving conversations as children get older and communicate verbally. Floortime most supports symbolic development (Weider & Greenspan, 2003);
- semi-Structured Problem Solving: 3–4 daily sessions. Activities include social games, ritualized learning, reading, 'work', 'getting ready', *etc.*;
- family Support and coaching;
- sensory Motor and Regulatory Activities: 4–6 daily sessions;
- play Dates and Social Groups: according to age and need;
- education and special education: School-based and hybrid programs;
- various Therapies: speech and language, occupational therapy, physical therapy, visual-spatial cognitive therapy, creative arts, and assistive technologies;
- biomedical and medication support.

In conclusion, it is important to emphasize that every child's journey is a family's journey, too, and in DIR we join families and work together. Parents know their children, develop with their children, and want to learn more. The family remains the constant support, but when one member is challenged, the entire family is affected. The stress is continuous and it is important to support family coping and strengths while also recognizing challenges and transitions. We work together and we respect boundaries and reflection. Families need other families and have taken the lead in advocating for autism services and awareness in the United States.

Last, every child's journey is our journey as clinicians and researchers. Each individual we work with provides us with opportunity to learn and develop. This work requires ongoing reflective supervision and mentoring, and there is always more to learn as we embrace the complexity of ASD and search for a better understanding of the underlying causes of this disorder and the methods that will help every individual progress.

DIR outcome studies, long evidenced in practice-based evidence, are now getting supported by research-based evidence. A randomized control study on DIR *vs.* community service groups found significant gains in social interaction, initiation of joint attention, and changes in language interaction skills (Casenheiser *et al.*, 2011). The Social Emotional Growth Chart (SEGC), part of the Bayley Scales of Infant Development, was field-tested on 1,500 infants and young children as a surveillance and screening instrument for autism spectrum disorders, showing a sensitivity of 87 per cent and a specificity of 90 per cent (Greenspan, 2004). The P.L.A.Y. project pre-/post-ratings of videotapes by blind raters using the Functional Emotional

Assessment Scale (FEAS) showed significant increases ($p \leq 0.0001$) in child subscale scores; 45.5 per cent of children made good to very good functional developmental progress (Solomon *et al.*, 2007). This program is now completing a NIMH randomized control study. The original 200-case chart review identified sensory processing and modulation difficulties in all children described in the profiles and reported that after two years of intervention, 58 per cent of treated children no longer met the criteria for ASD (Greenspan & Wieder, 1997). DIR research has taken a seat at the research table and further research is under way (Casenheiser *et al.*, 2011; Kasari *et al.*, 2006, 2010; Solomon *et al.*, 2007). More than a decade ago the National Academy of Sciences recommended comprehensive approaches that work with the child and family in terms of unique profiles of strengths and weaknesses (Lord & McGee, 2001). DIR meets these criteria and more, offering a dynamic model for the 21st century.

Conflicts of interest: The author declares no conflicts of interest.

References

Casenheiser, D.M. Shanker, S.G. & Stieben, J. (2011): Learning through interaction in children with autism: preliminary data from a social communication based intervention. *Autism* **1**, 1–22.

Greenspan, S. (2004): *Greenspan Social-Emotional Growth Chart*. Bulverde, TX: The Psychological Corporation.

Greenspan, S. & Wieder, S. (1997): Developmental patterns and outcomes in infants and children with disorders in relating and communicating: a chart review of 200 cases of children with autistic spectrum diagnoses. *J. Dev. Learning Disord.* **1**, 87–141.

Greenspan, S. & Wieder, S. (1998): *The Child with Special Needs: Encouraging Intellectual and Emotional Growth*. Reading, MA: Perseus.

Greenspan, S. & Wieder, S. (2006): *Engaging Autism: The Floortime Approach to Helping Children Relate, Communicate and Think*. Cambridge, MA: DeCapo Press/Perseus Books.

Greenspan, S.I. & Wieder, S. (2011): Relationship-based early intervention approach to autistic spectrum disorders: the DIR Model 1068. In: *Autism Spectrum Disorders*, pp. 1068–1080, eds. D.G. Amaral, G. Dawson & D.H. Geschwind. New York: Oxford University Press.

Kasari, C., Freeman, S. & Paparella, T. (2006): Joint attention and symbolic play in young children with autism: a randomized controlled intervention study. *J. Child Psychol. Psychiatry* **47**, 611–620.

Kasari, C., Gulsrud, A., Wong, C. & Kwon, S. (2010): Randomized controlled caregiver mediated joint engagement intervention for toddlers with autism. *J. Autism Dev. Disord.* Published online.

Lord, C. & McGee, J. (2001): *Educating Children with Autism*. National Research Council, Washington DC: National Academy Press.

Solomon, R., Necheles, J., Ferch, D. & Bruckman, D. (2007): Pilot study of a parent training program for young children with autism: the P.L.A.Y. Project Home Consultation model. *Autism* **11**, 205–224.

Wieder, S. (2011): DIR: Developmental, Individual-Difference, Relationship-Based Model: a dynamic model for the 21st century. In: *Research-Based Principles and Practices for Educating Students with Autism*, pp. 82–98, eds. D. Zager, M. Wehmeyer & R. Simpson. New York: Routledge/Taylor & Francis.

Wieder, S. (2013): The DIR Model. In: *Encyclopedia of Autism Spectrum Disorders*, ed. F.R. Volkmar. New York/Heidelberg: Springer Reference.

Wieder, S. & Greenspan, S. (2003): Climbing the symbolic ladder in the DIR model through Floortime/interactive play. *Autism* **7**, 425–436.

Chapter 16

The DIR model in treating autism: an Italian experience

Filippo Muratori and Giulia Campatelli

Fondazione Stella Maris, viale del Tirreno 331, 56018 Calambrone (Pisa), Italy
filippo.muratori@inpe.unipi.it

Summary

This paper is the result of almost ten years of experience using the DIR model to treat autism and includes three main areas of interest: a general overview of the DIR model, focusing on active involvement of parents and recognizing the great importance of evaluating the child's sensory-motor profile; the models of treatment usually applied in Italy; and the current level of knowledge of Italian professionals on the DIR model and its perceived effectiveness. The Stella Maris Scientific Institute's research group worked to evaluate outcomes of treatments in children with autism spectrum disorders (ASDs), and we can now report some of the results of treatment. In order to gain a precise picture of knowledge and application of the DIR model in Italy, we collected data using a questionnaire given to the Italian Association of Occupational Therapists (ANUPI) and to those who participated in DIR programs at Stella Maris in the last ten years. In view of these data, it appears fundamental to find new ways of integrating different therapeutic approaches to ASD so that interventions can be tailored to the child's needs, actively involve the family, and take account of the child's own environment.

Introduction

More than ten years ago I visited the United States to attend one of the first American IMFAR conferences and later met Grace Baranek. She was trying to set up a centre for early diagnosis and treatment of autism (in Chapel Hill, NC), an endeavor close to Eric Schopler's area of activity.

During that time, I also met Stanley Greenspan and noticed how often he emphasized that the DIR (Developmental, Individual-Difference Relation-Based) model needs to be considered not as behavioural or psychotherapeutic treatment, but rather as a developmental model that focuses on *relationships* and *engagement* (Greenspan *et al.*, 1998, 2006). At that time Greenspan had been one of the several scientists who regarded autism as a *neurodevelopmental* disease, predicting the nosographic classification of the yet-to-be-published DSM-5. Meeting Greenspan inspired me to analyze the DIR model in depth and to translate into Italian his book *The Child with Special Needs*. For the translation, I divided the book into two parts so that both parents and professionals could have a quick, useful, and smart guide to the concept of Floortime, which was basically unknown at the time.

There is a common misunderstanding about Floortime. It does not consist in totally spontaneous play by the parent, but rather means that parents need to be trained in playing with their child, whose condition presents as having great difficulties in play. Parents therefore must be motivated to be actively involved in their child's treatment; they need to be one of the main players in intervention. I mention this point as it seems to be a forerunner of recent guidelines of the Italian National Institute of Health, which point to parent-mediated intervention as a first-line effective treatment for children with ASDs.

Review of the topic

The research in this chapter focuses on early treatment in ASD after first diagnosis. The sample consists of 70 children (57 males and 13 females) aged between 24 and 48 months who were diagnosed with ASD using the DSM IV-TR, and whose diagnosis was confirmed via ADOS–G (Autism Diagnostic Observation Schedule–Generic). Before treatment started, children with ASD showed a Performance Quotient of more than 50. After 6 months of treatment, outcome measures have been collected through ADOS–G, SCQ (Social Communication Questionnaire), Griffiths–MDS, VABS–II, the MacArthur test, the CBCL (Child Behaviour Checklist), and PSI (Parenting Stress Index). Several centres participated in this study on early treatment of ASD.

One of the main results concerns changes in functional developmental levels after 6 months of treatment in those children who were treated together with parents. Once again, active involvement of parents seems to be a key factor in good-quality intervention (Muratori et al., 2012). The degree of parental involvement seems to lead closely to meaningful intergroup differences in outcome between the children.

For this reason the recent European Project of Research COST, coordinated by Dr. Tony Charman and involving 18 European countries, has proposed focusing on individuation of technological instruments to evaluate modifications in social reciprocity after treatment. This latter concept, referring to the effect of treatment on parent–child interaction, is something still missing in research and is an object of European research efforts.

The literature contains several meta-analyses of treatments of ASD, classifying interventions into several main classes: applied behavioural analysis (ABA), communication-focused interventions [collecting computer-assisted instruction, picture exchange communication system, (PECS) and sign language training], developmental approaches (as DIR), approaches to environmental modification [as Treatment and Education of Autistic and Related Communication-Handicapped Children (TEACCH)] and sensory-motor interventions.

The first great contribution of the DIR model is doubtless the importance of parental involvement in treatment; the child's family needs to be trained to be an active participant in intervention. The 'R' of the DIR acronym stands for *Relationship-based* as the model has strongly supported the idea of active parental involvement as a key factor for good treatment results. Usually children spend most of their time with parents, learning sensory-motor, cognitive, and social abilities from them. Observing the kind of spontaneous relationship among a child and his parents allows clinicians to have useful information on the child's level of development and on the way it combines with the family's style of interaction. Unfortunately, we often see parents excluded from therapy rooms while the therapists work alone with the child for a few hours a week. Conversely, those parents who are trained to modulate everyday intensity and timing of interaction and learn how to join the child's activities, supporting his lead and timing in each single play session at home, are more likely to see better results in terms of quality of engagement.

Also, the DIR model brings to light the great contribution of A.J. Ayres' Sensory Integration Theory to comprehension of child behaviour. Because sensory profile evaluation is not included in the DSM-IV just as it is not considered in ADOS and ADI, nor an area of interest in almost all other intervention programs, it may seem that we almost forgot about this fundamental source of information. Contrary to other approaches, the DIR model is strongly oriented to evaluation of the sensory-motor profile of the child as it is considered the biological root of development: in the DIR acronym, the 'I' stands for *Individual differences*: all those individual, peculiar biologically-based qualities as sensory-motor profile, biological vulnerabilities, sensory thresholds, *etc.* The Sensory Profile Questionnaire of W. Dunn can be used by clinicians to analyze the child's sensory-profile, but regrettably this has not yet been translated into Italian.

In the DIR model, the child's self-regulatory capacities are considered to be strongly influenced by neurologic sensory thresholds: children with high sensory thresholds would show hypo-reactivity to stimulation or sensation-seeking behaviours to achieve the best level of arousal and regulation, rather than the hyper-reactive behaviours or avoidance to stimuli shown by low sensory–threshold children. There are some interesting papers about evaluation of sensory profile in children with ASD (Ben-Sasson, 2008; Rogers, 2003) as well as some instruments to evaluate it, as the Sensory Profile of W. Dunn mentioned before. Another instrument is the Sensory Experience Questionnaire of Grace Baranek (Baranek *et al.*, 2006). These latter authors suggested that, curiously, hypo-reactivity often leads to ASD, while hyper-reactivity is often linked to maturational delays in both typical developed and impaired children.

Using W. Dunn's Sensory Profile (Dunn, 1994; Kienz & Dunn, 1997) the Stella Maris group published an exploratory study on the sensory profile of children with ASD (Muratori *et al.*, 2011), comparing 40 children with PDD and 38 typically developed children, both groups aged from 3 to 6 years. Statistical analysis showed meaningful differences in auditory processing, tactile processing, multi-sensory processing, sensory input modulation relating to emotional reactions, behavioural outcomes of sensory processing, sensory thresholds, emotional reactivity, lack of attention, fine motor skills. Moreover, the correlation between sensory abilities and the three areas of interest of the ADOS-G seems to suggest the presence of an important link.

The importance of the sensory profile evaluation emerged also from our study on the Italian experience with the DIR model. Providing a questionnaire on the DIR model level of mastering and application effects to Italian occupational therapists of ANUPI and to all of those who participated in DIR practice at Stella Maris in last ten years, we collected data that show how valuable the DIR model is to the professionals evaluating the sensory profile. Such evaluation is considered to be one of the most positive elements of DIR/Floortime in involving parents in intervention with their children with ASDs. Our questionnaire also showed other positive elements of applying the DIR approach to the evaluation of child's functional-emotional developmental level as its focus on emotion and relationship, circles of communication, and the child's own spontaneous interests.

Because of our recognition of the need for sensory profile evaluation, we recently translated *Sensory Integration and the Child* by A.J. Ayres (1979) in an effort to provide concrete and useful information to parents and professionals to help them to understand the concept of sensory integration and sensory thresholds. This need for understanding by the scientific and clinical communities is world-wide and, thanks to Greenspan's contributions among others, the DSM-V will soon include the sensory profile as one of the fundamental elements to be evaluated in the diagnosis of ASD.

Beyond the positive contributions of the DIR model toward understanding the child's behaviour and inner world, we also wanted the questionnaire to help in determining the answer to the crucial question: Does the DIR model work? Data show that professionals using the model are generally satisfied and tend to consider it effective in intervention in children with ASD. Moreover, those professionals reported greater than 50 per cent parental satisfaction with Floortime therapy.

Finally, some recent studies on DIR's effectiveness (Pajareya & Nopmaneejumruslers, 2011; Solomon *et al.*, 2007) show the key factors of good outcomes in parental training with Floortime sessions and videotaping. In particular these are improvements in the child's functional-emotional developmental level (Pajareya & Nopmaneejumruslers, 2011; Solomon, 2007), the decrease of CARS score (Pajareya & Nopmaneejumruslers, 2011), the improvements in functional development in 45.5 per cent of cases (*ibid.*), parental satisfaction in 90 per cent (*ibid.*), and lowered economic costs (*ibid.*).

According to the national guidelines of the Italian Institute of Health (2011), effective intervention is likely to be intensive, early, and parent-mediated to better support communication, engagement, and relationship and to help develop the cognitive capacities of children together with satisfaction, empowerment, and emotional wellness of parents.

We selected 18 children with ASD (13 males and 5 females) who have been treated with the DIR model from our survey on effectiveness of ASD treatments. These children were aged from 24- to 48 months, showed a Performance Quotient higher than 50, and received DMS-IV-TR diagnosis of ASD through ADOS–G. To detect improvements in these children's functioning, we used instruments such as ADOS–G, SCQ, Griffiths–MDS, VABS–II, the MacArthur–Bates test, CBCL (Child Behaviour Checklist), and PSI (Parent Stress Index) right after diagnosis and after 6 months of treatment.

DIR model treatment was provided by educators, occupational therapists, speech therapists, special education at school, school programs and parent training dependently on the child's needs and community resources, taking up to an average of 11–15 hours weekly. The child's development trends are similar both in DIR-treated children and in non-DIR-treated children in communication; eye-hand coordination; performance quotients of Griffiths scales; SCQ values; MacArthur values in language production, comprehension, and gestures; and Vineland values on communication, daily life capacities, and motor abilities.

Beyond the information gained by instruments measuring outcomes, meaningful changes are seen in clinical evaluations. From the original sample of 18 DIR-treated children with ASD, 10 showed autism while 8 showed other ASDs. Of those who received a diagnosis of autism, after 6 months of treatment only 6 of these diagnoses were confirmed, while only 4 received confirmation of a diagnosis of another ASD. Of those 8 children who had another autism spectrum disorder, after 6 months of treatment, only 1 child worsened and was diagnosed with autism, whereas 5 of them have been confirmed to be affected by another ASD. Moreover, 2 children of the original 8 with ASDs completely left the spectrum. The survey indicates the percentage of changes as 33 per cent.

Comparing those results with 52 children not treated with DIR model approaches, but by other methods, including PACT [Preschool Autism Communications Trial], ESDM [Early Start Denver Model], and ABA [Applied Behavior Analysis], we found a 32 per cent change in clinical evaluation. In particular, at baseline 47 children have been diagnosed with autism, whereas 5 have been diagnosed with other ASDs. Of those 47 who showed autism after 6 months of non–DIR treatment, 29 were confirmed to be affected by autism, while 16 had other ASDs. Of the 5 children with ASDs at baseline, 4 were confirmed to have ASD after 6 months of non-DIR treatment, whereas 1 child completely exited from the spectrum.

What seems remarkable is the percentage close to 30 per cent of children showing improvements on diagnosis (or who even exited from the spectrum) in *every* kind of treatment of ASD (see Dawson *et al.*, 2010 for ESDM; Green *et al.*, 2010 for PACT; and Smith & Eikeseth, 2011 for ABA).

Some questions need to be formulated: Is it possible to improve this percentage? Are the children responsive to PACT, ABA, ESDM, DIR or the current treatments used in Italy the same kind of children? Is it possible to move toward individualization of treatment? And to achieve this, what are the criteria for child-tailored intervention? This latter topic is discussed by Stahmer, Schreibman, and Cunningham in recent work (2011) in which the authors try to combine different models and techniques into a general theoretical framework to allow the real tailoring of intervention to the child's needs. These authors present a continuum of approaches in which interactive techniques need to be the background to all other interventions, from academic skills training to behavioural analysis, to increase the child's socio-communicative capacities. In particular, following the child's lead, imitating the child, animating and emphasizing affect and empathy, and modeling and expanding language are the basis of second-level techniques as playful obstruction, balancing turn-taking, communicative temptations ['temptation' is the term used in DIR Model to indicate those communicative opportunities in which the child does want to communicate because of the great positive affect deriving from interaction], and of a third level consisting in prompting and reinforcement.

Integration of different approaches would seem necessary to tailor intervention to a particular child's needs and profiles, but our questionnaire on the DIR model mastering level and knowledge shows that 19 per cent of DIR-competent professionals are against the integration of the DIR model with other approaches; for example, 20 per cent of the occupational therapists belonging to ANUPI that completed our questionnaire are reported to be against such integration. The rest of the Italian professionals who completed our questionnaire, almost 80 per cent, do integrate the DIR model with such other treatments as TEACCH, occupational therapy, ESDM, and augmentative and alternative communication (AAC).

Conclusions

In the DIR model, intervention is individual-difference-based, but is not applied to the individual child alone; on the contrary, it involves parents and school and other areas of daily life. Even within the same treated child, the focus is always globally oriented to the emotional and relational world, sensory-motor profile, functional-emotional developmental levels, and family resources.

The great contribution of the DIR model in comprehension of child psychology and behaviour can be shown in the pithy phrase of Vasudevi Reddy: 'From third-person psychology to second-person psychology'.

Conflicts of interest: The authors declare no conflicts of interest.

References

Ayres, A.J. (1979): *Sensory integration and the child.* Los Angeles, CA: Western Psychological Services.

Baranek, G.T., David, F.J., Poe, M.D., Stone, W.L. & Watson, L.R. (2006): Sensory Experiences Questionnaire: discriminating sensory features in young children with autism, developmental delays, and typical development. *J. Child Psychol. Psychiatry* **47,** 591–601.

Ben-Sasson, A., Cermak, S.A., Orsmond, G.I., Tager-Flusberg, H., Kadlec, M.B. & Carter, A.S. (2008): Sensory clusters of toddlers with autism spectrum disorders: differences in affective symptoms. *J. Child Psychol. Psychiatry* **49,** 817–827.

Dawson, G., Rogers, S., Munson, J., *et al.* (2010): Randomized, controlled trial of an intervention for toddlers with autism: the Early Start Denver Model. *Pediatrics* **125,** 17–23.

Dunn, W. (1994): Performance of typical children on the Sensory Profile: an item analysis. *Am. J. Occup. Ther.* **48,** 967–974.

Green, J., Charman, T., McConachie, H., *et al.* & PACT Consortium (2010): Parent-mediated communication-focused treatment in children with autism (PACT): a randomized controlled trial. *Lancet* **375,** 2152–2160.

Greenspan, S.I. & Wieder, S. (2006): *Engaging Autism: using the Floortime Approach to Help Children Relate, Think, and Communicate.* Cambridge, MA: Da Capo Press.

Greenspan, S.I., Wieder, S. & Simon, R. (1998): *The Child with Special Needs: Encouraging Intellectual and Emotional Growth.* Reading, MA: Addison-Wesley.

Kientz, M.A. & Dunn, W. (1997): A comparison of the performance of children with and without autism on the Sensory Profile. *Am. J. Occup. Ther.* **51,** 530–537.

Muratori, F., Tancredi, R., Massagli, A., *et al.* (2012): Effetti a sei mesi dell'intervento precoce nei disturbi dello spettro autistico. *Giornale di Neuropsichiatria dell'età evolutiva* **32,** (2).

Muratori, F., Narzisi, A., Tancredi, R., *et al.* (2011): The CBCL 1.5-5 and the identification of preschoolers with autism in Italy. *Epidemiol. Psychiatr. Sci.* **20,** 329–338.

National Guidelines of the Italian Institute of Health [Linee guida nazionale/SNLG-ISS] (2011): Il trattamento dei disturbi dello spettro autistico nei bambini e negli adolescenti. Available at http://www.snlg-iss.it [The treatment of autism spectrum disorders in children and adolescents].

Pajareya, K. & Nopmaneejumruslers, K. (2011): A pilot randomized controlled trial of DIR/Floortime™ parent training intervention for pre-school children with autistic spectrum disorders. *Autism* **15,** 563–577.

Reddy, V. (2008): *How Infants Know Minds.* Cambridge, MA: Harvard University Press.

Rogers, S.J., Hepburn, S. & Wehner, E. (2003): Parent reports of sensory symptoms in toddlers with autism and those with other developmental disorders. *J. Autism Dev. Disord.* **33,** 631–642.

Smith, T. & Eikeseth, S. (2011): O. Ivar Lovaas: pioneer of applied behavior analysis and intervention for children with autism. *J. Autism Dev. Disord.* **41,** 375–378.

Solomon, R., Necheles, J., Ferch, C. & Bruckman, D. (2007): Pilot study of a parent training program for young children with autism: the PLAY Project Home Consultation program. *Autism* **11,** 205–224.

Stahmer, A.C., Schreibman, L. & Cunningham, A.B. (2010): Toward a technology of treatment individualization for young children with autism spectrum disorders [review]. *Brain Res.* **22,** 229–239.

Chapter 17

Imitation in autism spectrum disorders: from research to treatment

Giacomo Vivanti

*Olga Tennison Autism Research Centre, School of Psychological Science,
La Trobe University, 3086 Melbourne, Victoria, Australia
G.Vivanti@latrobe.edu.au*

Summary

Imitation, according to Lev Vygotsky (1931), is 'one of the basic paths of cultural development of the child'. Indeed children, by imitating adults, can perform tasks that are beyond what they can independently achieve. Children with autism spectrum disorders, however, show difficulties in imitation, and this deficit might interfere with learning processes, social development and adaptive behaviour. In this chapter we review current evidence on the imitation deficit in autism, documenting that while frequency and accuracy of imitative behaviour are often reported to be reduced in this population, under specific conditions individuals in the spectrum show intact imitation abilities. Differences in imitative behaviour appear to be associated with differences in both social and motor skills in this population; however, the nature of these associations is still not clear. Recent research that employed eye-tracking technology is providing us with new insight on the nature of imitative abnormalities in this population. These studies show that there are basic differences in the way children with autism attend to others' actions, which can influence the way demonstrated actions are 'internalized' and, consequently, imitated. The role of social attention in imitation is acknowledged as well by a number of recently-developed treatments that focus on the social context of imitation, with preliminary data showing promising results.

Introduction

In her original description of 'the triad of impairments' in autism spectrum disorders (ASDs), Lorna Wing suggested that one of the key-symptoms is a 'lack of imagination' (Wing & Gould, 1979). This concept originates from clinical observations and experimental studies reporting poor imaginative and creative play, as well as a lack of figurative language and literal interpretation of others' language in this population (Jarrold, 2003; Woodard & Van Reet, 2011). Given the importance of abstract thinking and symbolic reasoning for cognitive development, difficulties in 'imagination' are very likely to have developmental sequelae in different domains. However, typically-developing children are not only imaginative and creative: they also imitate what others do. Indeed, most of the learning in childhood and throughout the life-span does not originate from trials and errors, but rather from observing what other people do and by participating in social and play interactions in which reciprocal imitation plays a major role (Hurley & Chater, 2005).

Children with ASD have difficulties not only with creating, but also with imitating. As originally suggested by Rogers and Pennington (1991), such difficulties might have an impact on key-developmental areas, including social-cognitive and motor-executive abilities. In this chapter we review recent findings on imitation and imitative learning in ASD, with a focus on developmental and neuropsychological factors, as well as remediation strategies.

Imitation in typical development

From infancy on, humans are programmed to navigate the social world. We are very good at reading other people's minds – a quick look at another person is enough to allow us to read behind the surface and capture their underlying feelings. We like the feeling of being interconnected – the success of new social technologies such as Facebook or Twitter reflects this inclination. And we fear a lack of human contact – for example, solitary confinement affects a prisoner's mental health more severely than any other legal form of punishment. Moreover, from the very first hours of life, we have a natural inclination to imitate others' actions. Humans appear to engage in imitative behaviours for two reasons: acquiring knowledge about the world (*e.g.*, learning how to use a tool) (Bandura, 1977) and establishing/consolidating social/affiliative bonds (Nadel & Butterworth, 1999).These two functions are often referred to as the apprenticeship and the social function of imitation (Uzgiris, 1981). The developmental pattern of imitative behaviour involves an initial stage, in which newborns can imitate a limited number of actions (Meltzoff & Prinz, 2002), followed by the emergence of synchronic/reciprocal imitation in the framework of mother–child dyadic exchanges between 18 and 24 months (Trevarthen, 2001). During childhood, imitation appears to be a powerful learning and social tool, with research showing that children who imitate others more frequently tend to be more socially responsive and cognitively able (Strid *et al.*, 2006; Young *et al.*, 2011). Imitation plays an important role in a later stage of development: as adults, we continue to copy others' actions both in order to acquire knowledge and to promote feelings of social-affective relatedness and psychological intimacy (Tomasello & Moll, 2010). This is reflected in the inclination to participate in social (*e.g.*, dancing) and learning (*e.g.*, yoga lessons) activities, which involve the imitation of others' actions, and in the tendency to imitate others even as we do not intend to nor are we aware of doing so (*e.g.*, clapping in unison with a crowd).

Imitation in ASD

Compared to typically-developing peers, individuals with autism appear to imitate other people less frequently and less accurately. The observation that imitation might be an area of weakness in ASD dates back to 1953 (Ritvo & Provence, 1953). In the following decades, more than a hundred studies, employing a variety of research methods, have investigated different aspects of imitative behaviour in ASD, as well as the social/emotional, cognitive, and neuropsychological factors that might be associated with difficulties in imitation. The picture emerging from the current literature indicates that imitation is not an area of absolute inability in ASD; rather, imitative performance in this population tends to vary according to the type of task.

In particular, individuals with ASD show difficulties in the imitation of non-meaningful intransitive actions, that is, actions that do not involve objects, do not carry a specific meaning, and can only be described in terms of changes of limb postures in space (*e.g.*, a hand moving across a forehead or eyebrows lifting three times). Impairments in the re-enactment of these types of actions are reported consistently in the ASD population, across levels of severity and chronological age ranges (Bernier *et al.*, 2007; Jones & Prior, 1985; Vanvuchelen *et al.*, 2007; Vivanti *et al.*, 2008). Research looking at the imitation of transitive actions (actions that involve objects) provided less consistent findings. A number of studies found an intact ability to imitate meaningful transitive actions (*e.g.*, opening a box by removing the lid) (Beadle-Brown & Whiten, 2004; Hobson & Hobson, 2008; McDonough *et al.*, 1997, but see Bernier *et al.*, 2007 and Colombi *et al.*, 2009). This methodology, however, presents some problems, as the understanding of the end-state of the demonstrated action (*e.g.*, a box is open) or the specific affordance of the object (a closed box 'invites' itself to be opened) might be sufficient to elicit a behaviour in the observer that is similar to one used by the demonstrator (removing the lid from the box). Thus, this makes it difficult to establish whether the observer is actually 'internalizing' the demonstrator's actions. Other studies, however, have documented ASD-specific difficulties in the imitation of non-meaningful transitive actions, that is, unconventional actions that do not carry a semantic meaning (*e.g.*, using a book to lift a brush), suggesting that individuals with ASD have particular difficulties in reproducing actions that do not result in a familiar/meaningful outcome. Supporting this view, two studies have documented that children with ASD are more likely to imitate actions that result in a visible/motivating feedback (Ingersoll *et al.*, 2003; Rogers *et al.*, 2010). Similarly, individuals with ASD appear to show an impairment in the imitation of non-meaningful oral-facial movements (Bernier *et al.*, 2007; Freitag *et al.*, 2006; Page & Boucher, 1998; Rogers *et al.*, 2003); however, many studies report intact abilities to imitate meaningful facial movements, such as emotional expressions, in this population (Dapretto *et al.*, 2006; Loveland *et al.*, 1994; Stel *et al.*, 2008; but see Grossman & Tager-Flusberg, 2008).

Finally, a number of studies have reported that individuals with ASD, across age range and developmental level, have more difficulties imitating sequences of actions compared to single actions (Vanvuchelen *et al.*, 2007; Libby *et al.*, 1997).

This pattern of strengths and weaknesses points to the importance of both the social processing and motor demand involved in the demonstrated actions in the imitative performance of individuals with ASD.

Recent research on the mechanisms underlying imitative difficulties in ASD

Given that the imitative behaviour of people with ASD appears to be driven by the outcome of the demonstrated actions, rather than the specific demonstrator's acts, we conducted a series of experiments to investigate how actions and outcomes are visually encoded by individuals with ASD. In a study based on eye-tracking technology (a system of infrared cameras that allows for a fine-grained measurement of where a person is looking), we examined what children with autism and typically-developing children look at when actions are being demonstrated to them (Vivanti *et al.*, 2008). Participants in the study (20 children with autism, and 20 with typical development) were asked to observe video clips of a person demonstrating an action. After viewing each clip, the children performed the demonstrated action. The results confirmed previous research that shows that children with autism are less accurate in imitating people than are normally developing children. Analysis of gaze patterns showed that both the children with autism and those without looked at the demonstrator's actions for similar durations; however, typically-developing children looked at the demonstrator's face twice as long as the group of children with autism did. The analysis of the visual attention patterns showed that children without autism were constantly shifting their attention between the demonstrator's face and his actions, while children with autism were focusing on the action, with little or no attention to the demonstrator's face.

In a second experiment we investigated whether differences in the way children with autism visually attend to others' actions had a specific impact on the understanding of the demonstrator's intentions (Vivanti *et al.*, 2011). Once again, participants observed a series of videoclips. In these clips, an actor began to perform an action, but the video ended before the end of the action was completed. Participants were then asked to complete the action as the model would have. While participants viewed videos, their eye movements were recorded by the eye-tracking system. Through the analysis of participants' eye movements, we found again that typically-developing children focused their attention both on the model's actions and on her face, while children with autism were mainly focusing on her actions. By doing so, they were missing crucial information on the model's intentions. For example, in one of the clips the demonstrator is stacking blocks according to a colour pattern, and then turns her head toward a block that would discontinue the pattern. The majority of typically-developing participants noticed the demonstrator's head-turn and interpreted it as signalling her intention to pick up and stack the block to which she turned and looked, which would change the colour pattern of the stack. All participants with ASD except for 2 (10 per cent) did not notice the head turn, and consequently, completed the demonstrator's action based on the colour pattern instead. In other words they relied on the outcome suggested by the objects' properties rather than the one suggested by the demonstrator's intentions. These are two rather different strategies that, under certain circumstances, might lead to similar results, which possibly explains why imitation of meaningful transitive actions (for which the appreciation of the demonstrator's intention is not necessary) is reported to be intact in ASD in many studies. However, these processing strategies are qualitatively different, and are most likely based on distinct neural systems.

These studies show that there are basic differences in the way children with autism attend to others' actions, which can influence the way demonstrated actions are processed. Consistent with these conclusions, Hobson & Hobson (2007) documented a reduced tendency to establish eye contact with the demonstrator in a group of children with autism. The less the children with autism looked at the demonstrator's face, the worse their ability was to imitate the demonstrator's actions. In another study, the observation of the demonstrator's face facilitated imitation in typically-developing individuals, but not in a group of individuals with ASD (Pierno *et al.*, 2006). Taken together, these data suggest that when a child with autism and a typically-developing child are observing someone's action, they are both observing the action, but they are not encoding the same breadth of social information (Vivanti & Hamilton, in press). Therefore, differences in how children with autism imitate others appear to begin with the very first step of the process: with selective attention guiding the perceptual input to the rest of the system.

Other steps of the imitative process might be impaired as well. A number of studies suggested abnormalities in the neuropsychological mechanisms underlying the translation of the visual input into motor output (often referred as mirror mechanisms; see Colombi *et al.*, 2011; Iacoboni, 2009; Rizzolatti, 2005). Moreover, there is growing evidence that motor abnormalities (including planning and executive abilities) might explain in part difficulties in imitative performance in this population (Mostofsky *et al.*, 2006; Vanvuchelen *et al.*, 2007; but see Rogers *et al.*, 2003). Recent research suggests that difficulties in imitation, just like difficulties in executing gestures on command, might reflect a developmental dyspraxia, that is, a deficit in the execution of skilled movements caused by difficulties in forming the sensory representation of the motor plan that is necessary to execute the actions (Dziuk *et al.*, 2007; Mostofsky & Ewen, 2011). This model appears to be corroborated by abundant data on abnormal connectivity in the brain systems underlying motor planning and execution in autism (Esposito & Vivanti, 2013; Lloyd *et al.*, 2011; Nayate *et al.*, 2005; Qiu *et al.*, 2010).

Abnormalities in social/attentional and motor/executive components of the imitation process, rather than suggesting mutually exclusive explanations for the deficit, appear to reflect a system-level vulnerability. In other words, multiple areas of weakness across social/attention and motor/executive domains in this population all concur in making imitation of others' actions difficult, yet not impossible, for individuals with ASD. This perspective might help to account for the relative strength in the imitation of actions that require less social understanding (*i.e.*, 'self-explaining' actions resulting in familiar outcomes, or actions in which the outcomes might be inferred on the basis of the objects' properties, rather than the demonstrator's social cues) and less motor/executive demand (*i.e.*, single *versus* sequential actions) in the ASD population.

Intervention strategies

Early attempts to teach imitative skills in individuals with ASD were based on the principles of operant conditioning (Skinner, 1953) and involved the use of highly structured settings and external reinforcements (*e.g.*, food) (Lovaas *et al.*, 1967). While these strategies were successful in eliciting imitative behaviour 'on demand', other important aspects, such as the spontaneous use of imitation to learn and to socialize in the environment, were not specifically addressed. More recently, several treatment strategies were developed addressing imitation difficulties with an emphasis on the social context of imitation, as well as spontaneous generalization to untrained environments in the absence of external reinforcement.

The Reciprocal Imitation Training model (Ingersoll, 2010; Ingersoll & Gergans, 2007; Ingersoll *et al.*, 2007) is a naturalistic intervention that emphasizes the role of social reciprocity in imitation. During play sessions involving a variety of pairs of toys, the therapist imitates the child's behaviour, in order to get the child's attention and to create a turn-taking routine. The therapist then models an action and waits for the child's contingent imitative response; in case the child does not respond after three attempts, the therapist physically prompts the child. All the prompted and spontaneous imitative behaviours are systematically reinforced through verbal praise. Results from a randomized control trial indicate that children in the treatment group made significantly more gains in elicited and spontaneous imitation, as well as in joint attention and social functioning (Ingersoll, 2010, 2011).

Similarly, the Early Start Denver Model (ESDM) (Rogers & Dawson, 2010) focuses on the development of spontaneous imitative behaviour during play-based reciprocal social interactions. In the ESDM, imitation is targeted together with multiple aspects of social reciprocity (*e.g.*, joint attention, sharing of affect, verbal and nonverbal communication) and nonsocial skills (*e.g.*, fine-motor, nonverbal cognitive skills) in the framework of joint activity routines. Teaching techniques involve capturing and holding the child's attention and fostering his/her motivation by getting him/her to choose the material/activity, establish a joint play routine that involves shared control of the materials and turn-taking exchanges, and model actions that are meaningful in the context of the current activity (*e.g.*, gestures associated with a song routine; or actions associated with a Play-Doh game), so that the child would be naturally reinforced to take a turn in the imitative routine in order to get the activity to continue. A randomized control trial of the ESDM has demonstrated strong positive outcomes when employed in a one-on-one format with children between the ages of 18 to 30 months, documenting gains in cognitive and adaptive skills (Dawson *et al.*, 2010).

The Interpersonal Synchrony model, described by Landa and colleagues (2011), focuses on fostering imitation, as well as other social behaviours such as joint attention and affect sharing, in the context of play-based interactions within a group program. A randomized control trial documented gains in the treatment group in imitation and other social initiation measures which were maintained over a 6-month period (Landa *et al.*, 2011).

Conclusions

The drive to imitate others and the ability to do so rely on a number of processes, including social motivation to align one's own behaviour with others' behaviour, understanding of others' behaviour, the transfer of the visual input into a motor plan, and motor/executive control on one's own movements to replicate observed actions. All of these processes are impaired to different degrees in individuals with ASD; therefore, it is not surprising that imitation represents an area of weakness in this population. However, in order to develop effective remediation strategies, it is important to tease apart the role of the different deficits (*e.g.*, social *versus* motor) underlying imitation difficulties – a process that appears to be arduous, given that social, attentional, cognitive, and motor processes are interconnected both from a neuropsychological and a developmental point of view. Recently-developed treatments that focus on the social context of imitation appear to be promising. Future research needs be based on a fine-grained analysis of the different imitative strategies that may be used to copy others' behaviour (*e.g.*, copying the outcomes of the demonstrator's actions *versus* copying the demonstrator's acts), with a focus on developmental and neuropsychological mechanisms underlying both spontaneous occurrence of imitative behaviour and accuracy/precision of imitation in elicited situations. Moreover, advances in our understanding of the neurocognitive correlates of imitation might pave the way for the definition of more precise and biologically-based markers of intervention efficacy (*e.g.*, changes in fMRI or eye-tracking patterns).

Conflicts of interest: The author declares no conflicts of interest.

References

Bandura, A. (1977): *Social Learning Theory*. Englewood Cliffs, NJ: Prentice Hall.

Beadle-Brown, J.D. & Whiten, A. (2004): Elicited imitation in children and adults with autism: is there a deficit? *J. Intellect. Dev. Disabil.* **29,** 147–163.

Bernier, R., Dawson, G., Webb, S. & Murias, M. (2007): EEG mu rhythm and imitation impairments in individuals with autism spectrum disorder. *Brain Cognit.* **64,** 228–237.

Colombi, C., Liebal, K., Tomasello, M., Young, G., Warneken, F. & Rogers, S.J. (2009): Examining correlates of cooperation in autism: imitation, joint attention, and understanding intentions. *Autism* **13,** 143–163.

Colombi, C., Vivanti, G. & Rogers, S. (2011): Imitation in ASD. In: *The Neuropsychology of Autism*, ed. D. Fein, pp. 243–266. New York: Oxford University Press.

Dapretto, M., Davies, M.S., Pfeifer, J.H., Scott, A.A., Sigman, M., Bookheimer, S.Y., *et al.* (2006): Understanding emotions in others: mirror neuron dysfunction in children with autism spectrum disorders. *Nature Neurosci.* **9,** 28–30.

Dawson, G., Rogers, S., Munson, J., Smith, M., Winter, J., Greenson, J., *et al.* (2010): Randomized, controlled trial of an intervention for toddlers with autism: the Early Start Denver Model. *Pediatrics* **125,** e17–23.

Dziuk, M.A., Gidley Larson, J.C., Apostu, A., Mahone, E.M., Denckla, M.B. & Mostofsky, S.H. (2007): Dyspraxia in autism: association with motor, social, and communicative deficits. *Dev. Med. Child Neurol.* **49**, 734–739.

Esposito, G. & Vivanti, G. (2013): Gross motor skills in autism. In: *Encyclopedia of Autism Spectrum Disorders*, ed. F. Volkmar. New York: Springer.

Freitag, C.M., Kleser, C. & von Gontardf, A. (2006): Imitation and language abilities in adolescents with autism spectrum disorder without language delay. *Eur. Child Adolesc. Psychiatry* **15**, 282–291.

Grossman, R.B. & Tager-Flusberg, H. (2008): Reading faces for information about words and emotions in adolescents with autism. *Res. Autism Spect. Disord.* **2**, 681–695.

Hobson, J.A. & Hobson, R.P. (2007): Identification: the missing link between joint attention and imitation? *Dev. Psychopathol.* **19**, 411–431.

Hobson, R.P. & Hobson, J.A. (2008): Dissociable aspects of imitation: a study in autism. *J. Exp. Child Psychol.* **101**, 170–185.

Hurley, S.L. & Chater, N. (2005): *Perspectives on Imitation: From Neuroscience to Social Science*. Cambridge, MA: MIT Press.

Iacoboni, M. (2009): Imitation, empathy, and mirror neurons. *Annu. Rev. Psychol.* **60**, 653–670.

Ingersoll, B. (2010): Brief report: pilot randomized controlled trial of reciprocal imitation training for teaching elicited and spontaneous imitation to children with autism. *J. Autism Dev. Disord.* **40**, 1154–1160.

Ingersoll, B. (2011): Brief report: effect of a focused imitation intervention on social functioning in children with autism. *J. Autism Dev. Disord.* **42**, 1768–1773.

Ingersoll, B. & Gergans, S. (2007): The effect of a parent-implemented imitation intervention on spontaneous imitation skills in young children with autism. *Res. Dev. Disabil.* **28**, 163–175.

Ingersoll, B., Schreibman, L. & Tran, Q.H. (2003): Effect of sensory feedback on immediate object imitation in children with autism. *J. Autism Dev. Disord.* **33**, 673–683.

Ingersoll, B., Lewis, E. & Kroman, E. (2007): Teaching the imitation and spontaneous use of descriptive gestures in young children with autism using a naturalistic behavioral intervention. *J. Autism Dev. Disord.* **37**, 1446–1456.

Jarrold, C. (2003): A review of research into pretend play in autism. *Autism* **7**, 379–390.

Jones, V. & Prior, M. (1985): Motor imitation abilities and neurological signs in autistic children. *J. Autism Dev. Disord.* **15**, 37–46.

Landa, R.J., Holman, K.C., O'Neill, A.H. & Stuart, E.A. (2011): Intervention targeting development of socially synchronous engagement in toddlers with autism spectrum disorder: a randomized controlled trial. *J. Child Psychol. Psychiatry* **52**, 13–21.

Libby, S., Powell, S., Messer, D. & Jordan, R. (1997): Imitation of pretend play acts by children with autism and Down syndrome. *J. Autism Dev. Disord.* **27** (4), 365–383.

Lloyd, M., Macdonald, M. & Lord, C. (2011): Motor skills of toddlers with autism spectrum disorders. *Autism* **32**, 6525–6541.

Lovaas, O.I., Freitas, L., Nelson, K. & Whalen, C. (1967): Establishment of imitation and its use for development of complex behavior in schizophrenic children. *Behav. Res. Ther.* **5**, 171–181.

Loveland, K.A., Tunalikotoski, B., Pearson, D.A., Brelsford, K.A., Ortegon, J. & Chen, R. (1994): Imitation and expression of facial affect in autism. *Dev. Psychopathol.* **6**, 433–444.

McDonough, L., Stahmer, A., Schreibman, L. & Thompson, S.J. (1997): Deficits, delays, and distractions: an evaluation of symbolic play and memory in children with autism. *Dev. Psychopathol.* **9**, 17–41.

Meltzoff, A.N. & Prinz, W. (2002): *The Imitative Mind: Development, Evolution, and Brain Bases*. Cambridge, UK; New York: Cambridge University Press.

Mostofsky, S.H. & Ewen, J.B. (2011): Altered connectivity and action model formation in autism is autism. *Neuroscientist* **17**, 437-448.

Mostofsky, S.H., Dubey, P., Jerath, V.K., Jansiewicz, E.M., Goldberg, M.C. & Denckla, M.B. (2006): Developmental dyspraxia is not limited to imitation in children with autism spectrum disorders. *J. Int. Neuropsychol. Soc.* **12**, 314–326.

Nadel, J. & Butterworth, G. (1999): *Imitation in Infancy*. Cambridge, UK; New York: Cambridge University Press.

Nayate, A., Bradshaw, J.L. & Rinehart, N.J. (2005): Autism and Asperger's disorder: are they movement disorders involving the cerebellum and/or basal ganglia? *Brain Res. Bull.* **67**, 327–334.

Page, J. & Boucher, J. (1998): Motor impairments in children with autistic disorder. *Child Lang. Teach. Ther.* **14**, 233–259.

Pierno, A.C., Mari, M., Glover, S., Georgiou, I. & Castiello, U. (2006): Failure to read motor intentions from gaze in children with autism. *Neuropsychologia* **44**, 1483–1488.

Qiu, A., Adler, M., Crocetti, D., Miller, M.I. & Mostofsky, S.H. (2010): Basal ganglia shapes predict social, communication, and motor dysfunctions in boys with autism spectrum disorder. *J. Am. Acad. Child Adolesc. Psychiatry* **49,** 539–551, 551 e531–534.

Ritvo, S. & Provence, S. (1953): Form perception and imitation in some autistic children: diagnostic findings and their contextual interpretation. *Psychoanal. Study Child* **8,** 155–161.

Rizzolatti, G. (2005): The mirror neuron system and its function in humans. *Anat. Embryol.* **210,** 419-421.

Rogers, S.J. & Pennington, B.F. (1991): A theoretical approach to the deficits in infantile autism. *Dev. Psychopathol.* **107,** 147–161.

Rogers, S.J. & Dawson, G. (2010): *Early Start Denver Model for Young Children with Autism: Promoting Language, Learning, and Engagement.* New York: Guilford Press.

Rogers, S.J., Hepburn, S.L., Stackhouse, T. & Wehner, E. (2003): Imitation performance in toddlers with autism and those with other developmental disorders. *J. Child Psychol. Psychiatry Allied Discipl.* **44,** 763–781.

Rogers, S.J., Young, G.S., Cook, I., Giolzetti, A. & Ozonoff, S. (2010): Imitating actions on objects in early-onset and regressive autism: effects and implications of task characteristics on performance. *Dev. Psychopathol.* **22,** 71–85.

Skinner, B.F. (1953): *Science and Human Behavior.* New York: Macmillan.

Stel, M., van den Heuvel, C. & Smeets, R.C. (2008): Facial feedback mechanisms in autistic spectrum disorders. *J. Autism Dev. Disord.* **38,** 1250–1258.

Strid, K., Tjus, T., Smith, L., Meltzoff, A.N. & Heimann, M. (2006): Infant recall memory and communication predicts later cognitive development. *Infant Behav. Dev.* **29,** 545–553.

Tomasello, M. & Moll, H. (2010): The gap is social: human shared intentionality and culture. In: *Mind the Gap: Tracing the Origins of Human Universals*, eds. P. Kappeler & J. Silk, pp. 331–349. Berlin: Springer.

Trevarthen, C. (2001): The neurobiology of early communication: intersubjective regulations in human brain development. In: *Handbook on Brain and Behavior in Human Development*, eds. A.F. Kalverboer & A. Gramsbergen, pp. 841–882. Dordrecht, the Netherlands: Kluwer.

Uzgiris, I.C. (1981): Two functions of imitation during infancy. *Int. J. Behav. Dev.* **4,** 1–12.

Vanvuchelen, M., Roeyers, H. & De Weerdt, W. (2007): Nature of motor imitation problems in school-aged boys with autism: a motor or a cognitive problem? *Autism* **11,** 225–240.

Vivanti, G. & Hamilton, A. (2013): Imitation in autism spectrum disorders. In: *Handbook of Autism and Developmental Disorders*, 4th ed., eds. F. Volkmar et al. New York: Wiley.

Vivanti, G., Nadig, A., Ozonoff, S. & Rogers, S.J. (2008): What do children with autism attend to during imitation tasks? *J. Exp. Child Psychol.* **101,** 186–205.

Vivanti, G., McCormick, C., Young, G.S., Abucayan, F., Hatt, N., Nadig, A., et al. (2011): Intact and impaired mechanisms of action understanding in autism. *Dev. Psychol.* **47,** 841–856.

Wing, L. & Gould, J. (1979): Severe impairments of social interaction and associated abnormalities in children: epidemiology and classification. *J. Autism Dev. Disord.* **9,** 11–29.

Woodard, C.R. & Van Reet, J. (2011): Object identification and imagination: an alternative to the meta-representational explanation of autism. *J. Autism Dev. Disord.* **41,** 213–226.

Young, G.S., Rogers, S.J., Hutman, T., Rozga, A., Sigman, M. & Ozonoff, S. (2011): Imitation from 12 to 24 months in autism and typical development: a longitudinal Rasch analysis. *Dev. Psychol.* **47,** 1565–1578.

Chapter 18

Speech and language therapy intervention from the perspective of a multi-professional approach

Luciano Destefanis and Giuseppe Maurizio Arduino

*Centre of Autism and Asperger's Syndrome (CASA), ASL CN1,
Ospedale Regina Montis Regalis, via San Rochetto 99, 12084 Mondovì (CN), Italy*
luciano.destefanis@asIcn1.it
giuseppe.arduino@aslcn1.it

Summary

One of the criteria defining autism spectrum disorders (ASDs) is the qualitative impairment in communication. For parents of an autistic child the most important need is to become able to communicate with their child. For a spectrum of disorders, a range of interventions needs to be used, tailored to that child with his specific functional profile and communication difficulties. In the treatment approach of the Centre of Autism and Asperger's Syndrome (CASA) of Mondovì, a public health clinic in Italy, the development of communication is the overarching goal. The responsibility is not just that of a single professional, but involves the whole multi-professional team as well as the family and the school. A proposal of a multi-modal extension of PVB [Primo Vocabolario del Bambino, the Italian version of the MacArthur–Bates Communicative Development Inventory (CDI)] and a creative way of using personal computers (PCs) with children with ASDs are presented as aspects of good, competent practice by the speech and language therapist in this multi-professional team.

Introduction

Qualitative impairment in communication is one of the criteria that define autism spectrum disorders (ASDs). The ability to communicate with the autistic child is the most important need expressed by parents. It is also the necessary condition for starting an educational intervention and one of the most important variables for understanding and managing behaviour problems.

With regard to communication we can observe a spectrum of impairments. The qualitative impairment in communication can occur with 'delay in, or total lack of, the development of spoken language (not accompanied by an attempt to compensate through alternative modes of communication such as gesture or mime)' (DSM–IV; American Psychiatric Association, 1994), comprehension difficulties of various degrees, reduced communicative intentionality, difficulty in making requests, and development of an early 'autonomy' in obtaining what these children want or need. On the other hand, qualitative impairment in communication can occur with echolalia (immediate or 'deferred'), which in many cases is not related to communicative intent; stereotyped and repetitive language, with a tendency to repeat the same words and phrases, asking the same questions or talking about the same subject; and organized language, but with difficulty in initiating or sustaining a conversation.

In addition, the child also shows difficulty in pretend play and has an impaired ability to imitate.

For a spectrum of disorders, we have to employ a range of interventions, tailored to that child, with his or her specific functional profile and communication difficulties (Wetherby et al., 1997).

At a first level, intervention aims to build multiple modes of communication, expand the range of communicative functions, develop strategies to persist in the communication and, when useful, to introduce augmentative and alternative communication (AAC) systems. At this level it is important that the child learns to be more active in social interactions. The role of partners is very important in building communicative situations and routines that create the motivation and the need for communication on the child's part.

At the higher level of skill, the intervention aims to expand vocabulary and communicative functions, produce communicative acts, and increase the complexity of language and more 'conventional' use of echolalia to express intentions. For those children with good language abilities, the objectives of the intervention are to develop conversational skills and the use of language to plan and organize behaviour and to express and regulate emotions.

Review of the topic

In the treatment approach of the CASA of Mondovì, a public health clinic, the intervention for communication development is the overarching objective for all habilitation activities. Achieving the goal of developing communication skills is not the responsibility of only a single professional, but rather of the whole team (the speech and language therapist, the 'neuropsicomotricità' therapist (similar to an occupational therapist), and the educator, psychologist, and child psychiatrist). The family and the school are involved too.

How do these different professionals work on communication? *Psychologists* and *child psychiatrists* are responsible for assessment and follow both the family and the school, promoting the practice of the strategies used by therapists in the school and family context. The psychologist is also responsible for updating the assessment of child development and reviewing treatment outcomes. The *neuropsicomotricità* therapist works particularly in the first phase of treatment, especially with children of nursery and kindergarten age, with interventions aimed at promoting intersubjectivity, communicative intentionality, and the ability to play.

The *educator* works with children and adolescents, using visual strategies to develop learning ability, personal autonomy, and social skills.

The effectiveness of the communication can be verified through periodic evaluation of spontaneous communication in the context of treatment and daily life. The important role of the *speech and language therapist* is discussed later.

An example is Luigi, a 4 1/2-year-old boy with ASD. Luigi has partially developed communicative intentionality, and spontaneous communication and language remains limited to a few words. The use of visual aids to communication has been proposed by the speech and language therapist, with a good response by the child; however, the occasions in which the child uses language and, more generally, spontaneous communication in the context of speech therapy, are reduced. The speech and language therapist thinks that an environment more conducive to fun and physical activity may be more motivating for the child.

The treatment then continues with a 'neuropsicomotricità' therapist in a play setting where the proposed activities are more likely to engage the child. To monitor treatment and, in particular, the development of spontaneous communication, the spontaneous utterances of the child were recorded for five months. We divided the observations into three periods of four sessions each, and we used as a baseline two sessions of free play in which there was also a cousin of the child. Observer data are shown in Figs. 1 and 2 (for the methodologic aspects, see Watson *et al.*, 1997). Fig. 1 shows the number of reports divided by spontaneous communicative function, and Fig. 2 the number divided by semantic categories.

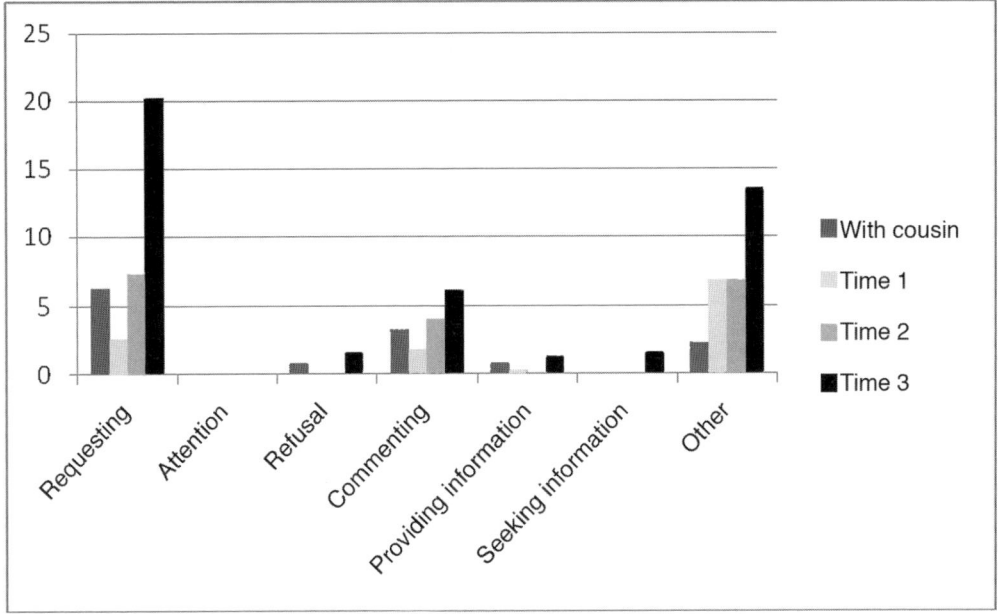

Fig. 1. Spontaneous communication distribution by communicative functions at the baseline and in three subsequent periods.

We can observe an increase in spontaneous communication between the first and the third observation and the difference between the average of the spontaneous reports of the first and third period is statistically significant. Luigi is an example of how different professionals can work with the speech and language therapist in the treatment of communication disorders in children with autism.

In the second part of this chapter we describe some of the specific roles the speech and language therapist in our team have in evaluating and treating children with autism. In particular, we will show the specific abilities of the speech and language therapist through the proposal of some new aspects/ideas of good practice regarding the assessment of communication and language and the use of technological tools for the development of communication.

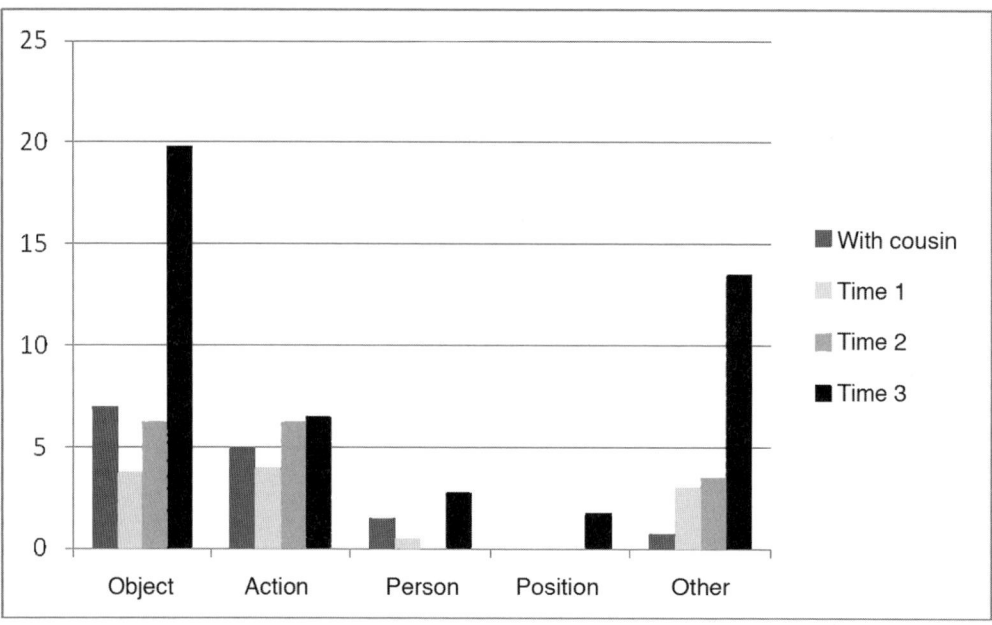

Fig. 2. Spontaneous communication distribution by semantic categories at the baseline and in three subsequent periods.

Proposal of a multimodal signal extension of the PVB inventory

The PVB (Primo Vocabolario del Bambino or First Vocabulary of the Child, Caselli & Casadio, 1995) is the Italian adaptation of the MacArthur–Bates CDIs (Fenson et al., 2007). These inventories allow us to assess the development of communication and language of children early in life (8–36 months of age). The PVB inventory consists of two forms: Words and Gestures (GP, or Gesti e Parole), for children aged 8 to 17 months and Words and Sentences (PF, or Parole e Frasi), with norms that range from 18 to 36 months in the latest version. A remake of the PVB second form (PF) is dated 2007 (Caselli et al., 2007) and also includes an abbreviated version. The reissue of the GP form for younger children, including a corresponding short form, is not out yet, but will be published in the future.

It should be pointed out that, at the vocabulary and sentence level, it is also possible to evaluate understanding with the GP form, and sentence production can mainly be evaluated with the PF form. Thus, in the PF form, while there are a few questions about sentence understanding too, mainly the PF inventory assesses vocabulary and sentence production. As well, in the GP form there is also a part that assesses a series of gestures and actions linked to the development of communication.

What are the positive aspects of the assessment made through the application of an inventory?

It is difficult to assess how younger children communicate, their verbal language, and their use of signals in general in some other way than with an inventory. The inventory tool allows the therapist to identify what parents and others who best know the child report. And a good correlation has been demonstrated between what is referred to in a questionnaire and data obtained with other types of standardized assessment. The presentation of the original version of the PVB questionnaire to the family allows us to provide necessary instructions about what information has to be reported and how to fill in the data; after about one week of observation, the parents can try to complete the questionnaire and return it. The first meeting with the parents after that may possibly be exhaustive in terms of attaining thorough completion of the questionnaire or it can indicate the need for subsequent in-depth meetings.

This, as will be seen, is an important aspect to the process of assessment, especially with the modified version (in the sense of an extension to multimodal signals) of PVB, which is introduced here and the presentation of which constitutes the object of this text.

The ideas that led to the extension were as follows:
(1) The PVB seemed, for the characteristics mentioned above, to be a useful tool to assess communicative and linguistic abilities of young ASD subjects.
(2) The scientific literature provides interesting references about the use of CDI in children with ASD. According to Luyster *et al.* (2007a) '[t]he CDI yielded scores that were predictive of outcome, suggesting that this parent report measure may be a quick and informative assessment of early verbal and nonverbal skills in children with ASD'. In another article, Luyster *et al.* (2007b) present work (modeled on that of Charman *et al.*, 2003) in which the CDI–Infant form is used. Results suggest that 'skills improve with increasing non-verbal mental age and chronological age but that most children with ASD are delayed in receptive and expressive vocabulary and non-verbal communication, functional object use and play skills'. A subsequent article (Smith & Mirenda, 2009) contains information that may be important for what we report; this shows 'the concurrent and predictive validity of both the CDI:WG and the CDI:WS for young children with ASD whose chronological ages exceed the test norms. The validity of the CDI for children who are older than the normative group is important information for clinicians in particular, who often experience the limitations of formal tests of language for children with ASD and other significant language impairments'.

However, it seemed like something was missing when relating to linguistic assessment of children with ASD. There was a need (1) to have more information about what the child does with types of signals other than verbal and be able to measure the evolution not only of verbal language, but also of multimodal types of signals; and (2) to make sure that this measure of evolution could be presented in a visual and understandable way even to those not strictly mastering the subject. Further, there was the desire to implement a computerized system in order to process data of this extension of PVB, displaying them in various ways and making them understandable, as mentioned, for parents, teachers and others involved in working with the children.

Fig. 3 shows one of the lexical categories (real/toy vehicles) as it appears in the original version of the PVB questionnaire in the Gestures and Words form. Notice how the lexical items appear with appropriate spaces to indicate whether the child understands and/or *says* as well as an area to record what the child says.

A first readapted version was simply aimed to allow calculation by computer, as shown in Fig. 4, in which the original grid of PVB was put into the Excel program. Then by adding other columns to the grid for other types of signaling, more and new data can be recorded, viewed, and compared (Fig. 5). We felt that additions of this type supplemented current psycholinguistic research. Information can be entered about how the child understands and produces a signal at a body-motor level (*e.g.*, to take the other's hand; to direct the other to an object or a place; going directly towards); at an object signaling system level (*i.e.*, where there are some signal objects which we conventionally refer to other real objects and events); at a

3. VEICOLI (veri o giocattoli)	Capisce	Dice			Capisce	Dice	
Aereo	O		O	Camion	O		O
Autobus	O		O	Motocicletta	O		O
Automobile	O		O	Passeggino	O		O
Barca	O		O	Treno	O		O
Bicicletta	O		O		O		O

Fig. 3. One of the lexical categories (Real/Toy vehicles) in the original version of the PVB–Gestures and Words questionnaire (Caselli & Casadio, 1995). Veicoli: vehicles*; capisce:* understands*; dice:* says.

gestural and sign language level; at a level of images (such as drawings, photographs, and visual symbols); and, of course, of words, oral or written (Watson *et al.*, 1997). We chose to consider no more than five categories at present so that the extended tool could be better visually apprehended. Other categories can be represented by alphanumeric coding in the columns when needed. A similar column structure has been added to all the parts of the PVB where this made sense, that is, to every part except the one called Actions and Gestures on PVB GP and except in some other parts of PVB PF. The result is a comprehensive grid whose data, provided by parents or others who know the child, once entered into the Excel spreadsheet, allow analysis at various levels of detail (Fig. 6).

3. VEHICLES (real or toy)	U.	P.	Articulation		U.	P.	Articulation
Airplane				Truck			
Bus				Motorcycle			
Car				Stroller			
Boat				Train			
Bicycle							

Fig. 4. Table in first readapted version of the original one in Fig. 3; this allows calculation in an Excel spreadsheet U: understanding*; P:* production.

	3. VEHICLES (real or toy)	Mot.		Obj.		Ges.		Img.		Ver.		Articulation			Mot.		Obj.		Ges.		Img.		Ver.		Articulation
		U	P	U	P	U	P	U	P	U	P				U	P	U	P	U	P	U	P	U	P	
1	Airplane												6	Truck											
2	Bus												7	Motorcycle											
3	Car												8	Stroller											
4	Boat												9	Train											
5	Bicycle																								

Fig. 5. A few columns have been added to the grid for types of signaling other than verbal in order to allow multimodal data to be recorded. The grid is still simple for data to be entered by parents or others who know the child. The multimodal signaling types (Watson et al.*, 1997) appear as follows: Mot.: motoric; Obj.:* object*; Ges.:* gestures and signs*; Img.:* images*; Ver.:* verbal.

	3. VEHICLES (real or toy)	Mot.		Obj.		Ges.		Img.		Ver.		Articulation
		U	P	U	P	U	P	U	P	U	P	
1	Airplane							1	1			
2	Bus							1				
3	Car							1	1			
4	Boat							1				
5	Bicycle							1				
		0	0	0	0	0	0	5	2	0	0	7

		Mot.		Obj.		Ges.		Img.		Ver.		Articulation
		U	P	U	P	U	P	U	P	U	P	
6	Truck							1				
7	Motorcycle							1				
8	Stroller											
9	Train							1				
		0	0	0	0	0	0	3	0	0	0	

Fig. 6. The extended grid transferred into an Excel spreadsheet with data that can be analyzed at various levels of detail. Some colours (here in greyscale) help to define different types of information and the cells that have already been filled. The other abbreviations are as those for Figures 4 and 5.

Currently this extended questionnaire is named PVB–ESTM (Extension to Multimodal Types of Signals). The data-processing computerised Excel form has been given the name Penelope's Patchwork.

As four columns are added to the one of verbal language and this is both for understanding and production in the GP extended version (and for production only in the PF extended version), the resulting paper questionnaire appears to be quite complex. It is important to meet the people who will fill in the extended version of the form to work through the data being collected, give explanations where necessary, and create at least part of the work together. At this meeting discussions can take place about the different possibilities and ways of communicating, ideas on different types of signal, and issues such as communicative intent, functions of communication, stereotyped communicative behaviours, and so on. During this meeting dialogue can take place on the subject of language and communication as a dynamic reference model is shared and changed accordingly. Data in the next part of this text refer to the version Extended to Multimodal Types of Signals of the Gestures and Words form of the PVB, which then refers to children between 8 and 17 months.

Before proceeding to some of the more complex and detailed charts, we present a general chart taken from the simplest level of electronic data processing (Fig. 7). The environment of communications that we interrogated through the questionnaire (the family in this case, but it could

	Mot.		Obj.		Ges.		Img.		Ver.		TOT. SIGNAL UNDERSTANDING	TOT. SIGNAL PRODUCTION
	U	P	U	P	U	P	U	P	U	P		
1. Sound Effects - Animal Sounds	0	0	1	0	0	0	0	0	10	2	11	2
2. Animal Names	0	0	0	0	0	1	16	5	1	0	17	6
3. Vehicles	0	0	0	0	0	0	8	2	0	0	8	2
4. Toys	0	0	0	0	0	0	3	0	1	0	4	0
5. Food and Drink	0	0	0	0	7	6	12	7	9	2	28	15
6. Clothing	0	0	0	0	1	0	8	0	6	0	15	0
7. Body Parts	0	0	0	0	0	0	13	0	5	0	18	0
8. Furniture and Rooms	0	0	0	0	1	0	1	1	11	0	13	1
9. Small Household Items	0	0	0	0	0	0	23	0	9	0	32	0
10. Outside Things - Places to Go	0	0	0	0	0	0	14	0	11	1	25	1
11. People	0	0	0	0	0	0	6	0	5	2	11	2
12. Routines	0	0	0	0	1	0	3	0	14	4	18	4
13. Action Words	0	0	0	0	2	1	4	0	29	0	35	1
14. Descriptive Words	0	0	0	0	4	0	3	0	11	0	18	0
15. Adverbs	0	0	0	0	0	0	2	0	3	0	5	0
16. Pronouns	0	0	0	0	0	0	0	0	0	0	0	0
17. Question Words	0	0	0	0	0	0	0	0	0	0	0	0
18. Prepositions	0	0	0	0	0	0	2	0	2	0	4	0
19. Articles and Quantifiers	0	0	0	0	0	0	0	0	0	0	0	0
TOT. NOUNS (2-10)	0	0	0	0	9	7	98	15	53	3	160	25
TOT. PREDICATES (13;14)	0	0	0	0	6	1	7	0	40	0	53	1
TOT. FUNCTORS (16-19)	0	0	0	0	0	0	2	0	2	0	4	0
TOTALS	0	0	1	0	16	8	118	15	127	11	262	34
TOT. VER. UNDERSTANDING									127			
TOT. VER. PRODUCTION									11			
TOT. NON VER. UNDERSTANDING					135							
TOT. NON VER. PRODUCTION					23							

Fig. 7. Table with information derived from the simplest level of electronic data processing. TOT. VER. UNDERSTANDING: total verbal understanding; TOT. VER. PRODUCTION: total verbal production; TOT. NON VER. UNDERSTANDING: total nonverbal understanding.

be the school or the therapist or other educational staff, for example) reported that the child understands 127 verbal signals, but produces only 11. In the signaling mode through images, around 118 signals appear to be understood and 15 are used for expression. Gestural mode signals being understood (those that the family declares the child totally understands among the signals they propose to her) are 16, 8 of which are used by the child in production. Only a signal object is reported as used by the child in production. No motor signals are reported.

At first glance you may correctly assume that the parents of this child trust verbal language, but that they also consider and explore the communicative use of images. What is proposed in our work with ASD patients, as already mentioned, is an open model with the use of signals in a multimodal sense, with different types of signal that are meant to increase the perceptibility of the functioning of communication and that make the communication process more feasible to the child both in understanding and in production.

In this global chart, which simply summarizes the information written in the inventory forms, there is a kind of overlap between the various data of the different signal types. Ultimately it cannot be known whether the words that the child understands in total at the verbal level are the same ones that he also understands through an image; the same is true for the production. In fact, the data suggest that the verbal items that get understood and the images that get understood are of a certain number, but they do not say how many and which lexical items are understood only verbally, and how many and which ones are understood through images only. At least some of the items understood in images may coincide with those understood verbally.

In any case, an immediate display of scrolling columns is given where the majority of raw scores can be seen, whether for understanding or for production and the kind of signaling. In addition, for each lexical category one can see the total number of scores and when the amounts are significantly different. You can get an idea of the preferred signal mode (*e.g.*, in category 3, vehicle items have 8 images and 0 verbal words in comprehension; you can infer here that the use of images allows a better chance of understanding). For category 10 (outdoor items), the comprehension scores are respectively 14 and 11, with a score of 1 for verbal production. Thus, there appear to be relatively better skills in the verbal mode for this semantic area compared to the previous one; we cannot say, at this level of analysis, whether the 14 positive answers obtained through the pictures coincide or not with those obtained through speech. There is, in any case, a gap of 3 points in favour of images.

You may say at a glance that this child has difficulty in using both words and images productively, with a low proportion between what he understands and what he produces in these signaling modes; these data need to be verified by observing other tables generated by Excel. It may be useful for amelioration of the child's communication competence to increase and make more systematic the category of gestures, along with improving the use of both the verbal and the visual modes.

The next two images (Figs. 8 and 9) show another type of graph that can be useful because of the visual impression of the 'lexical-semantic landscape'. The value of the personal computer is that once the data have been transferred to a computing environment, they can then be analyzed and displayed in various forms. In Fig. 8 the values of normative data, represented by columns in the background (the height of each bar shows the frequency with which the corresponding word is generally understood or produced in the age range explored by the test), appear in the same order (alphabetically) in which the words are used in the questionnaire. In Fig. 9 the normative data are sorted in descending order, giving an interesting result. Unlike Fig. 8, in which it was difficult to compare the presence of a column with the magnitude of the corresponding normative value, we can easily see that the words the child understands verbally and those that he understands through images are also words that are more frequently understood at the age span for which this form of the questionnaire refers. Some frequent words are not reported to be understood in terms of image or in any other way, and a considerable number of less common words are not understood at all. The information gained by these images can help the development of communication and language, especially with regard to bridging these gaps.

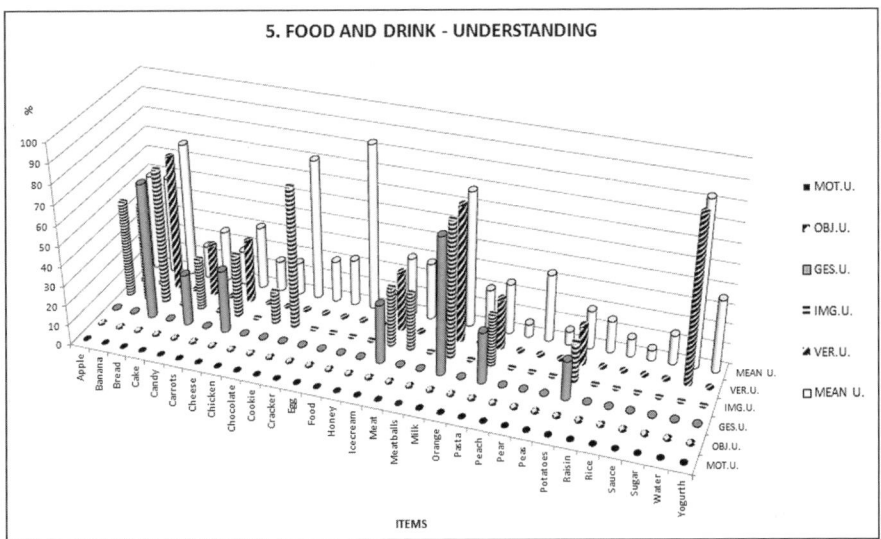

Fig. 8. 'Lexical-semantic landscape' with norm data for understanding (columns in the background) ordered according to alphabetical order of words in the Food and Drink category in children 8–17 months old. The norms are the ones of the PVB questionnaire (Caselli & Casadio, 1995). MOT. U.: motoric communication understanding; OBJ. U.: understanding through use of objects; GES. U.: gestural/sign understanding; IMG. U.: image understanding; VER. U.: verbal understanding; MEAN U.: norms for understanding.

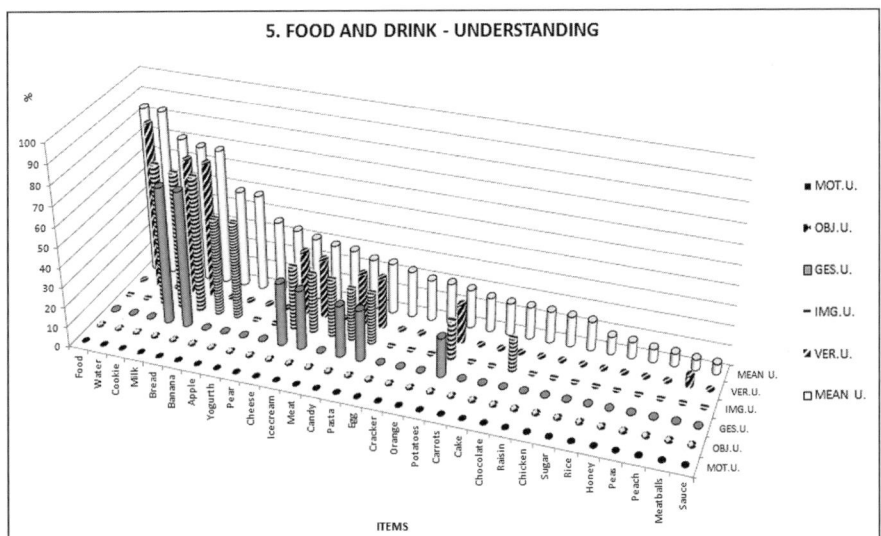

Fig. 9. 'Lexical-semantic landscape' with norm data for understanding (columns on the background) ordered from highest to lowest frequency of words in the Food and Drink category in children 8–17 months old. The norms are those of the PVB inventory (Caselli & Casadio, 1995). Abbreviations as in Fig. 8.

Figure 10 sets out the charts that are already present in some tables that analyze and compare the scores in the PVB manual, with a few additions. We see here a horizontal line called C.VER., which shows the raw score for the verbal comprehension. A second line was added, called C.VER. R + E (raw scores plus emergent scores for verbal comprehension), which shows the sum of items verbally managed, that is, the values of the verbal understanding we noted before, added to the items managed through the use of augmentative/alternative signaling mode. This second type of managed items was considered as 'Emerging' compared to the ones for which speech alone was sufficient. This form of the graph allows visual representation of a component of the potential for communication success (in this case for success in understanding) in relation to the use of multimodal signaling in support of verbal signaling alone.

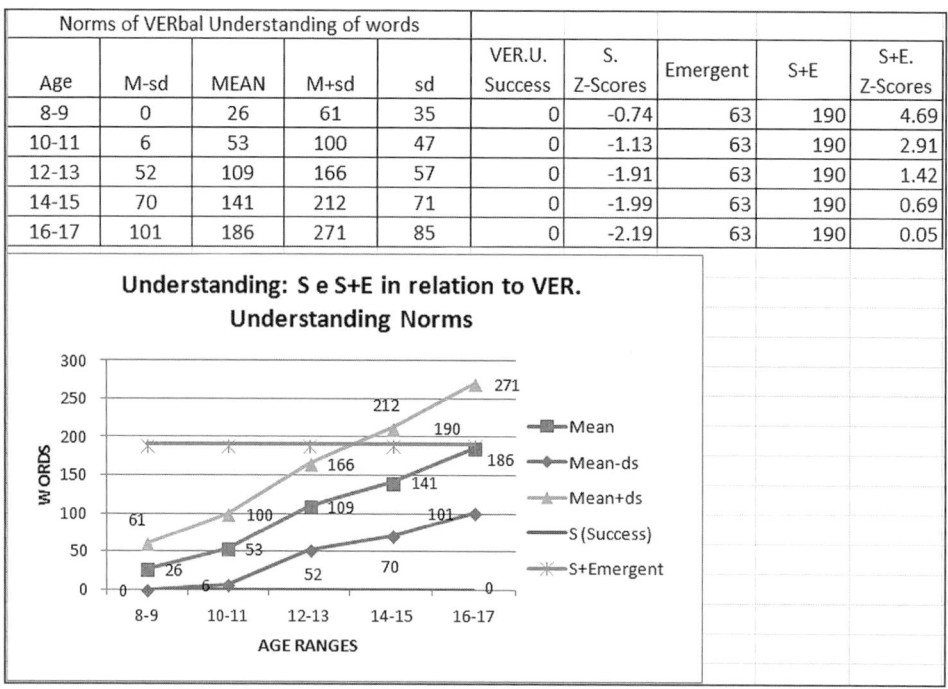

Norms of VERbal Understanding of words					VER.U. Success	S. Z-Scores	Emergent	S+E	S+E. Z-Scores
Age	M-sd	MEAN	M+sd	sd					
8-9	0	26	61	35	0	-0.74	63	190	4.69
10-11	6	53	100	47	0	-1.13	63	190	2.91
12-13	52	109	166	57	0	-1.91	63	190	1.42
14-15	70	141	212	71	0	-1.99	63	190	0.69
16-17	101	186	271	85	0	-2.19	63	190	0.05

Fig. 10. The norms of the PVB inventory (Caselli & Casadio, 1995) for verbal understanding allow a chart to be created in which the scores obtained through the use of multimodal signals can be compared. C. VER. R. represents the scores of verbal understanding success, while C. VER. R+E are the scores of verbal understanding success plus the ones obtained with other types of signaling. (Emergent). M-sd: mean minus standard deviation; MEAN: population mean; M+ds: mean plus standard deviation; ds: standard deviation; S+Z-Scores: z-score for success; E: emergent score; S+E: success score plus emergent score; S+EZ-Scores: z-score for success plus emergent.

In other words, next to the level of verbal understanding of the child we can consider that the child has an additional amount of vocabulary, but only when these meanings are communicated in a different signal mode than the verbal one. What we have considered is a semantic-lexical 'Emergence'. It is represented by a new line (C.VER. R + E), in this case appearing in a high-enough position compared with that relating to the verbal performance (C.VER. line).

The final part of the First Infancy inventory, relating to actions and gestures, has not been modified from the original form of the PVB. Some additional series of graphic representations and more data-processing capabilities can be obtained through the use of computing software.

It can be seen that whereas in Fig. 11 the columns of normative values appear in relative disorder, corresponding to the order in which items appear in the paper-form questionnaire, in Fig. 12 the same values are arranged in descending order and the visual result is again striking. In this case, the gestures that the child produces, compared with the norm, appear to be the more frequent.

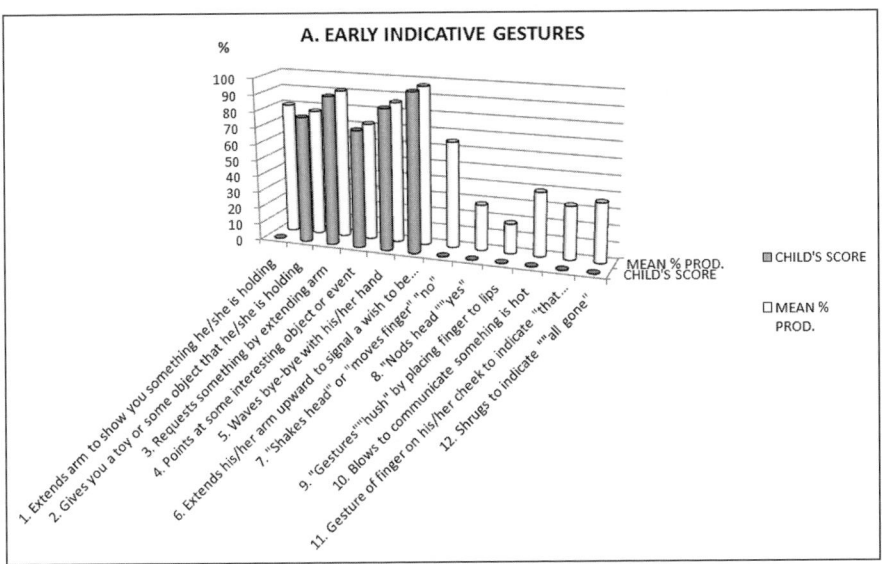

Fig. 11. Graph of one of the Actions and Gestures part of the inventory obtained by using Excel. Here the 'landscape' contains only two rows, one of the normative data (in the background) in the same order as the questionnaire items, and the other with the child's scores. MEAN % PROD.: mean per cent for production [open symbols]; CHILD'S SCORE [filled symbols]. At baseline, reading from left to right, the twelve areas listed describe communicative actions of varying complexity starting with showing an adult what he has in hand and giving it to the adult, to shrugging to indicate 'all gone'.

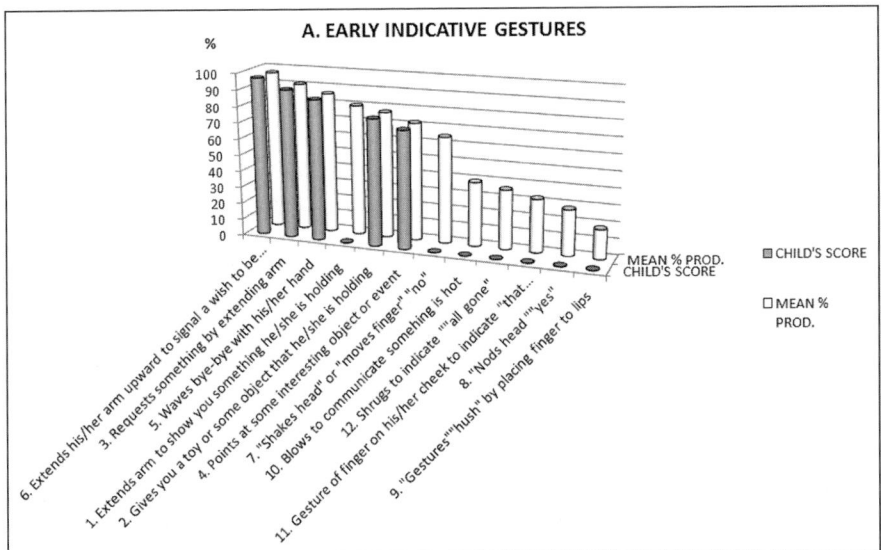

Fig. 12. The same graph of Actions and Gestures part of the inventory as shown in Fig. 11. Here the values in the row of normative data (in the background) are ordered from highest to lowest frequency. Open and filled symbols as in Fig. 11.

We are currently working on this extension of the already widely used and validated PVB. On one hand we are proposing some complementary aspects that appear to be useful in the communicative assessment and intervention programming for children with ASD and children with communication difficulties in general when multimodal signaling systems are used. On the other hand, we are showing how this method of assessment is 'helped' by the use of information technology.

Others working on this experimentation and development, as well as a network of collaborators in Italy and other countries working towards enlarging this multimodal extension to foreign versions of the inventory, are thanked in the Acknowledgments.

Creative use of the personal computer (CPC)

Creative PC (CPC) can be defined as a way to build situations of shared actions based on the creative use of a personal computer and software.

Although the principles underlying the practice that is going to be presented can guide the use of some excellent readily available educational or game software that can be purchased commercially or freely downloaded, I refer here, in the field of habilitation and rehabilitation, to the creation of small software applications made through the use of authoring programmes that are not too complex and most people can manage. They are known to permit the generation of units or slides which can be ordered or re-ordered into a sequence, put into multimedia materials, create links, relationships and constraints in the structures that allow for interaction with a user and that at a certain degree force him to behave with a preordered way.

We have used a variety of these tools in our speech and language therapy sessions with children who have had both language and above all communication difficulties, and for several years up to now our clinical experience has improved with individuals presenting with autistic spectrum disorders (ASD).

Currently we are concentrating on two of these authoring software packages – Microsoft PowerPoint and OpenOffice Presentation. We use these programs creatively, developing constructions, in real time or in a deferred way (that is, with the child or in her absence), with the aim of creating scenarios of shared action, according to a perspective inspired by the research of Jerome S. Bruner (1987). Within these sessions or 'formats' we negotiate progressively more shareable, more conventional, and functional systems of meanings and systems of signals.

Thanks to the personal computer and the use of these authoring software programs, we build situations that invite interaction and allow us to modulate its properties.

In practice we try to start from a position where the child is attracted by the computer. First. we turn it on so it is almost always available; we try to create a situation where we can do something together, for example, proposing to the child the use of an interactive game or the building of a simple application with the authoring software where we enter images and voice in real time. Examples include playing with some photos of animals and audio-recording a related children's song or onomatopoeia for the animals' sounds. Initially the child may be fully engaged or only gradually show an interest to want to do something together.

The basis of this approach is the development of situations where you can play together, you can share emotions, have fun, and share actions with the child. Using the ability to manipulate the software and being able to add and develop what you want and when and how it is needed, sometimes in real time or completing things at home and bringing them back to the next therapy session, you can help the child to progress in components of knowledge, social interaction, communication, and language acquisition.

As an example, we will show to the child different coloured balls on the screen (although in Fig. 13 they are shown in various shades of grey), and then say 'look, at the beautiful colours! Which one do you want to touch?'.

When a ball is touched, a bigger shape of the same colour appears in the middle of the screen (like the big cylinder in Fig. 13) and begins to go around, while a voice says simple key words like the colour name, 'ready... go!'; then the shape moves back to the starting point and the voice says 'stop' so it can be repeated over and over again.

In this example, the software was developed so that it would be as simple as possible because that particular child was very limited from a cognitive and interactive point of view. It was created so that the child's curiosity could be aroused to touch the splashes of color on the screen. This was a development of curiosity that had already appeared previously, when the child had played with coloured paper materials and thus the coloured shapes have been transferred to the personal computer.

From a communicative and linguistic point of view, at that time this child first needed to share with another person the pleasure of looking at the coloured shapes moving, and of being able to trigger the movement by himself, and in turn with the other person. Later on, he would improve his ability to make a request by pointing, on a simple paper communication panel, at

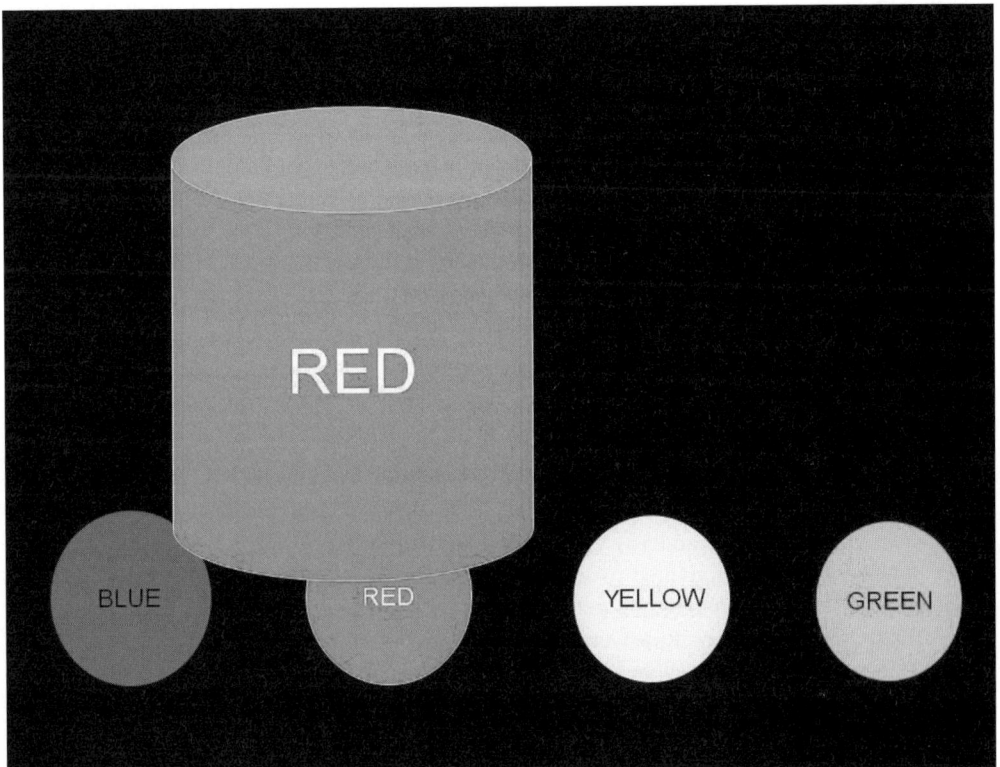

Fig. 13. Simple game made with the use of an authoring software; it consists of coloured shapes (in this case a big cylinder) that go around the screen when the circle of the same colour is clicked.

the colour he would touch afterwards on the screen in order to trigger the scene that he liked. It was useful for him to see that the adult also indicated the colour on the communication table just to anticipate what he would choose on his turn. The simple words that accompanied the movement of the shape on the screen represented a verbal model that at that moment the child could start to better understand if presented in a routine and in a clear and redundant way. Instead of the coloured shapes, other images, such as animals or familiar persons, could be provided and pointed at in a communicative table and named.

All these interactive situations (Bruner refers to them as 'formats' or 'scenarios') can be built by any one of us.

One of the key tricks is to prevent PowerPoint or Impress from progressing to the next slide in the presentation when the mouse is clicked. This is done by the use of buttons and action settings [in particular, in the 'presentation settings' menu the 'continuous presentation (full screen)' option should always be chosen] so that progression to different slides becomes strictly dependent on the button, shape or area of the screen that is clicked. This way you can have 'slides' set up for supposedly correct responses and 'other slides' for those not so. You can also force the way the person has to behave, for example, having her stay on a page until she did solve a problem, or making her go from one page to the other only after waiting for a certain amount of time, visualized in some way.

Clicking different buttons, shapes or areas of the screen can trigger an animation, sound or appearance of text or graphics.

It is important that the children are curious about what they see on the screen and that they consider they can influence it and have a chance to touch the screen when we propose that they do. We do not usually use touch screen displays, at least in a certain phase, turning the touch sensitivity off if necessary. Although there is no touch screen, we consider it very important to give the child the impression that they *could*; this way they can take the initiative and feel themselves to be an active and competent architect of change, when in fact we use a hidden mouse to click where they touch the screen, even if they do so imprecisely. The child has the impression that their shared action with the other person always works positively, that the cause-and-effect relationship is good. We are thus working on being in a relationship with a shared scene, of which adults are to some extent masters, and can manipulate it.

From our point of view we want to create chances for the child to act and interact, creating the opportunity both to build systems of shared meanings and to introduce signals through communication tables and various other augmentative and alternative modes, including speech if and when possible and as much as possible.

We could describe each of these software applications, but we consider it more important to see and use them, and to try and start to build some.

The next example (Figs. 14 and 15) was created for a child when she was in a certain phase of her development and motivated to share games of bingo with images on paper. The child was happy to ask for the images and get them in order to put them in her bingo folder, but she had difficulty using language to act out her request. She knew how to use a paper communication chart made up of images and was also able to manage when the images were progressively replaced by the corresponding written words. We wanted to make the procedure for making requests more elaborate and more fun, allowing her to be introduced to reading and writing in both a syllabic and a global way, while giving her the possibility of using language, thanks to the introduction of the personal computer. In this case the PC is used as a communication tool. Through each image of an on-screen communication chart, the child moves to a

Chapter 18 Speech and language therapy intervention in a multi-professional approach

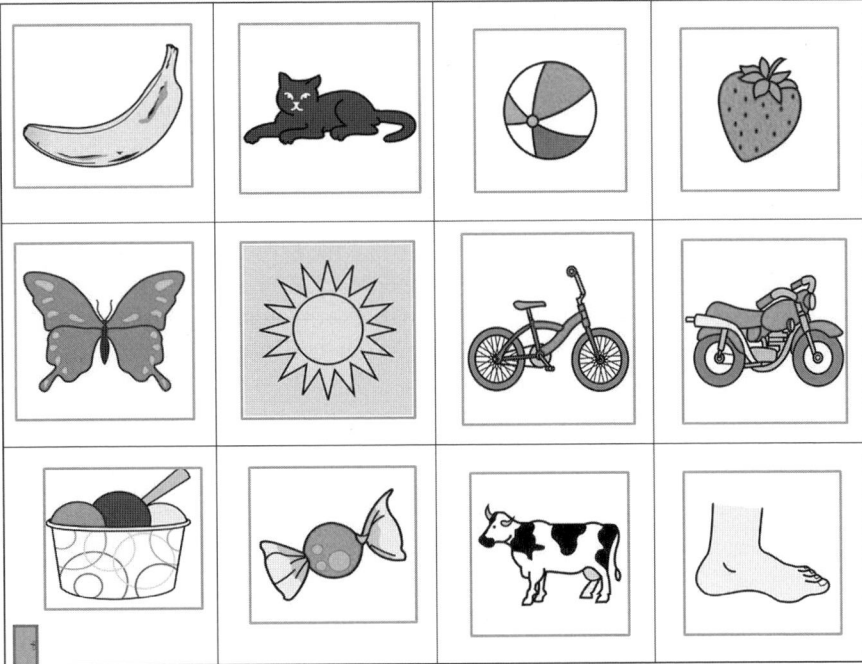

Fig. 14. An on-screen communication table of a Bingo game with images (see also Fig. 15); the game is partly played on paper and partly on the computer. When an image is clicked in order to communicate a request, a corresponding page opens to allow the child make the computer say the word (see Fig. 15).

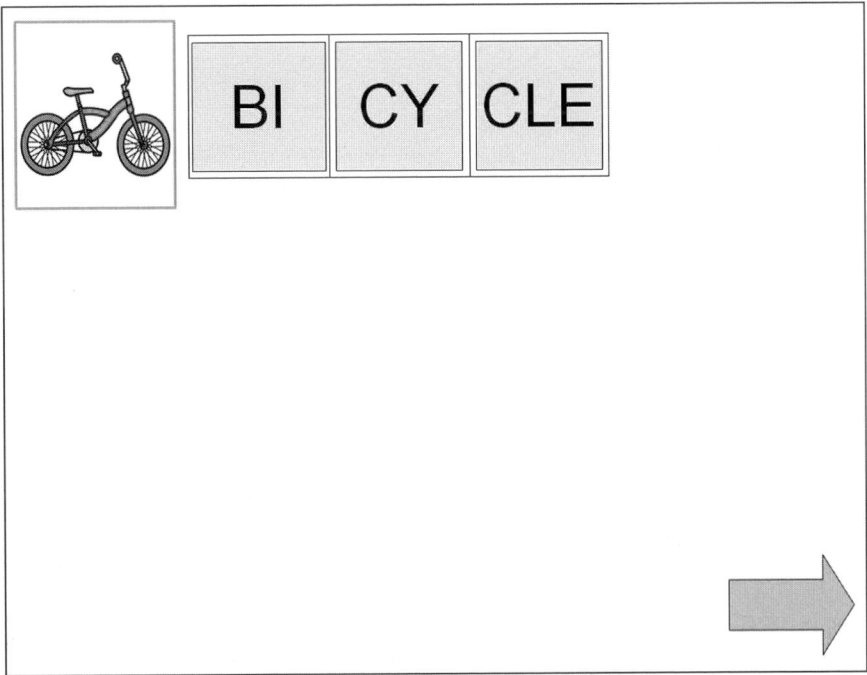

Fig. 15. The word of the image ('BICYCLE') that has been chosen in the communication table (Fig. 14) is pronounced by the computer when the syllables are clicked; the big arrow at bottom right allows return to the communication table.

page where the corresponding word appears written in syllables; she has to learn to click sequentially the syllables that compose the word from left to the right while hearing the corresponding syllable sounds. I stay behind the screen so I cannot see what she has selected, but I listen to the syllable sounds and offer her a picture of the requested image.

A third example (Fig. 16) shows a small cricket that either jumps and says 'Hop' when the child and I click on it, or sings a children's song. Playing in this way we establish an interaction where the computer is a tool of play and communication.

It is difficult if not impossible to find applications like these because each one is 'tailored' to an individual child, building on their strengths and developing skills to overcome their individual weaknesses. What it takes is time and a little bit of thought to prepare the applications, from the simplest ones to those for which more work is needed.

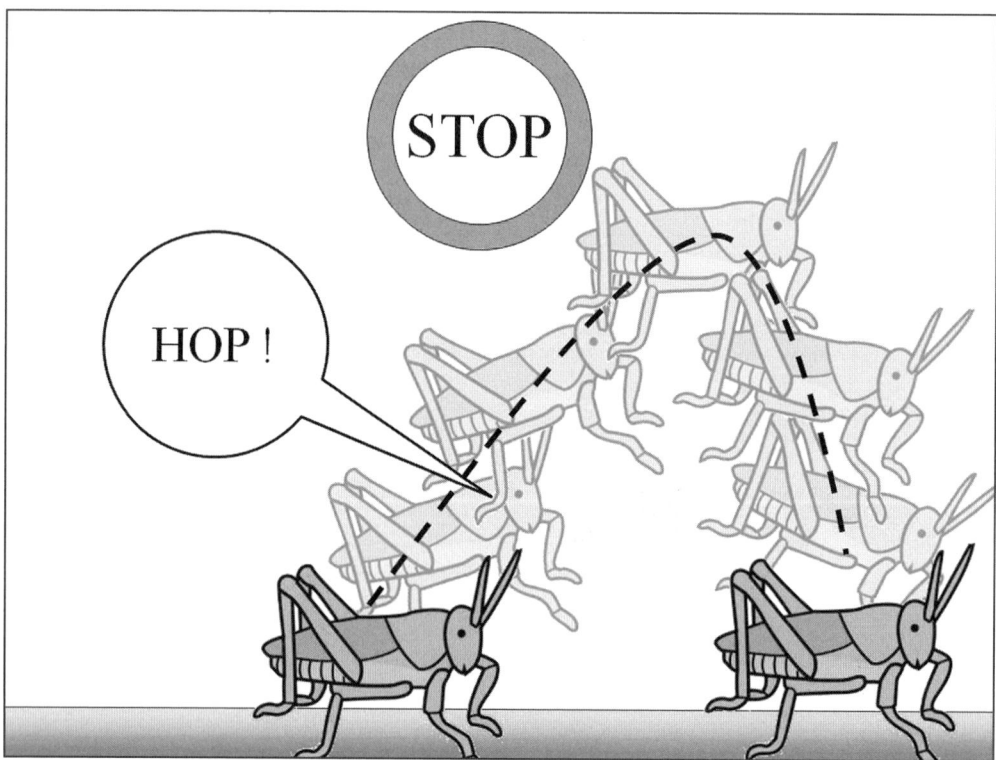

Fig. 16. The cricket jumps and says 'hop' when clicked. It is also possible to have him sing a song.

Conclusions

In this paper the model for communication intervention adopted in the Centre of Autism and Asperger's Syndrome in Mondovì is presented.

The protocol working with ASD children that the speech and language therapists in our team has recently used is called SCaN (Stimolazione della Comunicazione attraverso Negoziazione; or Activation of Communication through Negotiation). Its principles are based, among other work, on J.S. Bruner's perspective on the development of communication and language (Danna & Destefanis, 2004), in which a key component of the speech and language therapist's work is the construction of shared situations with an implicit emotionally positive interaction. In these jointly active situations, the necessary aid to the development and the use of coherent and conventional systems of shared meanings and signals is brought about in a number of ways. These include play; structuring the environment; augmentative and alternative means of communication; the use of information technologies; assessing skill levels and verifying evolution; and interprofessional planning of interventions.

The present work demonstrates an extension to Multimodal Types of Signaling of the well-known PVB assessment inventory tool (the Italian adaptation of the MacArthur–Bates CDI) and the CPC (Creative Personal Computer) method of using the computer as a means of interaction and communication development. From our perspective of speech and language therapy in children with ASD, the participation of adults and children in the growth of communication and language skills is seen as a process of active negotiation between the child and the communicative environment; different evidence-based tools and methods are used to aid in this process. This work is undertaken by the entire team – and this includes the family, the school and other social and educational institutions – working in concert to help the child achieve the greatest amount of communicative skills that he or she is able to attain.

Acknowledgments: We thank all those who have worked with us in development of and experiment with the multimodal signal extension of the PVB inventory, including Dr. Caterina Grillo, psycholinguist and music therapist (La Spezia); Dr. Debora Bonelli, speech and language therapist (Mondovì), who wrote a thesis on the subject for her degree in health professions and rehabilitation sciences; and Dr. Pasqualina Pace, psychiatric rehabilitation therapist (Reggio Calabria). We are also grateful to Dr. C. Caselli and Dr. O. Capirci, to whom we presented the idea of the extension and our first results with it, for their agreement to continue the project.

Conflicts of interest: The authors declare no conflicts of interest.

References

American Psychiatric Association (1994): *Diagnostic and Statistical Manual of Mental Disorders–IV*. Washington, DC: APA.

Bonelli, D. (2012): *Sperimentazione del Questionario MacArthur-Bates nella Versione Estesa a Tipi di Segnalazione Multimodale* [Experimentation of the MacArthur-Bates Questionnaire in the Version for Multimodal Signaling Types]. Thesis for degree in Health Professions and Rehabilitation Sciences, Turin University.

Bruner, J.S. (1987): *Il Linguaggio del Bambino: Come il Bambino Impara ad Usare il Linguaggio*. [In English *Child's Talk: Learning to Use Language*]. Rome: Armando.

Bruner, J.S. (2003): *La Ricerca del Significato: per una Psicologia Culturale*. [In English *Acts of Meaning*]. Turin: Bollati.

Caselli, M.C. & Casadio, P. (1995): *Il Primo Vocabolario del Bambino: Guida all'Uso del Questionario MacArthur per la Valutazione della Comunicazione e del Linguaggio nei Primi Anni di Vita*. [In English *Child's First Vocabulary: A Guide to the Use of the MacArthur Inventory for Communication and Language Assessment in the Early Years of Life*]. Milan: FrancoAngeli.

Caselli, M.C., Bates, E., Casadio, P., Fenson, J., Fenson, L., Sanderl, L. & Weir, J. (1995): A cross-linguistic study of early lexical development. *Cogn. Dev.* **10**, 159–199.

Caselli, M.C., Vicari, S., Longobardi, E., Lami, L., Pizzoli, C. & Stella, G. (1998): Gestures and words in early development of children with Down syndrome. *J. Speech Lang. Hear. Res.* **41**, 1125–1135.

Caselli, M.C., Pasqualetti P. & Stefanini, S. (2007): *Parole e Frasi nel 'Primo Vocabolario del Bambino': Nuovi Dati Normativi fra 18 e 36 Mesi e Forma Breve del Questionario* [In English *Words and Gestures in the 'Child's First Vocabulary': New Normative Scores for Ages between 18 and 36 Months and Short Version of the Inventory*]. Milan: FrancoAngeli.

Charman, T., *et al.* (2003): Measuring early language development in preschool children with autism spectrum disorder using the MacArthur Communicative Development Inventory (Infant Form). *Int. J. Child Lang.* **30**, 213–236.

Danna, E. & Destefanis, L. (2004): Una esperienza di logopedia con bambini autistici [In English *A speech and language therapy experience with ASD children*]. In: *Autismo* e *disturbi dello sviluppo*, Vol. 2, n. 1, gennaio. Trento: Erickson.

Fenson, L., Marchman, V.A., Thal, D.J., Dale, P.S., Reznick, J.S. & Bates, E. (2007): *MacArthur–Bates Communicative Development Inventories: User's Guide and Technical Manual*, 2nd ed. Baltimore, MD: Brookes Publishing.

Luyster, R., Qiu, S., Lopez, K. & Lord C. (2007a): Predicting outcomes of children referred for autism using the MacArthur–Bates Communicative Development Inventory. *Int. J. Speech Lang. Hear. Res.* **50**, 667–681.

Luyster, R., Lopez, K. & Lord, C. (2007b): Characterizing communicative development in children referred for autism spectrum disorders using the MacArthur–Bates Communicative Development Inventory (CDI). *Int. J. Child Lang.* **34**, 623–654.

Smith, V. & Mirenda, P. (2009): *Concurrent and predictive validity of the MacArthur-Bates communicative development inventory for children with autism*. Poster presented at the International Meeting for Autism Research (held by the International Society for Autism Research) in Chicago, Illinois on May 7–9, 2009. Poster V, 134.121. https://imfar.confex.com/imfar/2009/webprogram/Paper3765.html

Watson, L.R., Lord, C., Schaffer, B. & Schopler, E. (1997): *La Comunicazione Spontanea nell'Autismo* [In English *Spontaneous Communication in Autism.*]. Trento: Erikson.

Wetherby, A., Schuler, A.L. & Prizant, B.M. (1997): Enhancing language and communication development: theoretical foundations In: *Handbook of Autism and Pervasive Developmental Disorders*, 2nd ed., eds. D.J. Cohen & F.R. Volkmar. New York: John Wiley & Sons.

Chapter 19

Early psychomotor intervention in the treatment of young children with autism spectrum disorder

Roberto Militerni, Alessandro Frolli, Giovanna Gison, Guido Militerni and Ivana Sozio

Department of Child Neuropsychiatry;
Seconda Università degli Studi di Napoli, II Policlinico, via Pansini 5, 80131 Napoli, Italy
roberto.militerni@unina2.it

Summary

Early psychomotor intervention (EPI) is an Italian proposal to address the impairments that characterize the first stages of development of autistic spectrum disorders (ASDs). EPI is development-oriented, child-directed, and focused on natural interactions. The leading conceptual orientation of EPI is represented by a vision of development as an articulated and complex process in which manifold functions interact according to the theory of dynamic systems. The developmental perspective of EPI, which combines habilitation and rehabilitation needs, recognizes that play and interaction are the preferred modalities of approach. Thus, EPI falls within interventions indicated in the literature by the term *play-/interaction-based intervention*: 'These interventions use interactions between children and adults (either parents or researchers) to improve outcomes such as imitation or joint attention skills or the ability of the child to engage in symbolic play...' (AHRQ, 2011). EPI aims to teach children to attain pivotal skills that include a broad range of behaviours. According to ICF–CY these skills include: shared cooperative play (d8803), handling stress and other psychological demands (d2409), producing nonverbal messages (d335), and undertaking single tasks (d2109).

Early intervention is acknowledged as a key to treatment of infants with autism spectrum disorder (ASD). Early psychomotor intervention (EPI) is an Italian proposal to address the impairments that characterize the first stages of development of the autistic spectrum disorders.

The role of EPI in the treatment of infants with ASD

The key questions defining the role of EPI in the treatment of infants with ASD include the following:

1. What is early psychomotor intervention (EPI)?

2. What are the rehabilitation needs of the infant with ASD?

3. How can EPI answer the rehabilitation needs of children with ASD?

KQ.1 – What is early psychomotor intervention (EPI)?

EPI is a rehabilitation intervention, authorized by the Italian Office of Health (Ministero della Salute). The person trained to practice EPI is known as the 'Terapista della Neuro e Psicomotricità dell'Età Evolutiva' (Therapist of NPEE), who has obtained a triennial degree which is included in the formative offer of the Italian Office of the University (Ministero dell'Università) (OFF.F – MIUR, 1997/2001).

The leading conceptual orientation of EPI views development as an articulated and complex process in which manifold functions interact according to the theory of dynamic systems. The visible products of such interactions are represented by the emergence of a series of behaviours, included in well-defined functional areas: motor, communicative, socio-emotional, and cognitive.

In typical development, these behaviours play an 'instrumental' role in the realization of a much more complex process that is the full articulation of personality. The ability to move, to communicate, and to understand allows the child to fully realize himself as a person. In turn, to act and interact allows the enrichment and consolidation of the emerging abilities.

Neurodevelopmental disorders other than autistic disorders, such as mental retardation or cerebral palsy, are characterized, by definition, as the missed emergence of specific abilities – motor, communicative, and/or cognitive. Therefore, the failure of these 'instrumental' abilities interferes with the emergence of critical components of the personality – Self, Other, and Social Adjustment competencies.

EPI interrupts this situation and addresses both the treatment of the disability (rehabilitation) and the facilitation of those critical competencies for the full development of the person (habilitation). This developmental perspective, which combines habilitation and rehabilitation needs, recognizes play and interaction as the preferred modalities of approach.

Thus, EPI falls under the category of interventions indicated in the literature by the term 'play-/interaction-based intervention'. 'These interventions use interactions between children and adults (either parents or researchers) to improve outcomes such as imitation or joint attention skills or the ability of the child to engage in symbolic play...' (AHRQ, 2011).

Therefore, play and interaction are not the *aim* of the intervention, but rather the *means* by which they act on the impairment considered critical in the autistic behavioural phenotype, that is, joint attention deficit and impairment of the symbolic function (NAS, 2001). Within this frame of play and interaction, the therapist assumes the function of stimulus, regulation, and guidance in a developmental path that refers to a well-defined procedural framework (Militerni *et al.*, 1997).

Interventions that fall within the continuum of behavioural and developmental interventions have become the predominant treatment approach for promoting social, adaptive, and behavioural function in children with ASD based on efficacy demonstrated in empirical studies. These interventions may be viewed in terms of their position on a continuum from highly structured discrete trial training behavioural approaches guided by a therapist, to social pragmatic approaches, where teaching follows the child's interests and is embedded in daily activities in a natural environment (Ospina *et al.*, 2008). On the basis of the earliest reports, EPI falls within the developmental interventions and it shares a set of elements common to other forms of treatment widely diffused in the international panorama of interventions. In particular, points of convergence are found with DIR/Floortime (Greenspan & Wieder, 1998).

In conclusion, EPI is:
- *development-oriented*: It follows a developmental hierarchy of graded social and communication skills related to reciprocal social, pre-linguistic, pragmatic, and linguistic development;
- *child-directed*: Although parental involvement is a critical element of the whole rehabilitation project, the therapeutic work is aimed directly at the child to facilitate an adaptive reorganization of the impaired functions; and
- *focused on natural interactions*: It focuses on naturalistic teaching based on interactions between therapist and child. The regulatory role of the therapist, in all phases of the session, is extremely delicate because it is constantly negotiated and modulated by the experience of the child. Thus the child finds a form of continuity in the regularity of events. Moreover, in a perspective no longer tied to a single session, but referring to the entire course of treatment, the interactive experience in turning this into a possibility of recall of Self and Other, becomes an experience of historicity.

KQ.2 – What are the rehabilitation needs of the infant with ASD?

It is very important to intervene as early as possible, but it is also important to do this in as appropriate a way as possible. The quality of the intervention is related to two main factors: a diagnosis which meets the criteria of reliability and validity; and a treatment organized according to the biopsychosocial model of the World Health Organization.

The diagnosis must meet the criteria of reliability and validity
One problem is related to the stability of a diagnosis made at the age of 2 years. Recently, a systematic review of the diagnostic stability of ASD examined 23 studies with a total of 1,466 participants (Woolfenden *et al.*, 2012). Fifty-three per cent of children still had a diagnosis of autistic disorder (AD) and 14 per cent of children still had a diagnosis of another form of ASD at follow-up. Reading these data from a different perspective, it is possible to see that 33 per cent of children changed from having a diagnosis on the autism spectrum to either having a diagnosis of a non-autistic developmental disorder or having no diagnosis. Moreover, diagnostic stability is less strong for PDD-NOS. Forty-seven per cent of children initially diagnosed with PDD-NOS retained an ASD diagnosis. It means that the diagnosis was changed in 53 per cent of children, who were 'moving off' the spectrum (Daniels *et al.*, 2011; Kleinman *et al.*, 2008; Rondeau *et al.*, 2011).

Many factors can explain these changes in diagnostic categories. Among these may be considered an over-inclusive attitude that often tends to emphasize excessively, if not exclusively, behaviours related to the social component of the disorder ('he/she seems not to hear', 'he/she does talk', 'he/she prefers to play alone'). In this perspective, standardized tools based on a descriptive approach, such as the Autism Diagnostic Observation Schedules (Lord *et al.*, 2002), can only confirm what is already clinically obvious.

There is the need for a more interpretive approach that not only describes the observed behaviours, but also considers non-autistic factors that may affect the joint attention.

The treatment must be organized according to the biopsychosocial model of the World Health Organization
This is the second factor to be considered in order to confer 'quality' to the early intervention. If the diagnosis is the indispensable prerequisite for starting on the right foot, then you need to organize well the next steps.

Thus, the diagnosis should never be considered as a point of arrival, but rather as a *starting point* on which to formulate a treatment that takes into account the biopsychosocial originality of the person to whom it is addressed (WHO, 2007). In discussing the care of the person with ASD, the biopsychosocial model of the WHO emphasizes the need to implement 'good practices' as identified, discussed, and approved for years in the field of developmental rehabilitation.

Autism is a neurodevelopmental disorder so it shares with other neurodevelopmental disorders, such as mental retardation or cerebral palsy, a series of common features that guide the organization of the individualized rehabilitation program (IRP). The IRP is framework widely used in developmental rehabilitation, based on a combination of four specific intervention procedures, including (1) parental involvement in intervention, including ongoing parent coaching that is focused both on parental responsivity and sensitivity to the child's cues and on teaching families to provide interventions; (2) careful documentation of the child's unique strengths and weakness; (3) selection of appropriate goals for each child, according to age, developmental profile, and characteristics of the ecosystem; (4) focus on a broad rather than a narrow range of learning targets.

These four characteristics of efficacious interventions for infants and toddlers with other developmental challenges likely represent a solid foundation from which clinicians can build efficacious interventions for infants and toddlers at risk for or affected by ASD (Wallace & Rogers, 2010).

(1) Parental involvement can occur at multiple levels and should be supported through consistent presentation of information, ongoing consultation and individualized problem solving, and the opportunity to learn techniques for teaching their children new skills and reducing behavioural problems.

(2) Several principles underlie assessment for defining a young child's developmental profile (Sparrow, 1997):

Assessment of multiple areas of functioning is important. Assessment includes current intellectual and communicative skills, behavioural presentation, and functional adjustment.

A developmental perspective is critical. Given the strong association of mental retardation with autism, it is important to view results within the context of overall developmental level.

Variability of skills is typical. It is important to identify a child's specific profile of strengths and weaknesses rather than simply present an overall global score. Similarly, it is important not to generalize from an isolated or a 'splinter' skill to an overall impression of general level of ability since such skills may grossly misrepresent a child's more typical abilities.

Variability of behaviour across settings is typical. Behaviour of a child will vary depending on such aspects of the setting as novelty, degree of structure provided, and complexity of the environment. In this regard, observation of facilitating and detrimental environments is helpful.

Functional adjustment must be assessed. Results of specific assessments obtained in more highly structured situations must be viewed in the broader context of the child's daily and more typical levels of functioning and response to real-life demands. The child's adaptive behaviour (*i.e.*, capacities to translate skills into real-world settings) is particularly important.

(3) At the root of questions about the most appropriate goals lie differences in assumptions about what is possible and what is important to give children through intervention. The long-term goals for the rehabilitation program for children with ASD are the same as those for other children: personal independence and social responsibility. In children 6 years of age and younger, independence and responsibility are defined in terms of age-appropriate participation

in school and social activities to the maximum extent possible. These goals imply continuous progress in motor abilities, verbal and nonverbal communication skills, cognitive abilities, and adaptive skills.

Although the goals are common for all children, the functional profile defines for each child the ways in which goals must be prioritized. Furthermore, the functional profile allows the recognition for each child of the behaviours targeted for intervention and the instructional strategies.

(4) The rehabilitation needs of children with neurodevelopmental disorders require multiple interventions, included and systematically planned in the IRP. In the field of autism and ASD, IRPs are usually indicated as comprehensive programs or model programs.

There are many comprehensive programs for children with ASDs that differ in philosophy and practice. Strategies from various programs represent a range of techniques, including discrete trials, incidental teaching, structured teaching, and play-/interaction-based interventions. Some programs unilaterally use of one set of procedures, whereas others use a combination of approaches.

Overall, many of the programs are more similar than different in terms of levels of organization, staffing, ongoing monitoring, and structured teaching. Much more important than the name of the program attended is how the targeted behaviours and strategies selected allow implementation of the goals for the child and his or her family.

KQ.3 – How can early psychomotor intervention answer the rehabilitation needs of children with ASD?

EPI does not *have the intention* of representing itself as the treatment for ASD, as other techniques do. It proposes itself as one of the intervention within the IRP. Mainly, EPI is addressed to teaching children to attain 'pivotal skills', in the sense that their acquisition allows a child to learn many other skills more efficiently. The pivotal skills to be targeted as goals include a broad range of behaviours such as imitation, responding to natural and multiple cues, or learning to delay gratification (understanding 'first do this, then you get to do that').

The pivotal skills

According to the recommendation of the World Health Organization for a common language, the EPI is using the ICF–CY (International Classification of Functioning, Disability and Health) codes to describe the pivotal skills targeted for intervention. They fall in the component Activity and Participation.

Shared cooperative play (d8803, ICF–CY)
Joining others in sustained engagement in activities with objects, toys, materials, or games with a shared goal or purpose (WHO, 2007)

To teach cooperative play, EPI uses several naturalistic strategies that are designed to increase social responsiveness and intrinsic motivation. First, the adult contingently imitates the child's actions with toys, gestures, body movements, and vocalizations during play. Research indicates that contingent imitation enhances social responsiveness and coordinated joint attention (Escalona *et al.*, 2002; Ingersoll, 2012), which helps the child attend to the therapist of NPEE during modeling, increasing the likelihood of an imitative response. During contingent imitation, the therapist describes the actions that the adult and child are performing using simplified language. This form of indirect language stimulation has been shown to increase spontaneous and imitative language in young children with autism (Ingersoll & Schreibman, 2006). Once the child begins to show an awareness of the adult's contingent imitation, actions are modeled that are familiar and directly related to the child's current play. For example, if the child typically plays with a car by rolling it back and forth or spinning its wheels, the therapist might model rolling it back and forth, while the child is spinning the wheels. Once the child begins to imitate familiar actions, novel actions are introduced; however, at all times, imitation is taught around the child's current focus of interest.

Handling stress and other psychological demands (d2409, ICF–CY)
Carrying out simple or complex and coordinated actions to cope with pressure, emergencies or stress associated with task performance (WHO, 2007)

EPI facilitates the regulation of emotion by supporting, scaffolding, and modeling the child's emerging emotional understanding, emotional expression, and modification of these emotions. Using imitation, joint engagement, and pretend play, the therapist of the NPEE helps the child to be aware of the emotion and mental state.

During episodes of distress the therapist of NPEE engages in an array of strategies ranging from more active strategies (redirection, prompting, physical behaviour) to more vocal, comforting ones (vocal soothing and reassurance). More frequently, the therapist of NPEE redirects attention away from the source of the child's distress and reengages the child in an ongoing play activity. This appears to be an important regulatory skill. So, even within the first year of life, cognition and emotion work in concert to process information and guide action during emotional experiences. Self-regulation of emotions seems to be mediated by the development of cognitive regulatory abilities, specifically, attentional control (Sheese *et al.*, 2008).

Producing nonverbal messages (d335, ICF–CY)
Using gestures, symbols, and drawings to convey messages, such as shaking one's head to indicate disagreement or drawing a picture or diagram to convey a fact or complex idea (WHO, 2007)

Each session includes either a table-top training priming for the targeted communicative gestures (reaching, pointing, showing, and giving), and a floor play focusing on generalization of the skills within an optimized engagement setting.

During table-top training, the child was given opportunities to initiate and respond to the targeted behaviours within playful adult-driven activities. Teaching opportunities to encourage the initiation of gestures were created by using interesting toys (or objects), presenting the toys in, for example, a bag, or hidden to encourage gesture initiation, prompting gesture initiation when necessary by, for example, asking 'What do you have?', modeling gestures, or physical prompting, and by the therapist of NPEE exaggerating the interest in the shared toy. Brief moments of shared interest in the toys were established following each spontaneous or prompted child-initiated behaviour as the therapist joined the child's toy focus. Since the toys were appealing to the child, shared interest usually depended merely on the adult joining in. As an example of a teaching trial: the therapist of NPEE holds a bag with toys in front of the child. The child pulls out a car, and shows it to the therapist; with prompting if necessary. The therapist responds enthusiastically, 'Yeah, nice car!', and joins the child in play with the car for a few seconds and then says 'Bye, bye car'. Then the next trial starts. In contrast to table-top training, floor play was child-driven. Strategies applied included, for example, facilitating joint engagement, following the child's lead, creating play routines, talking about what the child was doing, prompting gesture skills, and responding to the child's requests.

Undertaking single tasks (d2109, ICF-CY)
Preparing, initiating and arranging the time and space required for a simple task; executing a simple task with a single major component, such as reading a book, writing a letter, or making one's bed (WHO, 2007)

Starting from the proposal of the child, it is important to teach the step necessary to plan an action. Carrying out simple or complex and coordinated actions, such as initiating a task, organizing time, space and materials for a task, and pacing task performance are related to the executive functions. Executive function refers to voluntary planned behaviour that is achieved by the representation of a goal in working memory (WM) and inhibition of automatic task-inappropriate responses. Executive function is critical to voluntary decision making. Essential to executive function is the ability to integrate cortical and subcortical systems that are widely distributed throughout the brain (O'Hearn *et al.*, 2010).

Conclusions

On the basis of the earliest reports, EPI falls within the definition of developmental interventions and it shares a set of elements common to other forms of treatment widely diffused in the panorama of the interventions defined as *play-/interaction-based intervention* (AHRQ, 2011).

Conflicts of interest: The authors declare no conflicts of interest.

References

AHRQ [Agency for Healthcare Research and Quality] (2011): *Therapies for Children with Autism Spectrum Disorders. Comparative Effectiveness Review* – Number 26, AHRQ Publication No. 11-EHC029-EF, www.ahrq.gov

Daniels, A.M., Rosenberg, R.E., Law, J.K., Lord, C., Kaufmann, W.E. & Law, P.A. (2011): Stability of initial autism spectrum disorder diagnoses in community settings. *J. Autism Dev. Disord.* **41,** 110–121.

Escalona, A., Field, T., Nadel, J. & Lundy, B. (2002): Brief report: imitation effects on children with autism. *J. Autism Dev. Disord.* **32,** 141–144.

Greenspan, S.I. & Wieder, S. (1998): *The Child with Special Needs: Encouraging Intellectual and Emotional Growth.* Reading, MA: Perseus Books [Italian translation, Rome: Giovanni Fiotiti Editore, 2005).

Ingersoll, B. (2012): Brief report: effect of a focused imitation intervention on social functioning in children with autism. *J. Autism Dev. Disord.* **42,** 1768–1773.

Ingersoll, B. & Schreibman, L. (2006): Teaching reciprocal imitation skills to young children with autism using a naturalistic behavioral approach: effects on language, pretend play, and joint attention. *J. Autism Dev. Disord.* **36,** 487–505.

Kleinman, J.M., Ventola, P.E., Pandey, J., Verbalis, A.D., Barton, M., Hodgson, S., Green, J., Dumont-Mathieu, T., Robins, D.L. & Fein, D. (2008): Diagnostic stability in very young children with autism spectrum disorders. *J. Autism Dev. Disord.* **38,** 606–615.

Lord, C., Rutter, M., DiLavore, P.C. & Risi, S. (2002): *ADOS, Autism Diagnostic Observation Schedule.* Los Angeles, CA: Western Psychological Services.

Militerni, R., Gison, G., Bravaccio, C., Cassese, S., Foria, E. & Mazzola, E. (1997): L'approccio diagnostico-terapeutico al bambino con disturbi relazionali precoci: un modello di intervento. *Psichiatria Infanzia Adolescenza* **64,** 611–617.

NAS [National Research Council] (2001): *Educating Children with Autism.* Committee on Educational Interventions for Children with Autism, eds. C. Lord & J.P. McGee. Washington, DC: National Academy Press.

O'Hearn, K., Asato, M., Ordaz, S. & Luna, B. (2008): Neurodevelopment and executive function in autism. *Dev. Psychopathol.* **20,** 1103–1132.

OFF.F MIUR: Classe di Laurea L/SNT2 - Professioni sanitarie della riabilitazione. http://offf.miur.it/pubblico.php/ricerca/show_form/p/miur

Ospina, M.B., Krebs Selda, J., Clark B, Karkhaneh, M., Hartling, L., Tjosvold, L., Vandermeer, B. & Smith, V. (2008): Behavioral and developmental interventions for autism spectrum disorder: a clinical. systematic review. *Plos ONE* **3,** e3755.

Rondeau, E., Klein, L.S., Masse, A., Bodeau, N., Cohen, D. & Guilé, J.M. (2011): Is pervasive developmental disorder not otherwise specified less stable than autistic disorder? A meta-analysis. *J. Autism Dev. Disord.* **41,** 1267–1276.

Sheese, B.E., Rothbart, M.K., Posner, M.I., White, L.K. & Fraundorf, S.H. (2008): Executive attention and self-regulation in infancy. *Infant Behav. Dev.* **31,** 501–510.

Sparrow, S. (1997): Developmentally based assessment. In: *Handbook of Autism and Pervasive Developmental Disorders*, 2nd ed., eds. D.J. Cohen & F.R. Volkmar. New York: John Wiley and Sons.

Wallace, K.S. & Rogers, S.J. (2010): Intervening in infancy: implications for autism spectrum disorders. *J. Child Psychol. Psychiatry* **51,** 1300–1320.

WHO [World Health Organization] (2007): *ICF–CY. International Classification of Functioning, Disability and Health: Children & Youth Version.* Geneva: WHO Press.

Woolfenden, S., Sarkozy, V., Ridley, G. & Williams, K. (2012): A systematic review of the diagnostic stability of autism spectrum disorder. *Res. Autism Spect. Disord.* **6,** 345–354.

Chapter 20

Social skill training in autism spectrum disorders

Massimo Molteni and Sara Forti

*Department of Developmental Psychopathology, Scientific Institute 'Eugenio Medea',
via don L. Monza 20, 23842 Bosisio Parini, Italy*
massimo.molteni@bp.lnf.it

Summary

Patients with autism are specifically impaired in social interaction. This difficulty could be related to specific problems in face processing or in oxytocin regulation. In social situations, mirror neurons of persons with autism spectrum disorders (ASDs) may be under-activated, along with problems of long-distance connectivity and attention impairments. Rehabilitation may follow two approaches: (1) a reactivation of mirror neurons through imitative practice; and (2) a gradual reactivation of long-distance connectivity through the simplification of stimuli to be processed.

Introduction

Poor social interaction is specific to autism and autism spectrum disorders (ASDs) (Carter *et al.*, 2005) and differentiates these patients from those with other developmental disorders (Klin *et al.*, 2007); indeed, even the most cognitively able individuals on the autism spectrum manifest social difficulties (Howlin, 2005). Social abilities are the core of inter-individual cooperation, and are thus fundamental for human development. Some human abilities can be deeply acquired only through cooperation, which in some cases represents the only possibility for learning those skills. Given the importance of the acquisition of social abilities and cooperation for human development, current research interests are focusing more and more on the social brain.

Also, the newest revision of the *Diagnostic and Statistical Manual of Mental Disorders* (DSM–5) is going to pay more attention overall to social impairments, and individuals showing social deficits with no associated symptoms will be included in a new self-standing diagnostic category: 'Social Communication Disorder'.

Discussion

The social brain

The identification of people from their faces and the comprehension of their mental state through facial expressions is at the origin of social communication. These skills are so important that human beings have a specialized neural network for face processing. This includes: right amygdala, inferior frontal cortex, superior temporal sulcus and face-related somatosensory and premotor cortex. A dysfunction of such network is supposed to be the origin of the difficulties in social skills shown by children with autism (Schultz *et al.*, 2006); in these patients, this is generally hypo-active when viewing faces (Hadjikhani *et al.*, 2007) with null activation of the fusiform gyrus, also called 'fusiform face area', which is specific and specialized for face-like stimuli (Pierce *et al.*, 2001).

However, poor sociality in autism has also been explained by declarative hypotheses, such as the theory of mind (Campbell *et al.*, 2006), the weak central coherence theory (Rippon *et al.*, 2007) and the hypothesis of low executive functioning (Happé *et al.*, 2006), that suggest different neural underpinnings of the disorder.

The role of oxytocin

Oxytocin represents the most important neuro-mediator for social interaction: it regulates sexual/maternal behaviour (Feldman *et al.*, 2007), processing of positive stimuli and processing of basic social stimuli. Indeed, oxytocin boosts positive social cues (such as romantic and attractive faces) by activating the social-reward mechanism of the amygdale and enhances then eye gaze (Guastella *et al.*, 2008). Also, brain activity evoked by the perception of 'animacy' (Allison *et al.*, 2012) is associated with the degree of OXTR methylation and high-level social processing, such as understanding actions and intentions, is facilitated when low-level perception is mediated by oxytocin (Pelphrey & Morris, 2006).

In fact, a variation in two common single nucleotide polymorphism (SNP) variants in the OXTR gene may explain part of individual variability in social behaviour: therefore social processes may be under epigenetic control.

As a consequence, oxytocin might play a role in mitigating the pathophysiology of autism (Bartz *et al.*, 2006). In fact, the infusion of synthetic oxytocin into adults with ASD improves their identification of facial expressions (Hollander *et al.*, 2007).

However, the oxytocin hypothesis needs to be supported by further research.

Mirror neuron system

The discovery of mirror neurons has unified perception and action processes: when we watch somebody moving, 'mirror neurons', coding for that action in our motor system are activated.

Mirror activation allows to predict the outcome of other people's actions without cognitive mediation (Rizzolatti et al., 2009); rather, mirror neurons make possible to experience the motor schema that is being observed. These findings have led to the 'embodied simulation theory' (Gallese & Sinigaglia, 2011). According to this hypothesis people make sense of others' actions through body representations of their own mental states. In this framework, mirror neurons are at the basis of motor competence, social competence and social behaviour: mirror neurons make it possible to predict other people's goals and to feel the individual's experience of others. In this respect, movements become the fundament for social actions, and represent the most direct way to communicate subjective feelings.

Visual attention

Although patients with ASD have been mainly characterized for social symptoms, evidence of dysfunctions in perception and attention is growing (for a review, see Mottron et al., 2006).

One example of attention problems concerns zooming, which is the ability to process some detailed information of stimulus leaving other information on the background. ASD patients show longer latencies in zooming-in to an object detail and, once engaged, in zooming-out from the local feature to the perceptual whole (Ronconi et al., 2012). Higher local connectivity and lower long-distance connectivity has been found in these patients (either due to a widespread alteration in synapse elimination or to local over-growth and distant under-growth of white-matter projections; Belmonte et al., 2004) and this neural functioning may explain attention behaviour. Indeed ASD patients may show reduced spatio-temporal integration, with advantages them in signal-detection tasks (Gomot et al., 2008) and disadvantages them when local features need to be integrated, such as for processing faces, emotions and biological motion (Klin et al., 2009). Even narrow interests in autism and what is clinically called 'need for sameness' may be determined by anomalous neural connectivity.

Moreover narrow attention/localized connectivity could explain motor anomalies of these patients, which are particularly evident in movement sequences (Forti et al., 2011; Nobile et al., 2011): individuals with autism are only partially able to plan movements, with problems in late movement phases and difficulties in integrating single motor acts in a motor chain for a goal-directed action (Fabbri-Destro et al., 2009).

And finally, localized connectivity may affect mirror functions, given those require the integration of multiple motor/auditory/visual channels.

Besides, also problems in the theory-of-mind may be explained by limited long-distance connectivity (Le Bell et al., 2009).

A neuro-constructivist approach to intervention

Within a neuro-constructivist framework, low-level deficits (Karmiloff-Smith, 1998) may affect higher functions: because perception is affected by attention (Forti et al., 2005) when attention to social stimuli is impaired social situation may be only partially processed, with consequences on social behaviour (for a recent review, see Mazer, 2011).

In these patients, the performance obtained at a perceptual task based on local-global integration (coherent dot motion task) correlated with the severity of social symptoms (Ronconi et al., 2012).

Attention mechanisms could also be at the basis of emotional processing: zooming in may be needed to process small local changes of facial posture in the global expression and perceive the expression dynamics for emotional meaning. In these terms facial expressions act as object affordances subtending emotions.

Moreover, face-processing areas belong to the mirror neuron network.

When looking at somebody's face, our mirror neurons may activate the corresponding emotional representation in our own limbic system, a mechanism that could be at the origin of empathy.

The big challenge for interventions in autism spectrum disorders is to be able to empower neural integration given by the mirror neuron system (MNS). One possibility could be through practicing mirror activities, where imitation is the mirroring task by definition (indeed children with autism are universally and specifically impaired in imitation; see Williams et al., 2004 for a review).

Imitation interventions have traditionally adopted a behavioural approach by breaking imitative behaviours up into a series of discrete sub-skills. These are taught in highly structured settings through prompting, shaping, and reinforcement. Recently, Ingersoll and colleagues have developed a more naturalistic intervention for imitation skills, called 'Reciprocal Imitation Training (RIT)'. In RIT, imitation is taught during play interactions with objects, with positive outcomes on spontaneous object imitation and gesture imitation (Ingersoll *et al.*, 2007) and improvements in language, play, and joint attention (Ingersoll & Schreibman, 2006).

However, imitation difficulties of children with autism are more common, evident, and severe when for movements without objects and with no symbolic meaning (Stone *et al.*, 1997; Vanvuchelen *et al.*, 2007; Ingersoll *et al.*, 2007). A specific intervention has been developed for the imitation of meaningless body gestures (Soundbeam Imitation Intervention) (Forti *et al.*, oral communication), by coupling sounds to body movements as feedback for imitation and significant improvements have been recorded in imitation and in social sustained attention.

Alternatively, we might facilitate neural integration through a step-by-step training on stimuli processing with increasing need for global integration of local features. We might suppose, for instance, that children with ASD could be trained to face processing starting from simplified face-like patterns (*e.g.*, static puppets).

Gradual training to integration through stimuli simplification is widely used: interventions like the Applied Behaviour Analysis (ABA), peer training, and video modeling through visual supports (such as social narratives, scripts, and visual activity schedules) are based on this methodology and have lead to significant improvements in social abilities (for a review, see Reichow & Volkmar, 2010). However, although these can be considered as an attempt to lessen the need for integrative processing, we cannot say that gradual training to integration is definitively successful, as in these techniques emotional reinforcement is always present as an external variable.

A similar approach may be represented by video-based instructions representing simplified communicative stimuli that could be useful to teach a wide range of adaptive social and communication skills. However, also in these cases, verbal correction of mistakes and immediate reinforcement are also added. Finally, we shall mention the potential utility of assistive technologies and portable multimedia devices (*e.g.*, iPads), both as stimuli for the development of age-appropriate leisure activities (listening to music, playing games) and as supporting media for video-based instructions (Kagohara, 2010); nevertheless, no effectiveness tests have been published.

Conclusions

People make sense of other people's actions through their own mental states in the form of body representations through the activation of mirror neurons. Poor social skills in autism might depend on low oxytocin mediation within such a network and there is evidence that persons with ASD show abnormalities at low-level attentive and perceptual processing, with slower attention zooming and higher local-, and lower long-distance connectivity. The hypothesis of narrow attention/localized connectivity can also explain the dysfunctions of the mirror neuron network, which is based on the integration of multiple motor/auditory/visual channels; as such, lower processing deficits (Karmiloff-Smith, 1998) may determine impairments in higher functions. Several interventions have been designed to improve social skills of individuals with autism; the aim today is to empower neural integration.

We have summarized two approaches: on the one hand, interventions grounded on activities involving the MNS, such as imitation; on the other hand, interventions based on progressive processing of stimuli needing global integration. Further research is needed: interventions based on imitation activities should mainly focus on not-meaningful body gestures; interventions based on stimuli simplification should be validated without external variables such as external prompting and support.

Conflicts of interest: The authors declare no conflicts of interest.

References

Allison, J., Connelly, J.J. & Morris, J.P. (2012): DNA methylation of the oxytocin receptor gene predicts neural response to ambiguous social stimuli. *Front. Hum. Neurosci.* **6,** 280.

Bartz, J.A. & Hollander, E. (2006): The neuroscience of affiliation: forging links between basic and clinical research on neuropeptides and social behaviour. *Horm. Behav.* **50,** 518–528.

Belmonte, M.K., Allen, G., Beckel-Mitchener, A., Boulanger, L.M., Carper, R.A. & Webb, S.J. (2004): Autism and abnormal development of brain connectivity. *J. Neurosci.* **24,** 9228–9231.

Campbell, R., Lawrence, K., Mandy, W., Mitra, C., Jeyakuma, L. & Skuse, D. (2006): Meanings in motion and faces: developmental associations between the processing of intention from geometrical animations and gaze detection accuracy. *Dev. Psychopathol.* **18,** 99–118.

Carter, A.S., Davis, N.O., Klin, A. & Volkmar, F.R. (2005): Social development in autism. In: *Handbook of Autism and Pervasive Developmental Disorders*, eds. F.R. Volkmar, A. Klin, R. Paul & D.J. Cohen, 3rd ed., pp. 312–334. Hoboken, NJ: Wiley.

Fabbri-Destro, M., *et al.* (2009): Planning actions in autism. *Exp. Brain Res.* **192,** 521–525.

Feldman, R., Weller, A., Zagoory-Sharon, O. & Levine, A. (2007): Evidence for a neuroendocrinological foundation of human affiliation: plasmaoxytocin levels across pregnancy and the post partum period predict mother-infant bonding. *Psychol. Sci.* **18,** 965–970.

Forti, S., Humphreys, G.W. & Watson, D. (2005): Eye movement in search in visual neglect. *Vis. Cognit.* **12,** 1143–1160.

Forti, S., Valli, A., Perego, P., Nobile, M., Crippa, A. & Molteni, M. (2011): Motor planning and control in autism: a kinematic analysis of preschool children. *Res. Aut. Spect. Dis.* **5,** 834–842.

Gallese, V. & Sinigaglia, G. (2011): What is so special about embodied simulation? *Trends Cogn. Sci.* **15,** 512–519.

Gomot, M., Belmonte, M.K., Bullmore, E.T., Bernard, F.A. & Baron-Cohen, S. (2008): Brain hyper-reactivity to auditory novel targets in children with high-functioning autism. *Brain* **131,** 2479–2488.

Guastella, A.J., Mitchell, P.B. & Mathews, F. (2008): Oxytocin enhances the encoding of positive social memories in humans. *Biol. Psychiatry* **64,** 256–258.

Hadjikhani, N., Joseph, R.M., Snyder, J. & Tager-Flusberg, H. (2007): Abnormal activation of the social brain during face perception in autism. *Hum. Brain Mapp.* **28,** 441–449.

Happé, F., Booth, R., Charlton, R. & Hughes, C. (2006): Executive function deficits in autism spectrum disorders and attention deficit/ hyperactivity disorder: examining profiles across domains and ages. *Brain Cognit.* **61,** 25–39.

Hollander, E., Bartz, J., Chaplin, W., *et al.* (2007): Oxytocin increases retention of social cognition in autism. *Biol. Psychiatry* **61,** 498–503.

Howlin, P. (2005): Outcomes in autism spectrum disorders. In: *Handbook of Autism and Pervasive Developmental Disorders*, eds. F.R. Volkmar, A. Klin, R. Paul & D.J. Cohen, 3rd ed., pp. 201–222. Hoboken, NJ: Wiley.

Ingersoll, B. & Gergans, S. (2007): The effect of a parent-implemented imitation intervention on spontaneous imitation skills in young children with autism. *Res. Dev. Disabil.* **28,** 163–175.

Ingersoll, B. & Schreibman, L. (2006): Teaching reciprocal imitation skills to young children with autism using a naturalistic behavioural approach: effects on language, pretend play, and joint attention. *J. Autism Dev. Disord.* **36,** 487–505.

Ingersoll, B., Lewis, E. & Kroman, E. (2007): Teaching the imitation and spontaneous use of descriptive gestures in young children with autism using a naturalistic behavioural intervention. *J. Autism Dev. Disord.* **37,** 1446–1456.

Kagohara, D.M. (2010): Is video-based instruction effective in the rehabilitation of children with autism spectrum disorders? *Dev. Neurorehab.* **13**, 129–140.

Karmiloff-Smith, A. (1998): Development itself is the key to understanding developmental disorders. *Trends Cogn. Sci.* **2**, 389–398.

Klin, A., Lin, D.J., Gorrindo, P., Ramsay, G. & Jones, W. (2009): Two-year-olds with autism orient to nonsocial contingencies rather than biological motion. *Nature* **459**, 257–261.

Klin, A., Saulnier, C.A., Sparrow, S.S., Cicchetti, D.V., Volkmar, F.R. & Lord, C. (2007): Social and communication abilities and disabilities in higher functioning individuals with autism spectrum disorders: the Vineland and the ADOS. *J. Autism Dev. Dis.* **37**, 748–759.

Le Bell, R.M., Pineda, J.A. & Sharma, A. (2009): Motor-auditory-visual integration: the role of human mirror neuron system in communication and communication disorders. *J. Commun. Disord.* **42**, 299–304.

Mazer, J.A. (2011): Spatial attention, feature-based attention, and saccades: three sides of one coin? *Biol. Psychiatry* **69**, 1147–1152.

Mottron, L., Dawson, M., Soulieres, I., Hubert, B. & Burack, J. (2006): Enhanced perceptual functioning in autism: an update, and eight principles of autistic perception. *J. Autism Dev. Disord.* **36**, 27–43.

Nobile, M., Perego, P., Piccinini, L., Mani, E., Rossi, A., Bellina, M. & Molteni, M. (2011): Further evidence of complex motor dysfunction in drug naive children with autism using automatic motion analysis of gait. *Autism* **15**, 263–283.

Pelphrey, K.A. & Morris, J.P. (2006): Brain mechanisms for interpreting the actions of others from biological-motion cues. *Curr. Dir. Psychol. Sci.* **15**, 136–140.

Pierce, K., Müller, R.A., Ambrose, J., Allen, G. & Courchesne, E. (2001): Face processing occurs outside the fusiform 'face area' in autism: evidence from functional MRI. *Brain* **124**, 2059–2073.

Reichow, B. & Volkmar, F.R. (2010): Social skills interventions for individuals with autism: evaluation for evidence-based practices within a best evidence synthesis framework. *J. Autism Dev. Disord.* **40**, 149–166.

Rippon, G., Brock, J., Brown, C. & Boucher, J. (2007): Disordered connectivity in the autistic brain: challenges for the 'new psychophysiology'. *Int. J. Psychophysiol.* **63**, 164–172.

Rizzolatti, G., Fabbri-Destro, M. & Cattaneo, L. (2009): Mirror neurons and their clinical relevance *Nat Clin. Pract. Neurol.* **5**, 24–34.

Ronconi, L., Gori, S., Ruffino, M, Franceschini, S., Urbani, B., Molteni, M. & Facoetti, A. (2012): Decreased coherent motion discrimination in autism spectrum disorder: the role of attentional zoom-out deficit. *PLoS One* **7**, e49019.

Ronconi, L., Gori, S., Ruffino, M., Molteni, M. & Facoetti, A. (2012): Zoom-out attentional impairment in children with autism spectrum disorder. *Cortex.* [E-pub ahead of print, 19 March].

Schultz, R., Chawarska, K. & Volkmar, F.R. (2006): The social brain in autism: perspectives from neuropsychology and neuroimaging. In: *Understanding Autism: From Basic Neuroscience to Treatment*, eds. S.O. Moldin & J.L. Rubenstein, pp. 323–348. New York: CRC Press.

Stone, W.L., Ousley, O.Y. & Littleford, C.D. (1997): Motor imitation in young children with autism: what's the object? *J. Abnorm. Child Psychol.* **25**, 475–485.

Vanvuchelen, M., Roeyers, H. & De Weerdt, W. (2007): Nature of motor imitation problems in school-aged males with autism: how congruent are the error types? *Dev. Med. Child. Neurol.* **49**, 6–12.

Williams, J.H., Whiten, A. & Singh, T. (2004): A systematic review of action imitation in autistic spectrum disorder. *J. Autism Dev. Disord.* **34**, 285–299.

Complementary
and alternative therapies

Chapter 21

A review of methods for facilitating speech in nonverbal children with ASD

Allison Landers, Gottfried Schlaug and Catherine Y. Wan

*Departments of Neurology, Music, Neuroimaging, and Stroke Recovery Laboratories,
Beth Israel Deaconess Medical Center, and Harvard Medical School,
330 Brookline Avenue, Boston, MA 02215, USA*
cwan@bidmc.harvard.edu

Summary

This chapter reviews the existing literature on effective methods and techniques that may be useful for eliciting speech in nonverbal children with autism spectrum disorders (ASD). A range of contemporary intervention approaches in ASD is outlined. While some of the interventions have resulted in improvements in aspects of behaviour other than speech, this review focuses specifically on evidence for improvements in speech outcomes. Specific strategies from the literature on speech and language pathology are also described. Although there are only a small number of studies (frequently, single-subject case studies, and a few randomized control studies) on nonverbal children with ASD, a number of promising techniques can be identified. Further research in this domain will help to elucidate the most effective strategies for individual nonverbal children with ASD.

Introduction

For children with autism spectrum disorders (ASDs), the ability to communicate verbally is a positive prognostic indicator for many quality-of-life outcomes (Lord *et al.*, 2006; Sherer & Schreibman, 2005). Little research, however, has been devoted to developing and evaluating methods that can facilitate speech in completely nonverbal children with ASD. This is especially surprising because a relatively large proportion of nonverbal children with ASD make little progress in speech through the usual and established interventions. While most of the studies examining new approaches have been pilot investigations, there appears to be a number of techniques that might help with speech acquisition in nonverbal children. This chapter presents existing research from the fields of ASD, developmental disability, and speech-language pathology regarding techniques that may be helpful in eliciting speech in nonverbal children with ASD. It is important to note that this review focuses on speech production as an outcome measure. Accordingly, while many of the approaches outlined below have yielded positive outcomes in non-speech measures (*e.g.*, language, behaviour), a summary of these studies is beyond the scope of this chapter. Instead, general descriptions of these popular interventions in ASD will be outlined, followed by a review of speech studies on nonverbal children. Finally, relevant techniques from the realm of speech language pathology, as well as novel treatment methods, will be highlighted.

Contemporary approaches in autism treatment

It is helpful to first consider contemporary approaches for ASD intervention. Many such approaches for ASD are enthusiastically supported by their developers, as well as by parents who hope to improve the quality of life of their children. Unfortunately, however, the efficacy of these treatment approaches in facilitating speech production has not been rigorously investigated. The following section outlines a number of popular treatment approaches for ASD and highlights evidence (if available) supporting their use in speech development in nonverbal children. It is also important to emphasise that most studies have focused on higher-functioning verbal individuals, thus making generalization to the nonverbal subgroup difficult. Nonetheless, more detailed descriptions of some of these and other methods, as well as their use in modifying non-speech outcomes (*e.g.*, language, behaviour), can be found elsewhere in this volume.

Applied Behavioural Analysis (ABA)

ABA is one of the most widely-known treatment approaches for ASD, and is often implemented in school settings (Choutka *et al.*, 2004; Hess *et al.*, 2008). A defining feature of ABA is the experimental analysis of behaviour, in particular, by examining how environmental events interact to influence a behavioural outcome. Within this framework, discrete trial training is often used to break down complex skills, and to teach each subskill through high-structured, massed teaching trials. Each trial consists of a direct instruction for a response, such as the imitation of the therapist's model and responding to a verbal request. Through the use of explicit prompting, shaping, and chaining techniques, learning occurs when target behaviours are systematically reinforced.

Within the ABA approach, teaching trials are often delivered intensively for up to 40 hours per week, for 2 or more years. A relatively large number of case studies (*e.g.*, Wolf *et al.*, 1964) support the use of prompting and reinforcing speech attempts as a means of teaching speech to nonverbal children with ASD. In a recent study, use of the rapid motor imitation (RMI) approach within an ABA framework was shown to be effective in eliciting first words in three nonverbal preschoolers (Tsiouri & Greer, 2003). Participants were taught to first imitate motor actions (*e.g.*, clapping, touching their nose) to get them into 'imitation mode', after which they were expected to imitate speech sounds. This highly didactic instruction took place in a highly structured setting (*e.g.*, at table-top) and was therapist-directed. This approach was also shown to be effective in eliciting vocal imitation in five nonverbal children with autism aged 5 to 7 years (Ross & Greer, 2003). This study was limited by the fact that it was preceded by varying amounts of motor imitation training for each participant and that the number of opportunities for response during intervention varied greatly between sessions. Whilst ABA has been successful in modifying behaviours in children with ASD, including vocal behaviours (*e.g.*, Tsiouri & Greer, 2003), some researchers believe that the adult-directed instructions, highly structured teaching environment, and the use of artificial reinforcers lead to cue dependency and rote responding, which can limit generalization as well as spontaneous and functional use of skills (*e.g.*, Horner *et al.*, 1988; Schreibman, 1997a, 1997b).

Pivotal Response Training (PRT) model

The PRT model (Arick *et al.*, 2005; Koegel *et al.*, 1999; Mundy & Stella, 2000) aims to implement evidence-based behavioural strategies in naturalistic environments. Similar to ABA, PRT is based on the following sequence: cue – child response – consequence. However, the sequence is embedded into a functional context within the natural environment. Ideally, it is implemented during a preferred activity (*i.e.*, an object or activity that a child has selected) and the reinforcer is a natural consequence of the prompted behaviour. For instance, if the therapist is playing with a toy that the child wishes to access, the therapist would cue the child to make a request (*e.g.*, 'my turn!') and then reinforce the request by handing over the desired toy (*i.e.*, the natural reinforcer).

As opposed to the drill-based intervention of traditional ABA, PRT allows therapists and/or caregivers to engage the child over the course of the entire day, and is thus designed to increase the child's motivation to communicate. Research is regrettably limited on the efficacy of PRT for nonverbal children. It has been shown that parental implementation of PRT leads to gains in functional utterances in preschoolers with ASD. However, these results do not necessarily apply to all nonverbal children because all participants in these studies had at least some functional speech sounds prior to participation (Coolican *et al.*, 2010; Minjarez *et al.*, 2011). One exception was a study that examined the effects of individualized orienting cues on facilitating first words in three nonverbal children with ASD through the use of PRT (Koegel *et al.*, 2009). The study found that the presentation of an attention-evoking cue (*e.g.*, 'high five' gesture, kisses, hugs, novel sounds) immediately prior to the verbal model resulted in an increased number of words produced according to parent reports.

Treatment and Education of Autistic and Related Communication-Handicapped Children (TEACCH)

The TEACCH approach focuses on 'Structured Teaching', which takes into account characteristics relating to the 'culture of autism', such as relative strength in processing visual details, variability in attention, communication deficits, the difficulty with concepts of time, adherence to routines, intense interests and impulses, and marked sensory preferences (*e.g.*, Ozonoff *et al.*, 2005). The TEACCH approach uses four kinds of structure to make activities clearer and easier to perform: (i) *physical structure*, such as rearrangement of furniture; (ii) *sequencing events* through the use of visual schedules; (iii) *individual tasks* to enable students understand where to be and what is required; and (iv) *work systems* to increase engagement in activities. In addition, TEACCH often incorporates the student's special interests (*e.g.*, favourite cartoon characters) and the use of visual schedules to enhance learning.

Whilst there is no specific curriculum for language, TEACCH considers receptive understanding as the foundation for expressive communication. Presumably, structure makes the student's environment understandable and predictable, so that spontaneous communication can emerge. For minimally verbal individuals, TEACCH begins by associating actual objects with activities (*e.g.*, a spoon for mealtime, a roll of toilet paper for going to the bathroom), followed by associating symbolic objects with activities (*e.g.*, a toy car for going home). These objects are then paired with spoken words (Mesibov *et al.*, 2005; Mesibov & Shea, 2010). Scaffolding, the provision of supports to facilitate successful learning, is also an important element of TEACCH. The goal is for the student to communicate independently, and the premise is that understanding object-based communication is a foundation for developing object-based expressive communication.

To date, no studies have specifically tested the effectiveness of TEACCH in facilitating speech in nonverbal children. However, Delprato (2001) compared eight studies on higher-functioning children that used discrete trial approaches (such as ABA) with those that used more naturalistic, 'normalized' approaches (that appear to share some elements of the TEACCH), and concluded that the normalized approaches are more effective for teaching language. However, it remains unclear what the impact of TEACCH is on speech development in nonverbal children with ASD.

Denver Model

The Denver Model is an intervention that adopts a developmental framework for children with ASD. Rather than focusing on behavioural deficits alone, the Denver Model views ASD as a complex disorder that affects many domains of functioning, thus requiring an interdisciplinary approach to address the associated challenges (*e.g.*, Dawson *et al.*, 2010; Rogers & Lewis, 1989). Accordingly, the Denver Model derives its teaching goals by constructing developmental profiles based on several sources, including: clinical observations of child-caregiver and child-therapist interactions, a developmental history and profile of current functioning, a review of current intervention programs, ongoing consultation with specialists from many disciplines (*e.g.*, speech-language pathologists, occupational and physical therapists, educators, psychologists), as well as biomedical evaluation. The Denver Model emphasizes the importance of incorporating teaching strategies into a child's natural environment (*e.g.*, typical family routines such as meals, bathing, playtime, outings), paying particular attention to the child's affect, attention, and arousal within a relationship-based context. Although teaching strategies are often consistent with the principles of ABA, each child's developmental curriculum is individualized, and there is a strong emphasis on the participation of parents and family in shaping behaviour. A recent study demonstrated acquisition of first words in five young boys with ASD after participating in the Denver Model intervention (Rogers *et al.*, 2006).

Social Communication, Emotional Regulation and Transactional Support (SCERTS)

The SCERTS model is another developmentally-based approach that prioritizes Social Communication, Emotional Regulation, and Transactional Support as primary targets for intervention in individuals with ASD (Prizant *et al.*, 2003). In addition to research on child development, the SCERTS model also draws heavily from current research on behavioural supports and ABA (*e.g.*, Fox *et al.*, 2000) and research on family-centred intervention and family systems theory (Prizant & Meyer, 1993). Specific goals are identified within each realm (social communication, emotional regulation, and transactional supports) and subsequently implemented with children with ASD and their families. Social communication goals include enhancing joint attention and increasing symbol use. Emotional regulation goals including increasing self-regulation capacities, enhancing abilities to seek supports from others to maintain regulation, and increasing abilities to recover from periods of dysregulation. Transactional supports include use of educational or learning supports (*e.g.*, visual supports), interpersonal supports (*e.g.*, adjusting the interaction partner's language level and level of communicative support, creating teachable moments), family supports (*e.g.*, emotional/educational support for parents), and professional supports (*e.g.*, continued education for professionals working with children with ASD). Goal selection is guided both by child development research and by individual family priorities and functional needs of the child. At present, no studies have specifically tested the effects of the SCERTS model on speech in nonverbal children with ASD.

Developmental, Individual-Difference, Relationship-Based (DIR)/Floortime

Another approach that draws from knowledge regarding development in typical children is the DIR/Floortime model (Greenspan & Wieder, 1997), which advocates individualized intervention that focuses on the developmental level, affective interaction, and individual strengths and weaknesses of each specific child. Spontaneous use of meaningful communication (*e.g.*, spoken language, gestures) is a main goal of intervention, as is development of relationships with caregivers, therapists, and other communication partners. Special attention is also paid to the development of social skills. DIR/Floortime also recognizes sensory, motor, biological, cognitive, and emotional differences within individuals and works to help develop these capacities in harmony with one another. Specifically, DIR/Floortime aims to foster development through six Functional Developmental Levels: (i) mutual attention; (ii) mutual engagement; (iii) interactive intentionality and reciprocity; (iv) representational/affective communication; (v) representational elaboration; (vi) representational differentiation, self-regulation, and interest in the world. Targets of intervention are based on an individual's current developmental functioning. For example, for a child who displays no interest in interacting with others, interventionists join a child in a preferred activity and work to maintain engagement with the child during that activity. If, however, the child displays difficulty expressing wants and needs, interventionists work to provide forms of communication (*e.g.*, words, gestures) that help the child access desired objects during a preferred activity. Intervention sessions are typically unstructured and occur within a child's natural setting (*e.g.*, during play) and focus on 'following the child's lead.' Presently, no studies have been conducted expressly examining the effects of DIR/Floortime on speech in nonverbal individuals.

Prompts for Restructuring Oral Muscular Phonetic Targets (PROMPT)

PROMPT draws from literature suggesting that speech deficits in ASD may be partially due to difficulties with oral motor control, similar to difficulties observed in apraxia of speech (*e.g.*, Adams, 1998), including oral motor planning and imitation. PROMPT was developed for use with both children and adults and is based on knowledge of neuromotor speech production [Chumpelik (Hayden), 1984; Hayden, 2006]. Specifically, PROMPT posits that touch is an important sensory modality that can be used for a variety of purposes including developing and/or re-establishing motor control of speech mechanisms, integrating sensory modalities (*e.g.*, audition, vision) to develop receptive and expressive language, and enhancing social-emotional interaction. To that end, PROMPT uses tactual-kinesthetic cues to facilitate speech production along with a variety of other motor-speech strategies including repeated practice of targets and planning goals/activities based on motor restructuring. PROMPT also recognizes the importance of cognitive-linguistic language intervention and also advocates for naturalistic teaching environments, social interaction, and functional use of speech. In Chumpelik (Hayden) & Sherman's 1980 study (as cited in Rogers *et al.*, 2006), a nonverbal 8-year-old child with ASD was shown to acquire 30 functional words over 4 months while receiving PROMPT intervention. More recently, a study reported useful speech in five young nonverbal boys with ASD after participating in PROMPT intervention (Rogers *et al.*, 2006).

Augmentative and Alternative Communication (AAC)

AAC strategies, originally developed for use with individuals with motor impairments such as cerebral palsy, are frequently provided to nonverbal children with ASD in the hope of increasing their communicative competency. AAC strategies are broadly classified into unaided strategies (*e.g.*, gestures, sign language) and aided strategies (*e.g.*, picture exchange systems, speech-generating devices). Aided strategies may be further classified into lite-tech (*e.g.*, communication notebooks, picture exchange systems) and high-tech (*e.g.*, speech-generating devices). While access to AAC undoubtedly increases a nonverbal child's ability to communicate (*e.g.*, Light *et al.*, 1998), the impact of AAC on speech development remains somewhat unclear. Regarding unaided strategies, evidence on the use of sign language is, regrettably, limited. While at least one study has shown that use of sign language neither positively nor negatively affects speech production in nonverbal children with ASD (Yoder & Layton, 1988), a number of single-subject studies show an improvement in speech in nonverbal children with ASD after the introduction of sign language (Schwartz & Nye, 2006). More research is clearly needed to further elucidate the relationship between sign language and speech.

Regarding lite-tech aided strategies, mixed evidence also exists for the positive impact of picture exchange systems, the most frequently utilized of which is the Picture Exchange Communication System (PECS). PECS integrates behavioural and pragmatic strategies, at the basic level, to instruct a child to utilize pictorial symbols to request desired objects or actions. Whilst single-case studies have reported an increase in the use of speech with PECS in children with ASD (*e.g.*, Charlop-Christy *et al.*, 2002; Ganz *et al.*, 2009; Ganz & Simpson, 2004; Kravits *et al.*, 2002; Tincani *et al.*, 2006), a recent meta-analysis showed that gains in speech in many studies were actually small to negative (Flippin *et al.*, 2010). A more recent randomized control trial of 84 school-aged children described as having little to no functional speech prior to participation showed an increase in spontaneous speech that persisted to 9 months post intervention after training in PECS (Gordon *et al.*, 2011). Studies of non-PECS picture exchange programs are limited, but some case studies also report slight but inconsistent increases in vocalizations after intervention (*e.g.*, Nunes & Hanline, 2007). While participants in all of the above-cited studies were described as nonverbal or lacking functional speech, the heterogeneity of the label 'nonverbal' also makes it difficult to determine the effects of such strategies on completely nonverbal individuals. Further research could help elucidate specific profiles of individuals likely to benefit from such strategies.

Evidence regarding impact of high-tech AAC devices on speech in nonverbal children is also mixed: many studies show an increase in speech for some but not all participants (*e.g.*, Olive *et al.*, 2007; Schlosser *et al.*, 2007). While not all participants in such studies were shown to make improvements in speech production, reports of decrease in speech production have not been noted. Similarly, computerized visual feedback has been shown to increase vocal imitation in nonverbal children with ASD to a significantly greater degree than traditional play interaction (Bernard-Opitz *et al.*, 1999). A systematic review of available studies revealed that access to AAC in general (all strategies, both aided and unaided) did not impede speech in nonverbal children with ASD, but instead led to modest gains in speech production (Schlosser & Wendt, 2008). Although research comparing types of AAC strategies is limited, some evidence indicates that nonverbal preschoolers with ASD are more likely to pair verbalizations with sign language than with PECS [Anderson (2002) as cited in Schreibman & Ingersoll, 2005; Tincani, 2004]. Again, the above studies are limited by the lack of a precise definition of 'nonverbal' children, making it difficult to pinpoint precise verbal abilities of participants. Thus, it is possible that these findings may not apply to completely nonverbal individuals. Future research should investigate the precise impact of AAC systems on acquisition of functional speech in contrast to direct intervention, be it didactic, naturalistic, or based on typical developmental approaches.

Comparing the efficacy of different interventions

Studies examining the efficacy of some of the above intervention approaches in facilitating speech production have yielded mixed results (*e.g.*, Schlosser *et al.*, 2007; Ganz *et al.*, 2009). In addition, controlled studies *comparing* the effectiveness of different interventions have, to date, been very limited. One study compared the Denver Model to PROMPT (Rogers *et al.*, 2006). In that study, 10 nonverbal children aged 2 to 5 years were randomized into one of the two target interventions and all of them had received at least 9 months of intensive therapy prior to enrolment. After 12 weeks of intervention, 80 per cent of children produced five or more novel words, but no differences in outcomes were observed between the two interventions. While this treatment study showed improvements in speech production in nonverbal children, it was conducted on relatively young children, and therefore, the possibility that some of the improvements were due to delayed speech development could not be ruled out.

Another study compared the effects of PECS to those of Responsive Education and Prelinguistic Milieu Teaching (RPMT), a treatment approach that shares many features with PRT and other naturalistic teaching methods (Yoder & Stone, 2006). Thirty-six preschoolers described as being nonverbal or low verbal (defined as having 20 or fewer functional words) participated in 24 hours of treatment over a 6-month period. Results indicated that PECS was more successful in teaching nonimitative communicative speech. Again, because these children were relatively young, delayed speech development cannot be ruled out as a cause for improvement. Furthermore, some children already had a degree of functional speech, thus complicating the generalisation of findings to completely nonverbal individuals. Further research is clearly warranted to elucidate differential effects of specific treatment approaches.

Speech-language pathology techniques applicable to the treatment of nonverbal children with ASD

General principles

Beyond specific intervention approaches, it is also useful to consider a variety of techniques from the realm of speech-language pathology that are frequently used to elicit speech in nonverbal children with ASD (*e.g.*, American Speech-Language-Hearing Association, 2005; Paul, 2007; Paul & Sutherland, 2005). At present, there is no 'gold standard' for speech and language intervention that targets nonverbal children with ASD. However, speech and language pathologists typically employ a wide range of strategies, as outlined below.

Speech and language pathologists view spoken language as consisting of three components: form (*i.e.*, speech sounds, parts of words, words), content (*i.e.*, semantics, meanings of words and phrases), and use (*i.e.*, pragmatic use of sounds, words, and sentences) (Bloom & Lahey, 1978; Paul, 2007). Sounds and words are not merely motor acts, but are viewed as part of a cognitive-motor-linguistic task involved in communication (Paul, 2007). Thus, the focus of the intervention is primarily use of functional sounds and words (*i.e.*, those that the child can use in his or her day-to-day life and words that he or she wants to use.). Thus, motivating words such as 'no', 'mommy', and 'drink' are better targets for an individual's first words than less motivating words such as 'thank you' or those representing colours or numbers. Similarly, therapeutic activities are frequently activities which the child is already interested in and is therefore motivated to communicate during intervention. For instance, a typical 3-year-old is more likely to want to talk about bubbles than about line-drawing photos of objects and actions.

By selecting activities that are inherently motivating (*i.e.*, activities the child enjoys), the child's motivation to communicate is increased. Speech and language therapy aims to increase the communicative *forms* (*i.e.*, signs, sounds, words) and communicative *functions* (*i.e.*, protesting, requesting, directing, commenting, questioning, organizing, socializing) to help the individual become a more efficient and effective communicator (*e.g.*, American Speech-Language-Hearing Association, 2007; Shane *et al.*, 2009). Consider, for example, a child who only produces the phoneme /m/ to request 'more'. Intervention targeting number of *forms* could include encouraging him to use the manual sign for *more* in conjunction with the sound or shaping the sound /m/ to /mo/ to have a word approximation closer to the target. Intervention targeting number of *functions* could include using vocalizations to gain the attention of others (*e.g.*, to get their mother to attend to them) or to greet peers entering the room.

Teaching foundational communication skills

Speech-language pathologists have long advocated for the teaching of foundational communication skills such as anticipation of routine, imitation, and joint attention to nonverbal children with ASD (Paul, 2007). Routines provide a unique opportunity for speech and language intervention, as they provide key points of communicative temptations for participants (Paul, 2007). Routines provide a predictable sequence of actions and words within the context of a pleasurable activity. Repetition provides for many learning opportunities, while pleasurable anticipation increases the child's motivation to participate. Routines could include games such as 'peek-a-boo'. After many rounds of the game with the parent saying 'peek-a-boo!' and revealing his or her face, the child can be encouraged to say 'peek-a-boo!' by the adult delaying his or her action. No specific research studies are presently available regarding the impact of such strategies on speech production.

Regarding imitation, children with autism have been shown to have significant impairment in imitation abilities, including oral-facial imitation, manual actions, and actions on objects, as compared with typically developing children and children with other developmental disorders (Rogers *et al.*, 2003). Thus, deficits in imitation may directly contribute to speech dysfunction in children with ASD. Intervention targeting imitation skills typically begins with teaching the concept of imitation, achieved by first imitating the child's actions and vocalizations to introduce the concept. Parents and therapists can be encouraged to imitate everything that a child does, from banging toys on the table to playing with speech sounds. Gazdag and Warren (2000) showed specifically that the imitation of vocalizations led to greater imitation in infants with developmental disabilities. While the above studies did not test nonverbal children with ASD, some of the strategies may be applicable to this subgroup.

Joint attention refers to the concept of two individuals attending to the same object or event and recognizing that the other person is attending to the same object or event. Typically-developing children frequently point out interesting objects in their environment to their parents and friends, seeking to share enjoyment. Encouraging a child with ASD to first look at a preferred object (*e.g.*, bubbles), then to their mother, then back to the preferred object may help foster development of joint attention skills. Drew *et al.* (2002), for example, reported results of a randomized control study that indicated that very young children with ASD showed a significantly greater increase in number of words produced (6.8 words pre-treatment *vs.* 96.6 words post-treatment) after 12 months of parent-based interventions aimed to promote joint attention skills as compared to a treatment-as-usual control group. While these results are encouraging, they were not replicated by Oosterling *et al.* (2010), whose participants at an average age of 34.4 months were approximately 1 year older than the participants in Drew *et al.* (2002) study and also appeared to be cognitively lower functioning. These results may suggest that joint attention intervention may be most effective for younger children. Another study showed an increase in use of vocalizations to communicate following early intervention targeting eye contact, use of gesture, and use of vocalization/words as compared to a control treatment-as-usual condition in children aged 17–36 months (Wong & Kwan, 2010). Importantly, these improvements were observed following only a 2-week intervention that comprised 10 half-hour sessions. One additional study compared the effects of interventions targeting joint attention with no-treatment controls in 3- and 4-year-old children with ASD (Kasari *et al.*, 2008). Results showed greater increase in expressive language for participants in the joint attention condition than in the control condition. More research is clearly warranted, particularly in older children, to specifically identify the relationship between joint attention intervention and speech production.

Applications of typical speech sound development to speech intervention for nonverbal children with ASD

Current knowledge of speech sound development can also be directly applied to interventions for nonverbal children with ASD. For instance, speech-language pathologists who work with children with speech sound disorders have long focused on first eliciting those words that contain sounds that the child can already produce (Paul, 2007). For example, if a nonverbal child independently produces phonemes such as /m/, /o/, and /g/, then excellent targets for word approximations could include /mo/ for 'more', while requesting more Goldfish crackers during snack time, or /go/ for 'go' while racing toy cars. One study showed that young children with specific language impairment were more likely to produce words with speech sounds that they had already mastered than those they had not (Leonard *et al.*, 1982). In addition, it is important to consider the 'teachability' of sounds in selecting initial phonemic targets (Fey, 1986). Sounds that are teachable are easily demonstrated, easily taught, and frequently used in natural contexts. Thus /m/ may be an appropriate primary speech sound to target as it has a salient mouth position that is easy to model on the therapist and on the child (*e.g.*, by holding his or her lips together) and occurs in a variety of naturally motivating words (*e.g.*, 'mommy', 'mine'). Speech and language therapy also often utilizes the shaping of existing sounds to create functional words (Paul, 2007). For example, if a child independently produces /d/, he or she might be sequentially encouraged to say /d/, /da/, /dadi/ for 'daddy'. First, /d/ would be accepted as 'daddy', and as the child became proficient at that level, they would then need to say /da/ to successfully gain Daddy's attention, and so on. This approach is similar to language-based approaches of expanding on the child's utterances, which has been shown to increase the child's imitation of the adult's utterance (Scherer & Olswang, 1984). Further, new sounds targeted in speech and language therapy sessions for children with speech sound disorders are typically informed by developmental norms indicating the course of speech sound acquisition, which identifies early-developing sounds (*e.g.*, /m/, /b/, /j/, /n/, /w/, /d/, /p/, /h/) and late-developing sounds (*e.g.*, /sh/, /th/, /s/, /z/, /l/, /r/) (Shriberg, 1993). It is likely useful to first target early-developing sounds in nonverbal children with ASD because these sounds may be inherently easier to produce.

Decisions regarding syllable shape of target words can also be informed by typical speech sound development and speech- and language-therapy practices. The first syllables produced by typically-developing children are open syllables (CV) such as /ba/ for 'ball' or /ti po/ for 'teapot', while closed syllables (CVC) such as 'ball' or 'pot' typically develop later (Bauman-Waengler, 2008). Thus, it may be helpful to target production and imitation of open syllables prior to closed syllables with nonverbal children with ASD. Similarly, first multi-syllabic sounds are typically reduplicated (*e.g.*, /mama/) instead of variegated (*e.g.*, /mami/), indicating that reduplicated words may be easier to learn prior to variegated words.

Minimal speech approach

Another approach to facilitating speech in nonverbal children, including those with autism, is the minimal speech approach (MSA), as described by Potter & Wittaker (as cited in Paul & Sutherland, 2005). MSA is designed to reduce dependence on prompts, and requires therapists to reduce their speech to one- to two-word utterances and to pause for 5 to 10 seconds at critical moments in interaction. For instance, a therapist could hold up a desired object (*e.g.*, a ball) in front of the child and wait expectantly. After the child has made a nonverbal attempt to request the object (*e.g.*, by pointing or reaching), the therapist would say 'ball' and hand the ball to the child. Similar procedures are encouraged while using 'proximal communication' strategies such as imitating the child and initiating sensory and gross-motor play. Again, the therapist models one- to two-word utterances (*e.g.*, 'Tickle!' 'Again!') only after the child has made a nonverbal attempt to communicate. By only providing simple, concrete linguistic information, the intent is to map specific words onto communicative intent. Although Potter and Whittaker have provided a theoretical rationale for using MSA, no formal studies have investigated its impact on speech production.

Strategies for children who do not imitate speech sounds

For children who do not readily imitate speech sounds, six evidence-based techniques for facilitating speech have been outlined by DeThorne *et al.* (2009). These include: (i) providing access to AAC; (ii) minimising the pressure on the child to speak in order to decrease the demand placed on the motor speech system in high-pressure situations; (iii) imitating the child; (iv) using slow tempo and exaggerated prosody; (v) augmenting auditory, visual, tactile, and proprioceptive feedback through use of tools such as PROMPT, computerized auditory visual feedback, touch cues (*e.g.*, a light touch on the child's lips during production of /b/), amplification of the child's productions through echo microphones, visual feedback through mirror and/or puppet play, and the use of flavored swabs and/or snacks to cue articulator placement; and (vi) employing caution against the use of non-speech oral motor exercises (*e.g.*, tongue wagging, blowing), and focusing instead on movement of articulators *in conjunction* with functional speech sounds (*e.g.*, to encourage tongue placement on the alveolar ridge, tongue clicking may be more appropriate than tongue protrusion). All of the above recommended techniques, typically applied with children who do not readily imitate speech (and present with diagnoses as varied as developmental delay to apraxia of speech), should be considered while planning an intervention for a nonverbal child with ASD.

Auditory-Motor Mapping Training (AMMT)

Related to the strategy of reducing the rate of speech and using exaggerated prosody (DeThorne *et al.*, 2009), singing has been used to promote speech sound production in nonverbal children with ASD as well as in a variety of other neurologic causes of speech impairment (Wan *et al.*, 2010a). A case study of a 3-year-old nonverbal boy showed that an adapted version of Melodic Intonation Therapy, which uses singing to emphasize prosody at a slow rate in conjunction with hand-tapping, was effective in helping him to respond to questions and to combine words (Miller & Toca, 1979). However, because of to his relatively young age, delayed typical language development cannot be ruled out as causative. But another study of a 6-year-old girl with autism also reported success in eliciting speech through a singing procedure (Hoelzley, 1993), suggesting that singing may help facilitate speech production in older children as well. More recently, the use of slow rate of speech and exaggerated prosody has been incorporated into a novel intervention, called Auditory-Motor Mapping Training (AMMT), which is specifically designed to facilitate speech output in nonverbal children with ASD (Wan *et al.*, 2011). AMMT aims to promote speech production directly by training the association between sounds and articulatory actions using intonation and bimanual motor activities (Wan *et al.*, 2010b). Notably, the age of the six children in the AMMT study was significantly older than many previously cited studies, ranging from 5 years and 9 months to 8 years and 9 months at the commencement of therapy. Moreover, all children were completely nonverbal despite having received extensive (> 2 years) speech therapy before enrolment. Results showed that after 8 weeks of AMMT, all children showed significant improvements in their ability to articulate words and phrases, with generalization to items that were not practiced during therapy sessions. Most importantly, these skills were maintained during the 8-week follow-up assessment. As AMMT is one of the only interventions that have been shown to be effective in eliciting speech in older children with autism, it clearly bears consideration for inclusion in interventions for nonverbal children with ASD.

Conclusions

For children with ASD, the ability to speak early is associated with improved quality-of-life outcomes (Howlin *et al.*, 2000). At present, available interventions that specifically aim to promote speech production in completely nonverbal children with ASD are extremely limited. Novel, evidence-based approaches such as the ones outlined here may facilitate this critical step of language development. When designing effective intervention curricula for nonverbal children, it is important to consider the behavioural heterogeneity of these children, because one specific approach may not work for everyone. Thus, larger-scale clinical studies that test the efficacy of novel treatment approaches may help to identify characteristics of better responders. This would allow the design of treatment plans that incorporate evidence-based techniques appropriate for an individual's strengths and weaknesses, thereby maximizing the speech and language outcomes in nonverbal children with ASD.

Acknowledgments: We gratefully acknowledge support from the Nancy Lurie Marks Family Foundation, the Deborah Munroe Noonan Memorial Research Fund, and Autism Speaks.

Conflicts of interest: The authors declare no conflicts of interest.

References

Adams, L. (1998): Oral-motor and motor-speech characteristics of children with autism. *Focus Autism Other Dev. Disabil.* **13**, 108–112.

Anderson, A.E. (2002): Augmentative communication and autism: a comparison of sign language and the picture exchange communication system [doctoral dissertation, University of California, 2001]. *Dissertation Abstr. Int.* **62**, 4269B.

American Speech-Language-Hearing Association (2006): Guidelines for speech-language pathologists in diagnosis, assessment, and treatment of autism spectrum disorders across the life span. Available from www.asha.org/policy.

Arick, J.R., Krug, D.A., Fullerton, A., Loos, L. & Falco, R. (2005): School-based programs. In: *Handbook of Autism and Pervasive Developmental Disorders*, eds. F.R. Volkmar, R. Paul, A. Klin & D. Cohen, vol. 2, pp. 1003–1028. Hoboken: Wiley.

Bauman-Waengler, J. (2008): *Articulation and Phonological Impairments: A Clinical Focus* (2nd ed.). Boston, MA: Pearson Education, Inc.

Bernard-Opitz, V., Sriran, N. & Sapuan, S. (1999): Enhancing vocal imitations in children with autism using the IBM Speech Viewer. *Autism* **3**, 176–180.

Bloom, L. & Lahey, M. (1978): *Language Development and Language Disorders*. Somerset, UK: Wiley.

Charlop-Christy, M.H., Carpenter, M., Le, L., LeBlanc, L.A. & Kellet, K. (2002): Using the picture exchange communication system (PECS) with children with autism: assessment of PECS acquisition, speech, social-communicative behaviour, and problem behaviour. *J. Appl. Behav. Anal.* **35**, 213–231.

Choutka, C.M., Doloughty, P.T. & Zirkel, P.A. (2004): The "discrete trials" of Applied Behaviour Analysis for children with autism: outcome-related factors in the case law. *J. Spec. Educ.* **38**, 95–103.

Chumpelik (Hayden), D. (1984): The PROMPT system of therapy: theoretical framework and applications for developmental apraxia of speech. *Semin. Speech Lang.* **5**, 139–156.

Chumpelik (Hayden), D. & Sherman, J. (1980): Using a tactile approach in the acquisition of functional oral communication in a non-verbal, eight year old autistic child: a case study. Unpublished research.

Coolican, J., Smith, I.M. & Bryson, S.E. (2010): Brief parent training in pivotal response treatment for preschoolers with autism. *J. Child Psychol. Psychiatry* **51**, 1321–1330.

Dawson, G., Rogers, S., Munson, J., *et al.* (2010): Randomized, controlled trial of an intervention for toddlers with autism: the early start Denver model. *Pediatrics* **125**, e17–e23.

Delprato, D.J. (2001): Comparisons of discrete-trial and normalized behavioural language intervention for young children with autism. *J. Autism Dev. Disord.* **31**, 315–325.

Dethorne, L.S., Johnson, C.J., Walder, L. & Mahurin-Smith, J. (2009): When 'Simon Says' doesn't work: alternatives to imitation for facilitating early speech development. *Am. J. Speech Lang. Pathol.* **18**, 133–145.

Drew, A., Baird, G., Baron-Cohen, S., *et al.* (2002): A pilot randomised control trial of a parent training intervention for pre-school children with autism: preliminary findings and methodological challenges. *Eur. Child Adolesc. Psychiatry* **11**, 266–272.

Fey, M. (1986): *Language Intervention with Young Children*. San Diego, CA: College-Hill Press.

Flippin, M., Reszka, S. & Watson, L.R. (2010): Effectiveness of the Picture Exchange Communication System (PECS) on communication and speech for children with autism spectrum disorders: a meta-analysis. *Am. J. Speech Lang. Pathol.* **19**, 178–195.

Fox, L., Dunlab, G. & Bushbacher, P. (2000): Understanding and intervening with children's challenging behaviour: a comprehensive approach. In: *Autism Spectrum Disorders: A Transactional Developmental Perspective*, eds. A. Wetherby & B. Prizant, vol. 9, pp. 307–332. Baltimore, MD: Paul H. Brookes.

Ganz, J.B. & Simpson, R.L. (2004): Effects on communicative requesting and speech development of the picture exchange communication system in children with characteristics of autism. *J. Autism Dev. Disord.* **34**, 395–409.

Ganz, J.B., Parker, R. & Benson, J. (2009): Impact of the Picture Exchange Communication System: effects on communication and collateral effects on maladaptive behaviours. *Augment Altern. Commun.* **25**, 250–261.

Gazdag, G. & Warren, S.F. (2000): Effects of adult contingent imitation on development of young children's vocal imitation. *J. Early Interv.* **23**, 24–35.

Gordon, K., Pasco, G., McElduff, F., Wade, A., Howlin, P. & Charman, T. (2011): A communication-based intervention for nonverbal children with autism: what changes? Who benefits? *J. Consult. Clin. Psychol.* **79**, 447–457.

Greenspan, S.I. & Wider, S. (1997): Developmental patters and outcomes in infants and children with disorders in relating and communicating: a chart review of 200 cases of children with autistic spectrum diagnoses. *J. Dev. Learn. Disord.* **1**, 87–141.

Hayden, D. (2006): The PROMPT model: use and application for children with mixed phonological-motor impairment. *Adv. Speech Lang. Pathol.* **8**, 265–281.

Hess, K.L., Morrier, M.J., Heflin, L.J. & Ivey, M.L. (2008): Autism treatment survey: services received by children with autism spectrum disorders in public school classrooms. *J. Autism Dev. Disord.* **38**, 961–971.

Hoelzley, P.D. (1993): Communication potentiating sounds: developing channels of communication with autistic children through psychobiological responses to novel sound stimuli. *Can. J. Music Ther.* **1**, 54–76.

Horner, R.H., Dunlap, G. & Koegel, R.L. (1988): *Generalization and Maintenance: Life-style Changes in Applied Settings*. Baltimore, MD: Paul Brookes.

Howlin, P., Mawhood, L. & Rutter, M. (2000): Autism and developmental receptive language disorder-a follow-up comparison in early adult life. II: social, behavioural, and psychiatric outcomes. *J. Child Psychol. Psychiatry* **41,** 561–578.

Kasari, C., Paparella, T., Freeman, S. & Jahromi, L.B. (2008): Language outcome in autism: randomized comparison of joint attention and play interventions. *J. Consult. Clin. Psychol.* **76,** 125–137.

Koegel, L.K., Koegel, R.L., Harrower, J.K. & Carter, C.M. (1999): Pivotal response intervention: I. Overview of approach. *J. Assoc. Pers. Sev. Handicaps.* **24,** 174–185.

Koegel, R.L., Shirotova, L. & Koegel, L.K. (2009): Antecedent stimulus control: using orienting cues to facilitate first-word acquisition for nonresponders with autism. *Behav. Anal.* **32,** 281–284.

Kravits, T.R., Kamps, D.M., Kemmerer, K. & Potucek, J. (2002): Brief report: increasing communication skills for an elementary-aged student with autism using the picture exchange communication system. *J. Autism Dev. Disord.* **32,** 225–230.

Leonard, L.B., Schwartz, R.G., Chapman, K., *et al.* (1982): Early lexical acquisition in children with specific language impairment. *J. Speech Lang. Hear. Res.* **25,** 554–564.

Light, J.C., Roberts, B., Dimarco, R. & Greiner, N. (1998): Augmentative and alternative communication to support receptive and expressive communication for people with autism. *J. Commun. Disord.* **31,** 153–180.

Lord, C., Risi, S., DiLavore, P.S., Shulman, C., Thurm, A., *et al.* (2006): Autism from 2 to 9 years of age. *Arch. Gen. Psychiatry* **63,** 694–701.

Mesibov, G.B. & Shea, V. (2010): The TEACCH program in the era of evidence-based practice. *J. Autism Dev. Disord.* **40,** 570–579.

Mesibov, G.B., Shea, V. & Schopler, E. (with Adams, L., Burgess, S., Chapman, S.M., Merkler, E., Mosconi, M., Tanner, C. & Van Bourgondien, M.E.) (2005): *The TEACCH Approach to Autism Spectrum Disorders*. New York: Springer.

Miller, S.B. & Toca, J.M. (1979): Adapted melodic intonation therapy: case-study of an experimental language program for an autistic child. *J. Clin. Psychiatry* **40,** 201–203.

Minjarez, M.B., Williams, S.E., Mercier, E.M. & Hardon, A.Y. (2011): Pivotal response group treatment program for parents of children with autism. *J. Autism Dev. Disord.* **41,** 92–101.

Mundy, P. & Stella, J. (2000): Joint attention, social orienting, and nonverbal communication in autism. In: *Autism Spectrum Disorders: A Transactional Developmental Perspective*, eds. A.M. Wetherby & B.M. Prizant, pp. 55–77. Baltimore, MD: Paul H. Brookes.

Nunes, D. & Hanline, M. (2007): Enhancing the AAC use of a child with autism through a parent-implemented naturalistic intervention. *Int. J. Disabil. Dev. Educ.* **54,** 177–197.

Olive, M.L., De la Cruz, B., Davis, T.N., *et al.* (2007): The effects of enhanced milieu teaching and a voice output communication aid on the requesting of three children with autism. *J. Autism Dev. Disord.* **37,** 1505–1513.

Oosterling, I., Visser, J., Swinkels, S., *et al.* (2010): Randomized controlled trial of the focus parent training for toddlers with autism: 1-year outcome. *J. Autism Dev. Disord.* **40,** 1447–1458.

Ozonoff, S., South, M. & Provencal, S. (2005): Executive functions. In: *Handbook of Autism and Pervasive Developmental Disorders* (3rd ed.), eds. F.R. Volkmar, R. Paul, A. Klin & D. Cohen, vol. 1, pp. 606–627. Hoboken: Wiley.

Paul, R. (2007): *Language Disorders from Infancy through Adolescence: Assessment & Intervention* (3rd ed.). St. Louis, MO: Mosby Elsevier.

Paul, R. & Sutherland, D. (2005): Enhancing early language in children with autism spectrum disorders. In: *Handbook of Autism and Pervasive Developmental Disorders* (3rd ed.), eds. F.R. Volkmar, R. Paul, A. Klin & D. Cohen, vol. 2, pp. 946–976. Hoboken: Wiley.

Potter, C.A. & Whittaker, C.A. (2001): *Communication Enabling Environments for Children with Autism*. London: Jessica Kingsley.

Prizant, B.M. & Meyer, E.C. (1993): Socioemotional aspects of language and social-communication disorders in young children and their families. *Am. J. Speech Lang. Pathol.* **2,** 56–71.

Prizant, B.M., Wetherby, A.M., Rubin, E. & Laurent, A. (2003): The SCERTS model: a family-centered, transactional approach to enhancing communication and socioemotional abilities of young children with ASD. *Infants Young Child.* **16,** 296–316.

Rogers, S.J. & Lewis, H. (1989): An effective day treatment model for young children with pervasive developmental disorders. *J. Am. Acad. Child Adolesc. Psychiatry* **28,** 207–214.

Rogers, S.J., Hepburn, S.L., Stackhouse, T. & Wehner, E. (2003): Imitation performance in toddlers with autism and those with other developmental disorders. *J. Child Psychol. Psychiatry* **44,** 763–781.

Rogers, S.J., Hayden, D., Hepburn, S., *et al.* (2006): Teaching young nonverbal children with autism useful speech: a pilot study of the Denver Model and PROMPT interventions. *J. Autism Dev. Disord.* **36**, 1007–1024.

Ross, D.E. & Greer, R.D. (2003): Generalized imitation and the mand: inducing first instances of speech in young children with autism. *Res. Dev. Disabil.* **24**, 58–74.

Scherer, N. & Olswang, L. (1984): Role of mothers' expansions in stimulating children's language production. *J. Speech Lang. Hear. Res.* **27**, 387–396.

Schlosser, R.W., Sigafoos, J., Luiselli, J.K., *et al.* (2007): Effects of synthetic speech output on requesting and natural speech production in children with autism: A preliminary study. *Res. Autism Spect. Disord.* **1**, 139–163.

Schlosser, R.W. & Wendt, O. (2008): Effects of augmentative and alternative communication intervention on speech production in children with autism: a systematic review. *Am. J. Speech Lang. Pathol.* **17**, 212–230.

Schreibman, L. (1997a): Theoretical perspectives on behavioural intervention for individuals with autism. In: *Handbook of Autism and Pervasive Developmental Disorders* (2nd ed.), eds. D.J. Cohen & F.R. Volkmar, pp. 920–933. New York: Wiley.

Schreibman, L. (1997b): The study of stimulus control in autism. In: *Environment and Behaviour*, eds. D.M. Baer & E.M. Pinkston, pp. 203–209. Boulder, CO: Westview.

Schreibman, L. & Ingersoll, B. (2005): Behavioural interventions to promote learning in individuals with autism. In: *Handbook of Autism and Pervasive Developmental Disorders* (3rd ed.), eds. F.R. Volkmar, R. Paul, A. Klin & D. Cohen, vol. 2, pp. 882–896. Hoboken: John Wiley & Sons.

Schwartz, J.B. & Nye, C. (2006): Improving communication for children with autism: does sign language work? *EBP Briefs* **1** (2), 1–17.

Shane, H.C., O'Brien, M. & Sorce, J. (2009): Use of a visual graphic language system to support communication for persons on the autism spectrum. *Perspect. Augment. Altern. Commun.* **18**, 130–136.

Sherer, M.R. & Schreibman, L. (2005): Individual behavioural profiles and predictors of treatment effectiveness for children with autism. *J. Consult. Clin. Psychol.* **73**, 525–538.

Shriberg, L.D. (1993): Four new speech and prosody-voice measures for genetics research and other studies in developmental phonological disorders. *J. Speech Lang. Hear. Res.* **36**, 105–140.

Tincani, M. (2004): Comparing the picture exchange communication system and sign language training for children with autism. *Focus Autism Other Dev. Disabil.* **19**, 152–163.

Tincani, M., Crozier, S. & Alazetta, L. (2006): The Picture Exchange Communication System: effects on manding and speech development for school-aged children with autism. *Educ. Train. Dev. Disabil.* **41**, 177–184.

Tsiouri, I. & Greer, R.D. (2003): Inducing vocal verbal behaviour in children with severe language delays through rapid motor imitation responding. *J. Behav. Educ.* **12**, 185–206.

Wan, C.Y., Demaine, K., Zipse, L., Norton, A. & Schlaug, G. (2010a): From music making to speaking: engaging the mirror neuron system in autism. *Brain Res. Bull.* **82**, 161–168.

Wan, C.Y., Rueber, T., Hohmann, A. & Schlaug, G. (2010b): The therapeutic effects of singing in neurological disorders. *Music Percept.* **27**, 287–295.

Wan, C.Y., Bazen, L., Baars, R., *et al.* (2011): Auditory-Motor Mapping Training as an intervention to facilitate speech output in non-verbal children with autism: a proof of concept study. *Plos ONE.* **6**, e25505.

Wong, V.C.N. & Kwan, Q.K. (2010): Randomized controlled trial for early intervention for autism: a pilot study of the autism 1-2-3 project. *J. Autism Dev. Disord.* **40**, 677–688.

Wolf, M., Risley, T.R. & Mees, H. (1964): Application of operant conditioning procedures to the behaviour problems of an autistic child. *Behav. Res. Ther.* **1**, 305–312.

Yoder, P.J. & Layton, T.L. (1988): Speech following sign language training in autistic children with minimal verbal language. *J. Autism Dev. Disord.* **18**, 217–229.

Yoder, P. & Stone, W.L. (2006): A randomized comparison of the effect of two prelinguistic communication interventions on the acquisition of spoken communication in preschoolers with ASD. *J. Speech Lang. Hear. Res.* **49**, 698–711.

Chapter 22

Complementary and alternative medicine in treating autism: myths and reality

Laurence Robel

*Department of Child and Adolescent Psychiatry,
Hôpital Necker Enfants Malades, Paris, France*
Laurence.robel@nck.aphp.fr

Summary

A growing number of families uses complementary and alternative medical treatments to try to improve the condition of their autistic child. In this review, we discuss the hypothesis underlying some of these treatments, such as gluten- and casein-free diets, as well as the few studies concerning their efficacy, risks, and side effects. We also focus on diet-based and medical approaches. Since most treatments do not have evidence to support their use, except for the prescription of melatonin in sleep disorders, we propose recommendations that may help physicians to guide parents in a safer and more rational approach.

Introduction

Autism is a pervasive developmental disorder, starting during the first three years of life and characterized by an alteration of reciprocal social interactions, nonverbal and verbal communication, and the occurrence of restrictive, repetitive, and stereotypical behaviour and interests. Other symptoms, including feeding and sleeping problems, are often associated and they may be as disruptive for the child and his family as the core symptoms. Although several genetic conditions and mutations have been associated with autistic disorders, no genetic or neurologic aetiology has been identified in a majority of cases. Moreover, even when a cause is found, no specific aetiologic treatment is available: treatments are mainly educative and psychotherapeutic, with variable efficacy. Therefore, raising a child with autism is very challenging for the parents, who may look for alternative strategies in order to decrease their child's symptoms as well as their own distress. The most popular alternative and complementary strategies are exclusion diets and nutriment supplementation. Indeed, Witwer & Lecavalier (2005) have shown in 353 non-referred patients with autism spectrum disorders (ASDs) aged 3–21 that 15.5 per cent had a modified diet, and 17.3 per cent received vitamins or supplements. In another study, Wong & Smith (2006) estimated that 52 per cent of patients with autism used a complementary alternative medical (CAM) therapy *versus* 28 per cent in a control group. Of interest, Mercer *et al.* (2006) reported that 51.2 per cent of the parents of an autistic child believe that diet is one of the main contributory factor of autism. And Wong & Smith (2006) reported that 75 per cent of the parents using CAM therapy think it is beneficial. Indeed, we know that causal beliefs are associated with treatment choices (Dardennes et al., 2011). Thus, the questions we address in this article are the following: What are the hypotheses underlying these alternative measures and are they scientifically founded? Is there any proof of efficacy of these measures in studies using scientific methods of investigation? Are these methods safe for the patients? How can we understand the popularity of these measures?

Origins of exclusion diets in autism

Before autism, schizophrenia had been associated with gluten and casein digestion. In 1966, Dohan published a paper showing the lessening of schizophrenic symptoms when the patient was under a casein-free diet, and their worsening after reintroduction of these nutrients. In 1976, Singh & Kay demonstrated the worsening of schizophrenic symptoms after a 3-week change in gluten intake. However, these results were not confirmed and this hypothesis was later abandoned. At the same time, the implication of gluten in autism was proposed on the basis of association of coeliac disease with autism in a 6-year-old boy along with the mitigation of his autistic symptoms under a gluten-free diet (Goodwin & Goodwin, 1969; Goodwin et al., 1971). A few years later, Panksepp developed his opioid theory, implicating gluten (AFSAA, 2009).

The Panksepp theory

Panksepp (1979) postulated that behavioural disturbances in autism can result from an abnormal activation of the opioid system on account of an excess of agonists in the brain. Reichelt et al. (1981) and Knivsberg et al. (2002) further developed the idea that gluten and casein were the source of peptides with opioid activities, called exorphins. In summary, the Panksepp theory implied: (i) a partial degradation of gluten and casein, related to immune-allergic mechanisms like those in coeliac disease; (ii) the increase of gut permeability, provoking the absorption of these degradation products in the blood and in the brain through the blood–brain barrier; and (iii) an endorphin-like effect on the central nervous system of these degradation products. In order to examine the scientific validity of this theory, we will now address several questions and see what answers we can find in the literature.

Is there an elevated rate of coeliac disease in patients with autism, or an elevated rate of patients with autism in the cohorts of patients with a coeliac disease?

Since the description by Goodwin and Goodwin in 1969 of autism in a patient with coeliac disease, and the positive impact of a gluten-free diet on this patient's condition, several studies have been conducted to attempt to answer this question. Pavone and collaborators (1979) studied a group of 120 children with coeliac disease, whose age ranged from 2 years, 6 months to 16 years. They divided these children in three groups: one following a strict gluten-free diet, the second a 'gentle' (*i.e.*, with reduced gluten) diet, and the third a normal diet. They did not report any case of autism among the three groups. Zelnick et al. (2004) did not find any case of autism among 111 20-year-old patients with coeliac disease. Moreover, Wakefield et al. (2000) did not describe any serum or histologic abnormalities characterizing coeliac disease in 148 children with pervasive developmental disorder (PDD). In conclusion, the review of the literature does not support the hypothesis of an association between coeliac disease and autism.

Is there a link between autism and gut inflammatory diseases?

Fombonne (1998) and Fombonne *et al.* (1997) did not report any association between inflammatory diseases and autism on epidemiologic samples. Wakefield *et al.* reported for the first time in 1998 and further confirmed in 2000 an elevated rate of nodular lymphoid hyperplasia (NLH) in a referred group of children with PDD presenting with gastrointestinal symptoms, such as a severe constipation with major dilatation of the recto-sigmoid colon. The rate of NLH was higher than that in a control group of children without gut symptoms, or in children with ulcerative colitis. These authors concluded that children with a regressive form of autism starting after 18 months have a chronic inflammatory disease, possibly related to mumps and rubella vaccinations. However, the link between vaccinations and autism has not been confirmed in epidemiologic samples, and Wakefield's publication was retracted. Moreover, the occurrence of NLH is frequent in young children, and is not always associated with clinical symptoms (Riddlesberger & Lebenthal, 1980; Walker-Smith *et al.*, 1983; Williams & Nicholls, 1994; Colón *et al.*, 1991). Finally, in a later publication, Wakefield (2000) reported a similar frequency of moderate endoscopic and histologic abnormalities in 72 children with PDD and control subjects.

Are there changes in gut permeability in autism?

The modification of gut permeability is a nonspecific consequence of inflammation of the gut membrane. According to the Pankspepp theory, a modification in gut permeability elicited by the presence of abnormalities in the digestive tract may contribute to the passage of dietary exorphins into the blood. D'Eufemia and colleagues (1996) were the first to study gut permeability in 21 children with autism aged 4 to 16 years compared to normal paired controls. They found an increased lactulose/mannitol ratio for 43 per cent of the children with autism, and none in the control group. Horvath *et al.* (1999) also found a high proportion of patients with increased gut permeability in patients with autism, but they did not compare them to a control group, and included patients with gut symptoms as well. In two recent independent studies, Robertson *et al.* (2008) and Kemperman *et al.* (2008) did not find any increase in gut permeability in patients with autism, either in patients with or without gut symptoms (Table 1).

In conclusion, the later studies were made on small samples, sometimes without even a control group, and the presence of gut symptoms was not always studied together with gut permeability. In the end, the results are, not surprisingly, controversial.

Table 1. Gut permeability in children with autism

Authors	Population	PDD/Controls	Presence of gut symptoms	L/M elevated ratio
Study of population				
D'Eufemia *et al.* (1996)	$N = 61$	21/40	No	40% 0 %
Horvath & Perman (2002)	$N = 25$	25/0	Yes	75% ND
Robertson *et al.* (2008)	$N = 29$	14/15	Yes/no	0% 0%
Kemperman *et al.* (2008)	$N = 23$	23	No	0% 0%

Is there an elevated frequency of gastrointestinal disorders in patients with autism?

We have previously seen that there is no evidence of an increase in either the frequency of gut inflammatory diseases or a modification of gut permeability in patients with autism. However, several studies conducted by gastroenterologists describe a high prevalence of gut symptoms. Table 2 shows the conclusions of different studies in epidemiologic samples, clinical samples in patients with ASD, or clinical samples in patients with ASD and gut symptoms.

In epidemiologic samples, the prevalence of gut symptoms is 9 per cent in both controls and children with ASD aged 0 to 11 years. These results are based on the study of the number of consultations in gastroenterology reported on registers in a population of 21,480 children included after 1998 (Black *et al.*, 2002). In clinical samples of children with ASD, the prevalence of gut symptoms is between 17 per cent and 24 per cent. Unfortunately, there is no comparison group in these studies, and no mention about the feeding habits of these children. In referred samples of patients with ASD and gut symptoms, the prevalence of gut symptoms is much higher, with a huge heterogeneity (36 to 76 per cent). In conclusion, the high prevalence reported in referred samples is likely to represent a recruitment bias rather than a general feature of children with ASD.

Table 2. Gastrointestinal symptoms in epidemiologic, clinical, and referred samples of patients with ASDs

Authors	Population	PDD/Controls	Presence of a control group	Prevalence of gut symptoms PDD /controls
Study of population				
Black *et al.* (2002) Before diagnostic	Registers of the General Practice Research $N = 21,480$	96/449	Yes	9% 9%
Fombonne & Chakrabarti (2001)	Geographic zone $N = 15,000$	96/0	No	18.8% ND
Taylor *et al.* (2002)	5 different PDD clinics	473/0	No	17% ND
Molloy & Manning-Courtney (2003)	$N = 151,000$	137 (24 to 96 months)	No	24% ND
Gastroenterologic studies				
Horvath & Perman (2002; review)	?	112/44	Siblings	76% 30 %
Afzal *et al.* (2003)	Department of Paediatric Gastroenterology	103/29	Yes	36% 10 % Severe constipation

Is it possible to detect the presence of abnormally degraded peptides in the urine?

The detection of abnormal degraded peptides in the urine of patients is often used as a biological marker that justifies the prescription of casein- and gluten-free diets. However, since the first papers of Reichelt (1981) and Gillberg *et al.* (1982), the more recent techniques used in several independent and recent papers have shown that the compounds detected in the urinary profiles do not correspond to degraded opioid peptides (Table 3).

Table 3. Detection of peptides in the urine of patients with ASDs

Authors	Population	Controls	Method	Detection of opioid peptides
Reichelt (1981)	Autism Schizophrenia	No	?	Yes Specific urinary profile
Gillberg et al. (1982)	Autism Other psychiatric disorders Normal controls	Yes	Trygstadt	Autism : 54% Others : 17% Controls: 5%
LeCouteur et al. (1998)	Autism Mental retardation	Yes	Trygstadt	No
Gylroy et al. (1991)	Autism	No	HPLC	No
Hunter et al. (2003)	Autism	No	LC-MSMS	No
Dettmer et al. (2007)	Autism Normal controls	No	HPLC	No
Cass et al. (2008)	Autism	No	HPLC MALDI-TOF	No

In conclusion, none of the correlates of the Panksepp theory supporting the use of a gluten- and casein-free diet has been thus far clearly established.

We will now investigate the efficacy of these diets through the few studies published in the literature.

Efficacy of the exclusion diets on autistic symptoms

We were able to find nine publications related to the effect of gluten-free or gluten- and casein-free diets on the behaviour of patients with ASD. Four of these studies come from the same group (Knivsberg et al., 1990, 1995, 2002; Reichelt, 1990). The main characteristics of these studies are summarized in Table 4. Most of the studies are made on small samples of patients, except for the study of Cade et al. (2000) on 149 patients. The length of the diet is very different among studies, as is the way to evaluate the impact of the diet on the patient's symptoms. Control groups are not always present. Some studies use a period of charge, others do not. The food habits prior to the diet are never mentioned, nor are the presence or the absence of gut symptoms or the method used to recruit families. Other educative or therapeutic interventions are not taken into consideration in the interpretation of the behavioural changes. The main problem is that the parents and evaluators were aware of the diet in all the studies (Cade et al., 2000; Knivsberg et al., 1990, 1995, 2002; Lucarelli et al., 1995; Sponheim, 1991; Whiteley, 1999) but one. The only double-blind against placebo assay (Elder et al., 2006), did not show any positive effect of the gluten-free diet. However, it was performed in a short period (12 weeks) on a small sample (15 patients). Of interest, some of the parents in this test were willing to go on with the diet, even if no beneficial effect was demonstrated. The other studies showed positive effects on behaviour and cognition after 6 months for a variable proportion of the subjects, with more drop-outs occurring at the beginning of the diet and no adverse effect of the charge when used.

Table 4. Efficacy of gluten- and/or casein-free diets

Author	Population	Protocol	Measure	Results	Remarks
Reichelt (1990)	N = 15 Autism (DSM3) Peptiduria	1 yr 3 groups -L-G -L+/-G -G+/-L	Parent and teacher reports	50% positive	Small group No control group No double blind No statistics
Knivsberg (1990; 1995)	N = 15 Autism (DSM3) Age: 6–22	4 years 3 groups	Behaviour Cognition Standardized instruments	6 drop outs Positive impact at 6 mo, but not at 1 yr	Small group No control group No double blind No statistics
Sponheim (1991)	N = 4 (17–33) N = 3 (8–12)	6-mo exclusion diet Charge in gluten vs. placebo	Real-life rating scale Analogic scale	No effect	Small sample No double blind Heterogeneity
Whiteley et al. (1999)	N = 22 Autism Asperger's pragmatic dysphasia Dyspraxia	6: no diet 6: diet then charge 10: diet	Behaviour Cognition Standardized instruments	Worst at 3 wk Better at 6 mo No change with charge	Small sample No double blind Heterogeneity
Lucarelli et al. (1995)	N = 36 (8–13)	8 weeks Milk and charge	Behavioural Summarized Evaluation (BSE) Before- and after -diet after charge	Improvement (5 scales) No effect of the charge	No double blind No control of the diet No control group
Cade et al. (2000)	N = 149 Autism, Asperger's disease (3.5–16) DSM3	1 yr Diet in 70 children No gluten, no casein	Behaviour (parent, teacher and clinician reports)	57 positive 13 negative	No double blind No control of the diet No control group
Knivsberg et al. (2002)	N = 20 Autism 59–127 mo Peptiduria	1 yr 10: no diet 10: diet	Behaviour Cognition Standardized instruments	Improvement in behaviour and cognition	No double blind No valid statistics
Elder et al. (2006)	N = 15 (2–16) DSM 4	12 wk Double blind 6-wk diet; 6 wk placebo diet	Behaviour and language videos	No difference	Small sample

In conclusion, the many methodologic weaknesses in the available publications compromise the conclusions of the authors. The reported efficacy of the diets, when present, may be explained by a placebo effect, or by indirect effects through changes in parental attitude and interactions with their child. Indeed, a previous secretin-*versus*-placebo trial showed a significant improvement in 30 per cent of the children with ASD under placebo (Sandler, 2005).

We have seen that the efficacy of the diets is not clearly established. The following question then is: Are they safe?

Safety of the exclusion diets

The suppression of nutriments may be harmful for growth and nutritional status. However, children with autism are known to have selective food habits that may also be harmful. Therefore, it may be difficult to differentiate the impact of the exclusion diets from the impact of autism itself on nutritional status (AFSAA, 2009).

Spontaneous food intake and nutritional status of children with autism

According to Emond and collaborators (2010), children between 5 and 54 months with ASD ($N = 79$) have a less varied diet than do controls ($N = 12,901$). However, their intake of energy, total intake, and total fat and protein are similar. There is no difference in BMI, height, or in hemoglobin concentrations. However, children with autism spectrum disorders have lower vitamin C intake. Deficits in iron, calcium, and vitamin D, but not in minerals, have also been reported (Hemdon et al., 2009).

There are very few studies on the impact of exclusion diets on the nutritional status of children with autism. Hediger et al. (2008) has shown that children under casein-free diets had two times–higher differences in the thickness of cortical bone, compared to other autistic children, suggesting a deficit in calcium metabolism. Another study reports an amino acid deficiency on the basis of plasma concentration (Arnold et al., 2003).

Indirect data come from the study of gluten-exclusion diets in patients with coeliac disease. Folates and vitamin B6 deficiency have been reported in a third of the patients, as has a slight modification of body composition in fat masses (AFSAA, 2009).

The main problem of exclusion diets is that they are costly and difficult to follow. Indeed, these diets exclude a large proportion of industrially processed food products. Therefore, families have to prepare themselves or buy specific dietetic preparations, which are more expensive. Moreover, it involves major changes in the child's habits, which can affect his eating patterns, and interfere with social integration (Robel et al., 2005).

In conclusion, gluten- and casein-free diets do not seem to be harmful if they are properly conducted, but they are costly and may be a drawback for social integration.

Nutriment supplementations in autism

Supplements such as vitamin B6 and magnesium, omega-3 fatty acids, iron, and digestive enzymes may be used alone or in association with an exclusion diet. Their use is related to the hypothesis of a bad absorption of these nutriments due to the presence of inflammatory processes in the gut (Hjiej et al., 2007). We will now review some of the most frequently used dietary supplements.

Vitamin B6 and magnesium

Supplementation of vitamin B6 and magnesium may facilitate neurotransmission through different mechanisms (Lelord et al., 1981; Rimland et al., 1978). Rimland (1988) published a retrospective study showing that 43 per cent of 318 families reported a decrease *versus* 5 per cent an increase of autistic symptoms under a diet enriched in vitamin B6. This study reported the results of a previous vitamin-*versus*-placebo assay using different doses of vitamin B6 (75 to 3,000 mg) in 16 patients aged 4 to 19 years (Rimland et al., 1978). Very few secondary effects (irritability, enuresis) were noticed, especially when magnesium was associated with vitamin B6. However, the patient sample was small and heterogeneous. The positive effect of the association was further confirmed in 1981 by the study of Lelord *et al.* (1981) in a double-blind assay versus placebo on a small group of patients with various doses of magnesium and vitamin B6. This conclusion was not confirmed by the only randomized double-blind assay to be carried out, which was performed by Findling two years later (1997). However, according to Rimland's meta-analysis (2002), 50 per cent of the patients included in 11 different double-blind assays show a lessening of autistic symptoms without adverse effect, even with high doses. However, the most recent Cochrane Review identified only three studies between 1993 and 2002 with an appropriate methodology, including a total of 28 patients with contradictory results (Nye & Bryce, 2005).

In conclusion, the results concerning vitamin B6 and magnesium supplementation are controversial, with several limitations in the methodology of the different assays, but several authors described improvement without major side effects (Hjiej, 2007).

Omega fatty acid supplementation

Polyunsaturated fatty acids are important for brain development, and their presence depends on the ingestion of fish and fish oils. Therefore, omega acid supplementation has become popular in several neurodevelopmental disorders.

Amminger *et al.* (2007) showed a positive effect of omega-3 fatty acid supplementation in a 6-week placebo-controlled pilot trial in 13 children aged 5 to 13 presenting with severe tantrums, aggression, or self-injurious behaviours. The main effect was a reduction of hyperactivity without adverse effect. More studies need to be published to confirm this preliminary result.

Iron supplementation

Deficits in iron have been described in children with autism. Dosman *et al.* (2007) studied iron intake from food records in 33 children, and showed that 69 per of preschoolers and 35 per cent of those in school had low iron intake. They describe an improvement in sleep together with an increase in ferritin concentration after iron supplementation, and suggest screening children with autism for iron deficiency.

Digestive enzyme supplementation (secretin)

Since 1998, several publications have studied secretin supplementation as a treatment for the core symptoms of autism. Two recent publications have clearly concluded that there is no evidence supporting the use of secretin: Krishnaswami *et al.* (2011) identified seven randomized controlled trials reporting a lack of effectiveness of secretin on ASD symptoms such as impairment of language and communication skills, severity of symptoms, and deficits in cognitive and social skills. This was further confirmed by Williams and collaborators (2005, 2012) when they assessed randomized controlled trials of intravenous secretin compared to placebo treatment in children or adults diagnosed with an ASD, with at least a standardized outcome measure. Although a meta-analysis of data was not possible because of the disparity of the methodologies, their findings consistently demonstrated the absence of effectiveness of secretin administration on the core features of ASD.

Melatonin supplement

Rossignol & Frye (2011) published a meta-analysis of nine papers studying the impact of melatonin prescription on sleep in patients with ASD. Several papers have reported an abnormal melatonin circadian rhythm or below-average physiologic levels of melatonin and/or melatonin derivates positively correlating with autistic behaviours. Their conclusion is that melatonin administration in ASD is associated with improvements in sleep duration, sleep-onset latency, and better daytime behaviour, and it had minimal side effects.

In conclusion, the only nutriment supplementation that brings a clear benefit in autism is melatonin.

Other alternative medical treatments

Heavy metal chelators

The apparent increase in ASD prevalence has resulted in the search for potential environmental causes (Levy & Hyman, 2008). The implication of heavy metals such as mercury is linked to the hypothesis that ROR (MMR) vaccination is implicated in autism. Despite the fact that this hypothesis was contradicted by several studies, the implication of mercury in autism remains popular. Therefore, chelation treatments by DMPS or DMSA have been developed, aimed at the elimination of mercury and other heavy metals, such as mercury, lead, or cadmium.

Soden *et al.* (2007) studied the concentration of arsenic, cadmium, lead, and mercury in the urine of 15 children with ASD versus 5 controls, before and after DMSA treatment. None of the patients or controls had an excess of chelatable compounds. Adams *et al.* (2009) reported the impact of DMSA treatment in 65 children with autism, on heavy metal excretions, platelet count, glutathione concentrations, and autistic symptoms. However, their methodology is based on the comparison of one round *versus* several rounds of chelation treatment rather than 0 *versus* one round of chelation, with no comparison to a control group of children, nor a comparison between the effects of the treatment in children showing a high excretion of heavy metals *versus* those with no excretion of heavy metals. The positive correlations described in these two papers between DMSA treatment, platelet count, and autistic symptoms are thus very difficult to analyze. Obviously, this study needs to be confirmed with new data and replicated by an independent team. Moreover, it should be emphasized that chelation treatments can be dangerous if they are not properly monitored, as shown by the paper of Baxter & Krenzelok (2008) reporting the death of a 5-year-old autistic boy who went into cardiac arrest after use of edetate disodium rather than edetate calcium disodium.

In conclusion, results are contradictory and preliminary. The improvement-to-risk balance is not in favor of these treatments, except if there is proved intoxication of heavy metals and if the treatments are conducted under strict medical scrutiny.

Antibiotic and antifungal therapies

Reports of gut dysbiosis provoked by more frequent infectious episodes and subsequent use of antibiotics in the early years of children with ASD are inconsistent (Levy & Hyman, 2008). According to the consensus report on gastrointestinal disorders in individuals with ASD (Buie *et al.*, 2010), empirical antibiotic and antifungal therapies are not recommended in patients with ASD. These authors emphasize that an abnormal culture result from a duodenal aspirate or abnormal stool culture is required before starting any treatment designed to alter intestinal flora.

Conclusions

Despite the great popularity of alternative medical therapies for children and adults with autistic spectrum disorders, the scientific basis of these therapies and the demonstration of their efficacy is far from proven.

The Pansksepp theory, suggesting exclusion dietetic approaches in autism, has no scientific support. The measurement of opioid peptides in urine is not valid and should not have been used to promote these diets. Moreover, the efficacy of gluten- and casein-free diets has not been proved so far, and these diets may induce a loss of some nutriments, such as amino acids, calcium, iron or vitamins. These diets are constraining and expensive, and may interfere with social integration.

However, it must be emphasized that patients with PDDs have selective feeding behaviours. Their protein, fat, and carbohydrate intake is not different from that of the general population, but their intake in vitamins C, D and E, iron, calcium, and fibres may be too low. Children with PDD may also have gastrointestinal symptoms. The frequency of these symptoms is about 9 per cent, like that in the general population; they may also have food intolerance or allergies, as in the general population. Since patients with ASDs can hardly communicate about their perceptions, the pain related to gastrointestinal symptoms may aggravate behavioural symptoms such as withdrawal, aggressiveness, hyperactivity, and auto-mutilation.

Therefore, it is important to look for gastrointestinal symptoms (such as constipation and diarrhoea) and to investigate and treat these symptoms in the same way they would be treated in normal children (Buie *et al.*, 2010). It is also important to investigate the feeding habits and to evaluate the nutritional intake of children with PDDs, in order to make dietetic recommendations or supplement low values in some nutriments, such as vitamin C, vitamin B6, iron, calcium, vitamin D, or omega-3 fatty acids. Melatonin may also be used safely to treat sleep disorders.

Some treatments should not been used because they are not effective (such as secretin) and/or potentially dangerous, like heavy metal chelation, or antifungal and antibiotic therapies, except when intoxication or infection has been proved by adequate investigation.

The power of belief and the placebo effect may explain the discrepancy between the proved efficacy of diets and their promotion by parents. However, these diets may also help a subgroup of children who have unbalanced diets or gastrointestinal symptoms. The diets may also provide a frame in the relationship between the parents and their child that may be beneficial to both. In any case, it shows the need for parents to be active in the treatment of their child, and to find an explanation for the child's symptoms.

Therefore, exclusion diets should not be recommended to patients with ASDs, but rather respected if they are the parent's choice, with a monitoring of appropriate food intake. Other alternative medical approaches should be used with caution, guided by the evaluation of risk and benefit.

Conflicts of interest: The author declares no conflicts of interest.

References

Adams, J.B., Matthew, B., Geis, E., *et al.* (2009): Safety and efficacy of oral DMSA therapy for children with autism spectrum disorders: Part B: Behavioral results. *BMC Clin. Pharmacol.* **9**, 17–26.

AFSAA [Agence Française de Sécurité Sanitaire des Aliments] (2009): Efficacy and safety of gluten-free and casein-free diets proposed in children presenting with pervasive developmental disorders (autism and related syndromes). <www.afssa.fr.>

Afzal, N., Murch, S., Thirrupathy, K., Berger, L., Fagbemi, A. & Heuschkel, R. (2003): Constipation with acquired megarectum in children with autism. *Pediatrics* **112**, 939–942.

Amminger, G.P., Berger, G.E., Schäfer, M.R., Klier, C., Friedrich, M.H. & Feucht, M. (2007): Omega-3 fatty acids supplementation in children with autism: a double-blind randomized, placebo-controlled pilot study. *Biol. Psychiatry* **61**, 551–553.

Arnold, G.L., Hyman, S.L., Mooney, R.A. & Kirby, R.S. (2003): Plasma amino acid profiles in children with autism: potential risk of nutritional deficiencies. *J. Autism Dev. Disord.* **33**, 449–454.

Baxter, A.J. & Krenzelok, E.P. (2008): Pediatric fatality secondary to EDTA chelation. *Clin. Toxicol. (Phila).* **46**, 1083–1084.

Black, C., Kaye, J.A. & Hershel, J. (2002): Relation of childhood gastrointestinal disorders to autism: nested case-control study using data from the UK general Practice Research Database. *Br. Med. J.* **325**, 419–421.

Buie, T., Campbell, D.B., Fuchs, G.J., III, *et al.* (2010): Evaluation, diagnosis, and treatments of gastrointestinal disorders in individuals with ASDs: a consensus report. *Pediatrics* **125**, s1–s18.

Cade, R., Privette, M., Fregly, M., *et al.* (2000): Autism and schizophrenia intestinal disorders. *Nutr. Neurosci.* **3**, 57–72.

Cass, H., Gringras, P., March, J., *et al.* (2008): Absence of urinary opioid peptides in children with autism. *Arch. Dis. Child* **93**, 745–750.

Colón, A.R., DiPalma, J.S. & Leftridge, C.A. (1991): Intestinal lymphonodular hyperplasia of childhood: patterns of presentation. *J. Clin. Gastroenterol.* **13**, 163–162.

Dardennes, R.M., Al Anbar, N.N., Prado-Netto, A., Kaye, K., Contejean, Y. & Al Anbar, N.N. (2011): Treating the cause of illness rather than the symptoms: parental causal beliefs and treatment choices in autism spectrum disorder. *Res. Dev. Disabil.* **32**, 1137–1146.

Dettmer, K., Hanna, D., Whestone, P., Hansen, R. & Hammock, B.D. (2007): Autism and urinary exogenous neuropeptides: development of an on-line SPE-HPLC tandem mass spectrometry method to test the opioid excess theory. *Anal. Bioanal. Chem.* **388**, 1643–1651.

D'Eufemia, P., Celli, M., Pacifico, L., *et al.* (1996): Abnormal intestinal permeability in children with autism. *Acta Paediat.* **85**, 1076–1079.

Dohan, F.C. (1966): Cereals and schizophrenia: data and hypothesis. *Acta Psychiatr. Scand.* **42**, 125–152.

Dosman, C.F., Brian, J.A., Drmic, I.E., *et al.* (2007): Children with autism: effect of iron supplementation on sleep and ferritin. *Pediatr. Neurol.* **36**, 152–158.

Elder, J.H., Shankar, M., Shuster, J., Theriaque, D., Burns, S. & Sherril, L. (2006): The gluten-free, casein-free diet in autism: results of a preliminary double-blind clinical trial. *J. Autism Dev. Disord.* **36**, 413–420.

Emond, A., Emmett, P.C. & Golding, J. (2010): Feeding symptoms, dietary patterns, and growth in young children with autism spectrum disorders. *Pediatrics* **126**, e337–e342.

Findling, R.L., Maxwell, K., Scotese-Wojtila, L., *et al.* (1997): High dose pyridoxine and magnesium administration in children with autistic disorder: an absence of salutary effects in a double-blind, placebo-controlled study. *J. Autism Dev. Disord.* **27**, 467–478.

Fombonne, E. (1998): Inflammatory bowel disease and autism. *Lancet* **351**, 955.

Fombonne, E. & Chakrabarti, S. (2001): No evidence for a new variant of measles-mumps-rubella-induced autism. *Pediatrics* **108**, E58.

Fombonne, E., du Mazaubrun, C., Cans, H. & Granjean, H. (1997): Autism and associated medical disorders in a large French epidemiological sample. *Am. Acad. Child Adolesc. Psychiatry* **36**, 1561–1568.

Gillberg, C., Trygstad, O. & Foss, I. (1982): Childhood psychosis and urinary excretion of peptides and protein-associated peptide complexes. *J. Autism Dev. Disord.* **12**, 229–241.

Goodwin, M.S. & Goodwin, T.C. (1969): In a dark mirror. *Mental Hygiene* **53**, 550–563.

Goodwin, M.S., Cowen, M.A. & Goodwin, T.C. (1971): Malabsorption and cerebral dysfunction: a multivariate and comparative study of autistic children. *J. Autism Child Schizophr.* **1**, 48–62.

Gylroy, J.J., Ferrier, I.N. & Crow, T.J. (1991): Urinary chromatographic profiles in psychiatric diseases. *Br. J. Psychiatry* **158**, 288–289.

Hediger, M.L., England, L.J., Molloy, C.A., Yu, K.F., Manning-Courtney, P. & Mills, J.L. (2008): Reduced bone cortical thickness in boys with autism or autism spectrum disorder. *J. Autism Dev. Disord.* **38**, 848–856.

Hemdon, A.C., Di Guiseppi, C., Johnson, S.L., Leiferman, J. & Reynolds, A. (2009): Does nutritional intake differ between children with autism spectrum disorders and children with typical development? *J. Autism Dev. Disord.* **39**, 212–222.

Hjiej, H., Doyen, C., Couprie, K.K. & Contejean, Y. (2007): Approches substitutives et diététiques du trouble autistique de l'enfant: Intérêts ou limites ? *L'Encéphale* 10.1016/j.enceph.2007.10.011.

Horvath, K. & Perman, J.A. (2002): Autistic disorder and gastrointestinal disease. *Curr. Opin. Pediatr.* **14**, 83–587.

Horvath, K., Papadimitriou, J.C., Rabsztyn, A., Drachenberg, C. & Tyson Tildon, J. (1999): Gastrointestinal abnormalities in children with autistic disorder. *J. Pediatr.* **135**, 559–563.

Hunter, L.C., O'Hare, A., Herron, W.J., Fisher, L.A. & Jones, G.E. (2003): Opioid peptides and dipeptidyl peptidase in autism. *Dev. Med. Child Neurol.* **45**, 121–128.

Kemperman, R.F., Muskiet, F.D., Boutier, A.I., Kema, I.P. & Muskiet, F.A. (2008): Brief report: normal intestinal permeability at elevated platelet serotonin levels in a subgroup of children with pervasive developmental disorders in Curaçao. *J. Autism Dev. Disord.* **38**, 401–406.

Kanner, L. (1943): Autistic disturbances of affective contact. *Nerv. Child.* **2**, 217–250.

Knivsberg, A.M., Wiig, K., Lind, G., Nodland, M. & Reichelt, K.L. (1990): Dietary intervention in autistic syndromes. *Brain Dysfunction* **3**, 315–327.

Knivsberg, A.M., Reichelt, K.L., Nodland, M. & Torleiv, H. (1995): Autistic syndromes and diet: a follow-up study. *Scand. J. Educ. Res.* **39**, 223–236.

Knivsberg, A.M., Reichelt, K.L., Hoien, T. & Nodland, M. (2001): Reports on dietary intervention in autistic disorders. *Nutr. Neurosci.* **4**, 25–37.

Knivsberg, A.M., Reichelt, K.L., Hoien, T. & Nodland, M. (2002): Controlled study of dietary intervention in autistic syndromes. *Nutr. Neurosci.* **5**, 251–261.

Krishnaswami, S., McPheeters, M.L. & Veenstra-Vanderweele, J. (2011): A systematic review of secretin for children with autism spectrum disorders. *Pediatrics* **127**, e1322–e1325.

Le Couteur, A., Trygstad, O., Evered, C., Gillberg, C. & Rutter, M. (1988): Infantile autism and urinary excretion of peptides and protein-associated complexes. *J. Autism Dev. Disord.* **18**, 181–190.

Lelord, G., Muh, J.P., Barthelemy, C., et al. (1981): Effects of pyridoxine and magnesium on autistic symptoms-initial observation. *J. Autism Dev. Disord.* **11**, 219–230.

Levy, S.E. & Hyman, S.L. (2008): Complementary and alternative medicine treatments for children with autism spectrum disorders. *Child Adolesc. Psychiatry Clin. N. Am.* **17**, 803–818.

Lucarelli, S., Frediani, T., Zingoni, A.M., et al. (1995): Food allergy and infantile autism. *Panminerva Med.* **37**, 137–141.

Mercer, L., Creighton, S., Holden, J.J. & Lewis, M.E. (2006): Parental perspectives on the causes of an autism spectrum disorder in their children. *J. Genet. Couns.* **15**, 41–50.

Molloy, C.A. & Manning-Courtney, P. (2003): Prevalence of chronic gastrointestinal symptoms in children with autism and autistic spectrum disorders. *Autism* **7**, 165–171.

Nye, C. & Bryce, A. (2005): Combined vitamin B6-magnesium treatment in autism spectrum disorder. *Cochrane Database Syst. Rev.* CD003497.

Panksepp, A. (1979): A neurochemical theory of autism. *Trends Neurosci.* **2**, 174–177.

Pavone, L., Fiumara, A., Bottano, G., Mazzone, D. & Coleman, M. (1997): Autism and coeliac disease: failure to validate the hypothesis that a link might exist. *Biol. Psychiatry* **42**, 72–75.

Reichelt, K.L., Hoel, K., Hamberger, A., et al. (1981): Biologically active peptide-containing fractions in schizophrenia and childhood autism. *Adv. Biochem. Psychopharmacol.* **28**, 1279–1290.

Reichelt, K.L., Elkrem, J. & Scott, H. (1990): Gluten, milk proteins and autism: dietary intervention effects on behavior and peptide secretion. *J. Appl. Nutr.* **42**, 1–11.

Reichelt, W.C., Knivsberg, A.M., Nodland, M., Sensrud, M. & Reichelt, K.L. (1997): Urinary peptide levels and patterns in autistic children from seven countries, and the effect of dietary intervention after 4 years. *Dev. Brain Dysfunct.* **10**, 44–55.

Riddlesberger, M.M. & Lebenthal, E. (1980): Nodular colonic mucosa of childhood: normal or pathologic? *Gastroenterology* **79**, 265–270.

Rimland, B. (1988): Controversies in the treatment of autistic children: vitamin therapy. *J. Child Neurol.* **3,** 568–572.

Rimland, B. (2002): The use of vitamin B6, magnesium and DMG in the treatment of adults and children. In: *Biological Treatment of Autism*, ed. W. Shaw. Lenexa, KS: The Great Plains Laboratory, Inc.

Rimland, B., Callaway, E. & Dreyfus, P. (1978): The effect of high doses of vitamin B6 on autistic children: a double crossover study. *Am. J. Psychiatry* **135,** 472–475.

Robel, L., Beauquier-Maccotta, B., Bresson, J.L., Schmitz, J. & Golse, B. (2005): Autisme et gluten: mythes et réalités. *Psychiatr. Enfant* **48,** 577–592.

Robertson, M.A., Signalet, D.L., Holst, J.J., Meddings, J.B., Wood, J. & Sharkey, K.A. (2008): Intestinal permeability and glucagon-like peptide-2 in children with autism: a controlled pilot study. *J. Autism Dev. Disord.* **38,** 1066–1071.

Rossignol, D.A. & Frye, R.E. (2011): Melatonin in autism spectrum disorders: a systematic review and meta-analysis. *Dev. Med. Child Neurol.* **53,** 783–792.

Singh, M.M. & Kay, S.R. (1976): Wheat gluten as a pathogenic factor in schizophrenia. *Science* **191,** 401–402.

Soden, S.E., Lowry, J.A., Garrison, C.B. & Wasserman, G.S. (2007): 24-hour provoked urine excretion test for heavy metal in children with autism and typically developing controls, a pilot study. *Clin. Toxicol. (Phila)*, **45,** 476–481.

Sponheim, E. (1991): Glutenfri diet ved infantile autism. *Tiddskr. Nor. Laegeforen* **111,** 704–707.

Taylor, B., Miller, E., Lingam, R., Andrews, N., Simmons, A. & Stowe, J. (2002): Measles, mumps, and rubella vaccination and bowel problems or developmental regression in children with autism: population study. *Br. Med. J.* **324,** 393–396.

Wakefield, A.J., *et al.* (1998): Ileal-lymphoïd-nodular hyperplasia, non-specific colitis, and pervasive developmental disorder in children. *Lancet* **351,** 637–641.

Wakefield, A.J., *et al.* (2000): Enterocolitis in children with developmental disorders. *Am. J. Gastroenterol.* **95,** 2285–2295.

Walker-Smith, J.A., Hamilton, J.R. & Walker, W.A. (1983): *Practical Paediatric Gastroenterology*, pp. 245–255. Norwich: Butterworth.

Whiteley, P., Rodgers, J., Savery, D. & Shattock, P. (1999): A gluten-free diet as an intervention for autism and associated disorders: preliminary findings. *Autism* **3,** 45–65.

Williams, C.B. & Nicolls, S. (1994): Endoscopic features of chronic inflammatory bowel disease in childhood. *Baillères Clin. Gastroenterol.* **8,** 121–131.

Williams, K., Wray, J. & Wheeler, D.M. (2005): Intravenous secretin for autism spectrum disorder. *Cochrane Database Syst. Rev.* CD003495.

Williams, K., Wray, J.A. & Wheeler, D.M. (2012): Intravenous secretin for autism spectrum disorder. *Cochrane Database Syst. Rev.* CD003495.

Witwer, A. & Lecavalier, L. (2005): Treatment incidence and patterns in children and adolescents with autism spectrum disorders. *J. Child Adolesc. Psychopharmacol.* **15,** 671–681.

Wong, H.H. & Smith, R.G. (2006): Patterns of complementary and alternative medical therapy use in children diagnosed with autism spectrum disorders. *J. Autism Dev. Disord.* **36,** 901–909.

Zelnick, N., Patch, A., Obeid, R. & Lerner, A. (2004): Range of neurologic disorders in patients with coeliac disease. *Pediatrics* **113,** 1672–1676.

Mariani Foundation
Paediatric Neurology Series

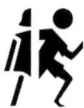

1: Occipital Seizures and Epilepsies in Children
Edited by: *F. Andermann, A. Beaumanoir, L. Mira, J. Roger and C.A. Tassinari*

2: Motor Development in Children
Edited by: *E. Fedrizzi, G. Avanzini and P. Crenna*

3: Continuous Spikes and Waves during Slow Sleep – Electrical Status Epilepticus during Slow Sleep
Edited by: *A. Beaumanoir, M. Bureau, T. Deonna, L. Mira and C.A. Tassinari*

4: Metabolic Encephalopathies: Therapy and Prognosis
Edited by: *S. Di Donato, R. Parini and G. Uziel*

5: Neuromuscular Diseases during Development
Edited by: *F. Cornelio, G. Lanzi and E. Fedrizzi*

6: Falls in Epileptic and Non-Epileptic Seizures during Childhood
Edited by: *A. Beaumanoir, F. Andermann, G. Avanzini and L. Mira*

7: Abnormal Cortical Development and Epilepsy – From Basic to Clinical Science
Edited by: *R. Spreafico, G. Avanzini and F. Andermann*

8: Limbic Seizures in Children
Edited by: *G. Avanzini, A. Beaumanoir and L. Mira*

9: Localization of Brain Lesions and Developmental Functions
Edited by: *D. Riva and A. Benton*

10: Immune-Mediated Disorders of the Central Nervous System in Children
Edited by: *L. Angelini, M. Bardare and A. Martini*

11: Frontal Lobe Seizures and Epilepsies in Children
Edited by: *A. Beaumanoir, F. Andermann, P. Chauvel, L. Mira and B. Zifkin*

12: Hereditary Leukoencephalopathies and Demyelinating Neuropathies in Children
Edited by: *G. Uziel, F. Taroni*

13: Neurodevelopmental Disorders: Cognitive/Behavioural Phenotypes
Edited by: *D. Riva, U. Bellugi and M.B. Denckla*

14: Autistic Spectrum Disorders
Edited by: *D. Riva and I. Rapin*

15: Neurocutaneous Syndromes in Children
Edited by: *P. Curatolo and D. Riva*
16: Language: Normal and Pathological Development
Edited by: *D. Riva, I. Rapin and G. Zardini*
17: Movement Disorders in Children: a Clinical Update, with video recordings
Edited by: *N. Nardocci and E. Fernandez-Alvarez*
18: Mental Retardation
Edited by: *D. Riva, S. Bulgheroni and C. Pantaleoni*
19: Perinatal Brain Damage: From Pathogenesis to Neuroprotection
Edited by: *L.A. Ramenghi, P. Evrard and E. Mercuri*
20: Genetics of Epilepsy and Genetic Epilepsies
Edited by: *G. Avanzini and J. Noebels*
21: Neurology of the Infant
Edited by: *F. Guzzetta*
22: Brain Lesion Localization and Developmental Functions
Basal ganglia – Connecting systems – Cerebellum – Mirror neurons
Edited by: *D. Riva and C. Njiokiktjien*
23: Lysosomal Storage Diseases: Early Diagnosis and New Treatments
Edited by: *R. Parini, G. Andria*
24: New Diagnostic and Therapeutic Tools in Child Neurology
Edited by: *E. Mercuri, E. Fedrizzi and G. Cioni*
25: Brain Lesion Localization and Developmental Functions
Frontal lobes – Limbic system – Visuocognitive system
Edited by: *D. Riva, C. Njiokiktjien and S. Bulgheroni*

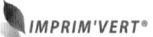

IMPRIM'VERT®